Prior to the nineteenth century, the practice of medicine in the Western world was as much art as science. But, argues W. F. Bynum, "modern" medicine as practiced today is built upon foundations that were firmly established between 1800 and the beginning of World War I. He demonstrates this in terms of concepts, institutions, and professional structures that evolved during this crucial period, applying both a more traditional intellectual approach to the subject and the newer social perspectives developed by recent historians of science and medicine. In a wide-ranging survey, Bynum examines the parallel development of biomedical sciences such as physiology, pathology, bacteriology, and immunology, and of clinical practice and preventive medicine in nineteenth-century Europe and North America.

Focusing on medicine in the hospitals, the community, and the laboratory, Bynum contends that the impact of science was more striking on the public face of medicine and the diagnostic skills of doctors than it was on their actual therapeutic capacities. He shows how even doctors who had little time for the claims of science within medicine benefited from the public status and credibility that science gave them and argues that by the end of the century, most were quite happy to be seen as marching in the steps of Welch and Osler, Lister and Virchow, Pasteur and Koch. And through the work of these and other prominent researchers, both the conceptual foundations and the practice of medicine were slowly transformed into a modern cast that still characterizes the profession today, even with the vast changes that further discoveries have wrought.

Science and the Practice of Medicine
in the Nineteenth Century

CAMBRIDGE HISTORY OF SCIENCE

Editors
GEORGE BASALLA
University of Delaware

OWEN HANNAWAY
The Johns Hopkins University

Physical Science in the Middle Ages
EDWARD GRANT
Man and Nature in the Renaissance
ALLEN G. DEBUS
The Construction of Modern Science: Mechanisms and Mechanics
RICHARD S. WESTFALL
Science and the Enlightenment
THOMAS L. HANKINS
Biology in the Nineteenth Century:
Problems of Form, Function, and Transformation
WILLIAM COLEMAN
Energy, Force, and Matter:
The Conceptual Development of Nineteenth-Century Physics
P. M. HARMAN
Life Science in the Twentieth Century
GARLAND E. ALLEN
The Evolution of Technology
GEORGE BASALLA
Science and Religion: Some Historical Perspectives
JOHN HEDLEY BROOKE
Science in Russia and the Soviet Union: A Short History
LOREN R. GRAHAM
Science and the Practice of Medicine in the Nineteenth Century
W. F. BYNUM

SCIENCE AND THE PRACTICE OF MEDICINE IN THE NINETEENTH CENTURY

W. F. BYNUM
Wellcome Institute for the History of Medicine

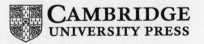
CAMBRIDGE
UNIVERSITY PRESS

Published by the Press Syndicate of the University of Cambridge
The Pitt Building, Trumpington Street, Cambridge CB2 1RP
40 West 20th Street, New York, NY 10011-4211, USA
10 Stamford Road, Oakleigh, Melbourne 3166, Australia

First published 1994
Reprinted 1994, 1995, 1996 (twice)

Printed in the United States of America

Library of Congress Cataloging-in-Publication Data is available

A catalogue record for this book is available from the British Library

ISBN 0-521-25109-5 hardback
ISBN 0-521-27205-X paperback

FOR JULIE

Contents

Illustrations

Preface

THIS volume has a thesis and a purpose. The thesis may be simply stated: in terms of concepts, institutions, and professional structures, the medicine of 1900 was closer to us almost a century later than it was to the medicine of 1790. In other words, modern medicine, by which I simply mean "our" medicine, was the product of nineteenth-century society. This is not to deny that vast changes have occurred in the twentieth century; rather, it is to argue that modern medicine has been built on foundations that were firmly established before World War I.

My purpose is to describe this transformation in a way that strikes a balance between an older intellectual approach to the history of science and medicine, and the newer social perspectives of the present generation of historians. It has become fashionable to discount the content of past scientific theories in medicine, and to stress their rhetorical uses. It is also common to point out that the translation of scientific knowledge into effective curative or preventive measures is never simple, instantaneous, or universal. Rather, in its creation, application, and dissemination, knowledge is (to use a currently fashionable word) negotiated.

These and other equally valuable insights have enriched our understanding of the history of medicine and made us skeptical about the easy assumption that the discovery of the tubercle bacillus by Robert Koch caused the decline in the prevalence of tuberculosis, or the invention of the stethoscope by R. T. H. Laennec led to dramatic new ways of treating heart disease. Nor would I wish my claim that medicine in 1900 was essentially modern to be taken as meaning that the practice of medicine at that time was unambiguously "scientific," or that all doctors sought to use contemporary scientific discoveries in their daily practices. That was true for neither the 1900s nor the 1990s. The ideas and ideals of science could mean one thing to one person, and something entirely different to another; clinicians who had little time for laboratory experimentation could still hold they were practicing "scientific" medicine; and the nature of science within medicine changed during the course of the century. Further, for many doctors, the practice of medicine was based on custom, tradition, individual experience, or cosmologies partially or completely alien to those of the high priests of scientific medicine. For others, science provided the rationale for theories and actions that, in the cold light of hindsight, appear anything but sensible or beneficial. One generation's science can be another generation's prejudice.

Nevertheless, I argue in this volume that science was one of the important influences in shaping the structure of medicine in the nineteenth century. The impact of science was more striking on the public face of medicine, and on the diagnostic skills of doctors, than it was on their therapeutic capacities. Nevertheless, most, though by no means all, doctors by the end of the century would have been happy to be seen marching in the shadow of Welch and Osler, Lister and Virchow, Pasteur and Koch. Even those members of the profession who had no time or inclination for the claims of science within medicine still benefited from the status and credibility that science gave them collectively.

I am conscious that by stressing the ideas of a number of traditional "heroes" within the medical pantheon, the volume acquires a traditional cast. Indeed, the bald thesis that I have stated could be seen as Whiggish: as seeking to view nineteenth-century medicine in terms that are defined by late twentieth-century values. Some of the valuable contributions of the social history of medicine have been to increase appreciation of the complexity and slowness of change, and to highlight what have been called the pitfalls of progress. At the same time, the work of individuals such as Billroth and Louis, Virchow and Helmholtz, Lister and Bowditch, Pasteur and Koch, did change both the conceptual foundations of medicine and its practice, and in this small book on a large subject, I make no apology for concentrating on such people.

In taking the relation between science and medicine as a dominant theme, I am aware that several important topics have been given short shrift, though I have tried to provide a reasonable number of references in the bibliographical essay. By way of apology I offer three such areas.

First, there is little in this volume on alternative medicine, either in the way of systematic challenges to the establishment such as homeopathy and osteopathy, naturpathy and hydropathy, or in the individualistic activities of patent medicine vendors, neighborly healers, druggists, and sharp-witted quacks. Much historical attention has been focused on these groups and individuals of late, partly because they form part of the rich texture of the medical world of the past, and partly because the threats that they posed to "orthodox" doctors had important ramifications on the latter's individual and collective behavior. We have now become even more conscious of the history of alternative medicine as the prestige of contemporary scientific medicine has declined in the past decade or two. History is always about the present as well as the past.

Second, I have not done full justice to the role of women within the fabric of nineteenth-century medicine: as healers, nurses, patients, and, eventually, as still marginal members of a male-dominated profession. Each of these themes could have been expanded beyond the brief treatment accorded them here but to do so would have changed the balance of the volume.

Finally, some readers may feel that I have written about medicine in the United States only as an afterthought. This relative neglect of American medicine was partly dictated by the fact that, before the last third of the century, American doctors were more consumers than producers of scientific ideas, and I do try to describe briefly the late-century transformation that permitted the emergence of American medicine on the world stage in the decades following World War I. More pragmatically, there already exist better teaching materials for American medicine of the period than for European. At the same time, I am conscious that my Europe is rather Anglocentric, and that at the level of institutions and professional values, a good deal of my account takes Great Britain as its principal focus; and that Europe, outside of France and the German-speaking lands, receives virtually no coverage. To do justice to developments in Spain and Italy, Holland, or the Scandinavian countries would take me beyond my competence and in any case would be impossible in a volume of this size.

There are many other gaps and idiosyncrasies, but not so many as there would have been without the careful reading of several friends mentioned in the Acknowledgments. And I hope that readers will find the volume useful for what it contains rather than deficient for what it does not.

Acknowledgments

THIS volume has been a long time in the making, and I have acquired many debts along the way. Few scholars would deny that the Wellcome Institute for the History of Medicine is a kind of Mecca for the discipline, and I have been privileged to work there for the past two decades. My thanks go to the Governors of the Wellcome Trust for supporting the Institute, and to Sir Henry Wellcome for his vision. More immediately, the Library staff who serve the public are models of courtesy and efficiency. Some of them have even tried patiently to initiate me into the mysteries of how to use a rather cumbersome computer catalogue of the Library's incomparable riches.

In the meantime, the various drafts of this book have been produced on a variety of machines, from an electric typewriter to a word processor to a sophisticated personal computer. The first version was, however, invariably written with pen and paper and I am grateful to the late Heather Edwards, Frieda Houser, Betty Kingston, and Sally Bragg for coping with the vagaries of my writing. Sally in particular was as eager as I to finish it. In addition, Janice Wilson and Caroline Overy have provided expert and cheerful research assistance. Special thanks also go to Chris Carter in the photography and Andy Foley in the photocopying departments.

A number of friends have read the manuscript and made useful comments. Among them are the late William Paton, Andrew Scull, Mike Neve, Chris Lawrence, Roy Porter, Tilli Tansey, John Harley Warner, and Gert Brieger. Stephen Lock and Jonathan Bynum went through the manuscript line by line and corrected many infelicities of style, grammar, and content. The referees for Cambridge University Press were also both generous and helpful. At the Press, John Kim, Alex Holzman, and Richard Ziemacki have been extraordinarily patient. Helen Wheeler has edited my manuscript with exemplary care, and Jean Runciman's full index will be appreciated by any user of this volume. Early on, the book was encouraged by the late Bill Coleman, who read a prior version of the first two chapters. His premature death was a blow to everyone in our discipline, and I hope he would have been satisfied with the result. The faults that remain are mine.

My son Jonathan deserves personal as well as professional thanks. He witnessed my losing many friendly bets with Bob Lamb on the book's probable completion date, fortunately on a standard double or quits basis. We can now quit. To Bob and Bron, to Dave Bonnett, and to Dr. R. Bag, my warm thanks. Finally, if anyone was more anxious than me to see the completion of this book, it was Julie, to whom the volume is dedicated.

1

Medicine in 1790

Every one nowadays pretends to neglect theory, and to stick to observation. But the first is in talk only, for every man has his theory, good or
bad, which he occasionally employs; and the only difference is, that weak
men who have little extent of ability for, or have had little experience in
reasoning, are most liable to be attached to frivolous theories.

William Cullen, "Introductory Lectures," in *Works*,
ed. J. Thomson (1827), I, p. 402

I

N 1790, as the poet Wordsworth was to recall, it was bliss to be alive,
while to be young was very heaven. Englishmen had hardly ceased
rejoicing at the mad King George III's recovery of his faculties when,
for a few of Wordsworth's countrymen, events across the Channel au-
gured the dawn of the bright new day. Most Englishmen shared the
poet's subsequent opinion that the French Revolution quickly soured,
but it brought in its train rapid changes in medical education and medical
thought. As Chapter 2 will examine, these may constitute a medical
revolution.

If Wordsworth's bliss did not last, his youthfulness was at least shared
by many, for the population of Europe and America in 1790 was much
younger than our own. The birthrate was high, but so was the deathrate,
and the biblical threescore years and ten was the exception rather than
the rule of life expectancy. Much of the wastage occurred among infants
and young children, but deathrates among all age groups were higher
than at present. Despite a 25-percent chance that an English child born
in 1790 would not survive to his or her fifth birthday, England's population, like that of much of Europe, was rising. Indeed, this was the
early stage of the sustained population growth that connects our contemporary world directly to the eighteenth century.

Demographers are still debating about the relative contribution of
increased fertility and reduced mortality in this early phase, but they
are more certain that, with the possible exception of smallpox inoculation, organized medicine had little to do with it. Medical schools, hospitals, medical societies and journals, medical knowledge, and energetic

doctors all existed in 1790. But these did not necessarily result in life-prolonging therapeutics.

This is our historical judgment. In 1790, many laymen, and most doctors, saw reasons, if not for contentment, then at least for optimism. Doctors claimed to understand, and to cure, disease. They looked upon their education and their institutions, their theories and their science, as important if sometimes ineffective bulwarks against the common diseases within their societies. As the backdrop to the vast changes that occurred within nineteenth-century medicine, we shall look briefly at the state of the medical professions, medical knowledge, prevalent diseases, and medical practice in the late eighteenth century.

I. THE MEDICAL PROFESSIONS AND THEIR EDUCATIONS

With their characteristics of specialized knowledge, autonomy, and an ethos of service, modern professions are often seen as products of nineteenth-century society. Many groups – architects, engineers, teachers, accountants – had achieved some degree of professional status by 1900. But the word profession, and some rudiments of the modern concept, have much longer histories. Medicine was one of the three traditional learned professions (other "professionals" being clergymen and lawyers), a status confirmed in medieval universities by separate faculties of theology, law, and medicine in addition to arts faculties. But formally educated medical men were part of a much larger group that included individuals, like surgeons and apothecaries, who were also concerned with the healing arts but commonly were untouched by the pretensions to learning, gentility, and position that universities conferred. Historically, however, the Church as often as the State was involved in conferring legitimacy on medical practitioners, and local clergymen were often entrusted with the cure of bodies as well as souls. In addition, wise women, herbalists, good samaritans, midwives, itinerant drug peddlars, ladies of the manor, mountebanks, and quacks also dispensed advice and recommended medicines. Further, neighborly consultations, family remedies, and self-medication have always been important, just as they are today. These informal aspects of medical care have begun to receive serious historical attention, although they can be dealt with only in passing in this book, which focuses primarily on the recognized medical "professions": physicians, surgeons, and apothecaries. Their positions and training in 1790 varied with national and social contexts in Britain, the European mainland, and the United States.

The physicians are the easiest to identify, since they were university graduates. In England, "university" meant only the ancient ones of Oxford and Cambridge. Both medical faculties had distinguished episodes in their past and bright futures, but in the eighteenth century they were often dead in the summer and moribund in the winter. Only a handful of young men took medical degrees at Oxford or Cambridge each year. Recruitment in general to the ancient universities was much lower in the eighteenth century than it had been the previous century, and this combined with the exclusion of all but communicants of the Church of England, the length and expense of an Oxbridge medical education, and the low esteem in which medicine was held by those whose sons went there, produced sleepy medical faculties. The education was broadly classical, for not only did medical students first pursue the ordinary B.A. degree, but their medical course still placed emphasis on classical medical authors like Hippocrates and Galen. The inculcated attitudes could be complacent, but many Oxbridge men were visible on the medical scene; the polish and contacts they acquired there undoubtedly helped.

So, too, did the fact that Oxbridge graduates dominated the Royal College of Physicians of London. Barring exceptional circumstances, only they were eligible for the Fellowship in the College. Although technically responsible just for regulating the practice of medicine in London and for seven miles around the city, the College of Physicians was a prestigious if introverted institution in 1790. Several earlier attempts to liberalize its policies so that medical graduates from other universities could be elected Fellows (instead of merely as Licentiates, nonvoting affiliates), and to turn it into a more egalitarian instrument of medical reform had failed. Like the universities, the College remained more concerned with privilege than responsibility. But neither the College of Physicians nor the universities was bereft of energetic sons. William Heberden (1710–1801) combined impeccable classical scholarship with original contributions to clinical medicine. His son, William Heberden, the younger (1767–1845), who in 1790 was still a student at his father's old college, St. John's, Cambridge, went on to edit his father's works and to make his own mark in the treatment of children's diseases. Thomas Young (1773–1829), remembered more for his wave theory of light and his work on color vision, was also a Cambridge medical graduate. Young, however, had already studied medicine in London, Edinburgh, and Göttingen before deciding in 1797 to spend two years as a mature student in Cambridge. His eclectic education reminds us of the flexibility and informality of earlier medical training, even among physicians.

For those who did not belong to the Church of England, or who, increasingly, desired medical experience rather than simply social polish, Oxbridge was out. Earlier in the century, the alternative was often the University of Leiden, where Hermann Boerhaave (1668–1738) offered clinical instruction in a twelve-bed ward. By the 1750s, however, the

Scottish universities had replaced the Dutch as the favorite destination for aspiring students without the desire, money, religion, or connections to get into Oxbridge. There were important medical faculties at the universities of Edinburgh and Glasgow. The University of St. Andrews offered cheap medical degrees but no medical instruction. Edinburgh was preeminent. Although Edinburgh's most famous medical teacher, William Cullen (1710–90), had finally retired in 1789, the University still had many attractions: reasonable tuition costs, a respected medical faculty, clinical lectures, successful extramural teaching, active student societies, and the general intellectual life associated with the city that the Scots loved to call the Athens of the North. Scotland's "democratic intellect" placed a high premium on literacy and education, and students from England, Ireland, Wales, and the United States gave Scottish universities an international flavor. Since teaching was in the vernacular, Edinburgh was never so cosmopolitan as Padua had been in William Harvey's time, or Leiden in Boerhaave's. But Scottish graduates leavened the medical scene all over the English-speaking world. Some, like John Coakley Lettsom (1744–1815), founded hospitals, dispensaries, and medical societies, like the Medical Society of London (1773). Others, such as James Lind (1716–94) and Gilbert Blane (1749–1834), worked to reform the medical services of the armed forces. Another Cullen pupil, John Morgan (1735–89), pioneered medical education in the United States.

There were even surgical students in the Scottish universities, many of whom pursued careers in the army or navy. Only a few of these bothered to take medical degrees since their ordinary mode of training was still through an apprenticeship with a master surgeon or practitioner. Rather, budding surgeons would come to Edinburgh or Glasgow for a year or two of their apprenticeship (normally seven years) to study anatomy, chemistry, and other subjects less easy to acquire with their master. The Monro family – son succeeding father – created an anatomical dynasty in Edinburgh lasting from 1720, when John Monro (1670–1740) arranged for his son Alexander Monro *primus* (1697–1767) to teach anatomy in the newly formed medical faculty, to 1846, when the incompetent Alexander Monro *tertius* (1773–1859) finally relinquished the stranglehold. Monro *primus* and Monro *secundus* (1733–1817) were particularly energetic and in the 1790s there were over 400 students enrolled each year in the latter's anatomy classes. Edinburgh encouraged its professors to become pedagogical entrepreneurs because most of their salaries came from the fees students paid to take their courses. Students from other faculties in the University and even townspeople often signed up for popular courses like anatomy, so class numbers must be treated with caution as an accurate guide to the size of the medical faculty. Nevertheless, many ambitious surgeons, like Sir Astley Cooper (1768–

1841) and Sir Charles Bell (1774–1842), spent at least part of their student days in Edinburgh.

By 1790, however, London had also become a major center for surgical education. From 1746 to his death William Hunter (1718–83) taught anatomy to generations of surgical and medical students, from 1769 at his private school in Great Windmill Street. The school survived under Hunter's nephew Matthew Baillie (1761–1823), Charles Bell, and others until 1832 and by the 1790s offered instruction in a whole range of medical subjects, including anatomy, physiology, chemistry, and the practice of medicine and surgery. Some half-dozen other private anatomy and medical schools competed with the Hunterian School for student patronage and although clinical facilities were limited in this private sector, students supplemented their training by "walking the wards" of the London hospitals. There, clinical instruction and some experience in patient care were available.

But for many young surgeons, London meant above all John Hunter (1728–93), William's younger brother and the most famous surgeon of the century. In 1790, a sick man suffering from the heart disease that was shortly to end his life, Hunter taught hundreds of students at St George's Hospital, where he was on the staff, and at his private surgical school in Leicester Square. An avid collector of anatomical and pathological specimens, an experimentalist of considerable talent, and an innovative operative surgeon, Hunter encouraged his fellow surgeons to think of themselves as scientific professionals instead of merely as craftsmen. They had already achieved formal separation from the Barbers in 1745, when the London Company of Surgeons was granted independent status. After Hunter's death, Parliament bought his vast collections and presented them to the Surgeons who, in 1800, received a royal charter establishing the Royal College of Surgeons, a tangible embodiment of the upward mobility they desired. Legally, however, surgery was still an apprenticed craft, and students' experience of metropolitan life was generally sandwiched between periods of articled apprenticeship, where the practical aspects of their occupation were learned. Except for élites in metropolitan centers, surgeons spent only a fraction of their time in what today would be considered surgery. Rather, they performed many functions of a general practitioner and might treat farm animals as well.

Even more numerous than surgeons were the apothecaries. In 1790, their London company, the Society of Apothecaries, still had its great days before it. Legally obliged to earn their livings through the sale of drugs, apothecaries technically practiced a trade. In actuality, they provided general medical care for many. Since the early eighteenth century they had had the right to prescribe without consulting with a physician, although prescriptions made by a physician would still be taken to an apothecary for compounding. Their apprenticeships were shorter and a bit cheaper than those of surgeons. Their social origins tended to be lower than those of physicians and surgeons but apothecaries ranged from solidly middle-class citizens to ill-paid, badly educated marginal men who combined selling drugs with general shopkeeping and a variety of other occupations. They were expected to know enough Latin to read prescriptions, and botany and chemistry were the sciences deemed most relevant to their occupation. The majority of eighteenth-century remedies were botanical, but preparations of mercury, antimony, phosphorous, arsenic, and iron were also popular. In London, the College of Physicians was conscious of the threat to physicians' practices from the apothecaries (who offered their services more cheaply), but in the provinces professional hierarchies were not so clearly defined and many apothecaries made substantial contributions to the intellectual and cultural life of the period. Some who subsequently took medical degrees, like John Fothergill (1712–80) and William Withering (1741–94), began their medical careers as apothecaries' apprentices. By dint of their very numbers, apothecaries provided most official medical care and by 1790 the Society of Apothecaries was only a generation away from the substantial educational role thrust upon it by the Apothecaries Act of 1815 (see Chapter 2).

Certain similarities between the organization and education of medical men in Britain and in France obscure important differences. For one thing, bureaucracy was more entrenched in French life, with a spate of regulations, statutes, and certificates governing medical qualification and practice. France also had more formal medical institutions: over twenty universities with medical faculties and colleges or guilds of medicine or surgery in many nonuniversity cities. The faculties of medicine in Paris, Montpellier, Toulouse, Strasbourg, and Rheims were most active in Enlightenment France. The Paris Faculty had a venerable history of cautious conservatism. It had opposed Vesalius in the sixteenth century, Harvey in the seventeenth, and remained one of the last bastions of Galenism. Chronically in debt throughout the eighteenth century, the Faculty had been left behind by events even before the Bastille had been stormed, and by its closure in 1793, it had recommended no new licentiates for over three years, and granted no doctorates since 1785. Its Dean and teachers had traditionally been chosen by lot, an obsolete vestige of the presumed equality of élites. Even though the Faculty continued to enjoy a monopoly on Paris medical teaching until the 1790s, it never recovered from the foundation, in 1778, of the Société Royale de Médecine. The latter, the outgrowth of the Royal Correspondence Society of Medicine, established two years earlier by François de Lassone (1717–88) and Félix Vicq d'Azyr (1748–94), became a focus of pre-Revolutionary medical reform (see Chapter 3).

For most of the Enlightenment, however, the Medical University at Montpellier was more vigorous than any other in France. The Scottish doctor and writer Tobias Smollett (1721–71) was scathing about the diagnosis and advice Antoine Firez (1689–1765), a leading Montpellier physician, gave him (by post) on Smollett's own case of consumption in 1763. However, the work of Théophile de Bordeu (1722–76) and his pupil Joseph Barthez (1734–1806) kept that ancient University a center of medical studies during the decades before the Revolution. Their theories of vitalism were to bear fruit in Bichat's physiological researches (see Chapter 2), and Montpellier graduates tended to dominate the medical appointments to the King's household at Versailles. Of equal consequence, Montpellier offered a combined doctorate in medicine and surgery, taken by more than 600 students between 1760 and 1794.

Quite apart from this formal university recognition of a unified medicine and surgery, surgery itself was a vigorous craft in Enlightenment France. Its internal hierarchical arrangement was more strikingly apparent than for medicine, with the premier surgeon to the King commanding vast powers within the occupational group. Eighteenth-century premier surgeons such as Georges Mareschal (1658–1736), François de la Peyronie (1658–1747), and G. P. de la Martinère (1696–1783) dedicated themselves to furthering the autonomy and prestige of surgery. La Peyronie left his enormous fortune to the College of Surgery of Paris, which between 1743 and 1750 achieved its independence from the Faculty of Medicine. The College's three-year course provided instruction in anatomy, physiology, pathology, therapy, obstetrics, and surgical operations. Its faculty included Antoine Louis (1723–92), Jacques Tenon (1724–1816), and others who frequently contributed to the Royal Academy of Surgery. The foundation of the Academy in 1731 by Mareschal and La Peyronie had helped to establish surgery's pretensions to learned status. French surgeons were encouraged to obtain university degrees, but surgical training remained practical and hospital-oriented. Young surgical students worked their way up a steep gradient of hospital posts, with only a few achieving that of resident surgical chief (*gagnant-maîtrise*). So important was this post as the springboard to power and status within the surgical community that the hospitals and the College of Surgery vied for control of these appointments. Surgery's guild origins were perpetuated by students learning practical skills under a master surgeon, but the importance of apprenticeships declined during the century, hastened by an edict of 1772 requiring pupils to attend surgical schools. As in Britain, demand for surgical training was also partly met by private schools often specializing in anatomy. One of these teachers, Pierre-Joseph Desault (1738–95), went on to participate in two of the major ancien régime experiments in surgical education, the Hospice of

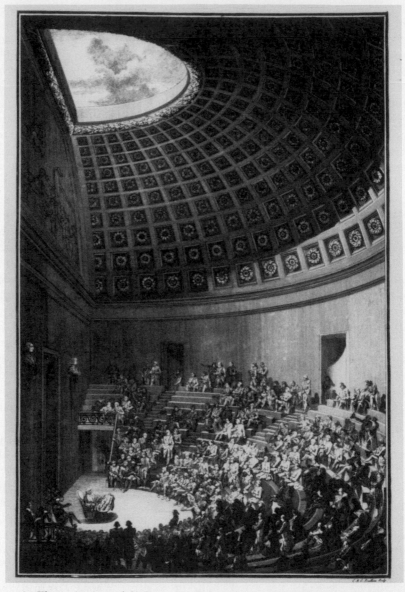

Figure 1. The aspirations of the Paris surgical community are well captured in this 1780 engraving of an anatomical demonstration in the Lecture Theater of the College of Surgery. M. Gondouin, Description des écoles de chirurgie *(Paris: P. D. Pierres et Cellot, 1780), Plate xxix.*

the College of Surgery and Desault's own surgical service in the *Hôtel-Dieu.*

The Hospice, established in 1774 as a small teaching and research hospital, broadened Desault's clinical experience. He often assisted its chief Tenon in operations and learned there the value of routine post-mortem examinations. Cases at the Hospice were also actively discussed by leading College surgeons. In 1782 Desault was appointed chief surgeon at the *Charité;* in 1785 he moved to the *Hôtel Dieu.* In 1791 Bichat claimed that the surgical school there was the best in Europe.

Under Desault's impetus, surgical students were placed in charge of wards, caring for patients and keeping medical records. A new surgical amphitheater permitted operations to be discussed and performed in front of large numbers of students. This was supplemented by clinical lessons in the outpatient clinic. Autopsies became routine as ways of correlating clinical symptoms with pathological findings.

Desault's innovations were not accepted without protest from religious groups, from the nursing sisters, and from some patients, who objected to the loss of nursing control over matters of diet and convalescence, protested against the indignity of disrobing for examination and operation in front of so many male students, and insisted that Desault's long surgical lessons left patients inadequately cared for. Matters came to a head in 1789, when the hospital authorities backed Desault against the formal complaints of the nurses. Their decision was a turning point in the history of the teaching hospital, and it was taken even as the Bastille was being stormed.

The Hospice and *Hôtel Dieu* were not the only experiments in "hospital medicine" before the Revolution, but they were the most striking. Although these innovations were primarily surgical, it is no accident that two of Desault's most distinguished pupils – Bichat and J. N. Corvisart – turned, as we shall see in Chapter 2, from surgery to medicine.

Just as the surgeons were working for social status, so, too, were the apothecaries or pharmacists. Traditionally, the teaching of pharmacy was the responsibility of the faculties of medicine, but in 1777 Parisian apothecaries secured a royal declaration creating their own College of Pharmacy. Many of their élites – for instance, J. J. Virey (1775–1846) – became men of substance, and Revolutionary notions of equality were to grant them, briefly at least, a measure of official patronage. But, like most surgeons outside the famous hospitals and institutions of Paris and other major French cities, most apothecaries were concerned primarily with earning a living through the provision of drugs and medical services to the populace. As the progenitor of the general practitioner, the apothecary was much more important in England than in France, where surgeons tended to fill that niche.

In the German-speaking lands, the story is even more complex, for a ed Germany under the leadership of Prussia was still in the future the Austrian Empire was developing its own medical traditions. rtheless, by 1790 the emergence of a great national literature, centered above all on Goethe (1749–1832), helped elevate the German language to European status. This encouraged German-speaking doctors and naturalists to use the vernacular in writing and teaching, as their colleagues in Britain and France were already doing.

A distinctive feature of medical education and the medical profession in Northern Europe was a university system that contained some vigorous pockets of activity. Most of the German principalities had their own universities, many of them of Medieval and Renaissance origin but others (e.g., Königsberg, 1735; Göttingen, 1737) had been established more recently. Early in the century, the Prussian University of Halle (f. 1694) was preeminent among medical faculties. There, Friedrich Hoffmann (1660–1742) and Georg Ernst Stahl (1660–1734) were expounding their medical theories, which rivaled Boerhaave's in European influence. Hoffmann, working in the mechanistic tradition, developed theories of the role of the nervous system in health and disease, which Cullen put to systematic use. Stahl (equally famous for his work on phlogiston theory) stressed the importance of the soul in physiological functions. Stahl's physiological notions were much admired by the Montpellier vitalists in the second half of the century. By the 1720s Halle had some 500 medical students, including many from Italy and France. Few British students wandered as far afield as Halle, but the foundation of the University of Göttingen by the British monarch George II (who was also Elector of Hanover) brought a German university closer to home. Albrecht von Haller (1708–77) taught there from its foundation until 1753, and from 1777 the dominant figure in its vigorous medical faculty was J. F. Blumenbach (1752–1840). His concept of the "life force" (*nisus formativus; Bildungstrieb*) was assimilated into German Romantic biology and medicine, but Blumenbach was also a careful comparative anatomist and physiologist whose works on these subjects gained cosmopolitan significance.

Various universities in German-speaking areas also established teaching clinics, on the model of Boerhaave's in Leiden. In 1753, a Boerhaave pupil, Gerhard van Swieten (1700–72), took charge of one such clinic in Vienna, and by the century's end clinical instruction was obligatory in Erlangen, Altdorf, Kiel, Göttingen, Jena, Tübingen, and Leipzig.

The easier availability of university-based medical education made the physician more visible on the German landscape. At the same time, surgeons had also become more integrated into the universities, again following the Dutch lead. Most important were the surgical clinics in Vienna and Göttingen. This movement away from the apprenticeship and the colleges of surgery led to professional equality between physicians and surgeons with intraprofessional tension being shifted to that between educated élites and more lowly practitioners with less prestigious training. It was still easy to buy doctorates in many German universities, and religious and secular authorities granted them as tokens of favor or sources of income. This made the M.D. degree easy to acquire in Germany and meant that physicians were more important than apothecaries in providing general medical care. By contrast, apothecaries busied themselves more with keeping shops and filling prescriptions than in England, where they served as general practitioners as well.

Britain provided the major influence on early American medical education; indeed, many colonial physicians actually trained in British universities, particularly Edinburgh. However, the formation of indigenous medical schools, like that at the University of Pennsylvania (1765) and King's College, New York (1767: later Columbia University) created a native medical ethos. In addition to these formal institutions, apprenticeships with local physicians and surgeons provided another route for the medical student. The regulation of medical practice was in the hands of state legislatures, and although most states in the young Republic instituted licensing laws, little attempt was made to regulate the quality of medical training. Such neglect was to result in a spate of proprietary medical schools early in the nineteenth century, each offering cheap, quick doctorates. Some of the schools attached to universities maintained reasonable standards, but throughout the nineteenth century, many ambitious American doctors supplemented their medical educations with European study. In 1790, this study abroad was still primarily in Britain, although later Americans went to France, Germany, and Austria to absorb more systematic clinical and scientific training.

II. MEDICAL KNOWLEDGE

The existence of such diverse backgrounds, educations, and social functions among eighteenth-century medical men inevitably led to wide variations in explaining, diagnosing, and treating disease. The age's individualism encouraged many to tout their own special claims to the public, and differences of medical opinion tended to increase, rather than diminish, the polemicism of much medical writing. Nevertheless, some sense of what counted as knowledge, and the order in which it was to be learned, can be gained from the systematic expositions of leading medical educators. Cullen provides a good example. Not only were his works translated into many European languages, but his teaching also spanned a wide range of medical subjects: chemistry, physiology, materia medica, pathology, and the practice of medicine. He argued that medicine ("the art of preventing and of curing disease") rested on three pillars, collectively known as the Institutions (or Institutes) of Medicine: "The first treats of life and health [physiology]. The second delivers the general doctrine of disease [pathology]. The third delivers the general doctrine concerning the means of preventing and curing diseases [therapeutics]."[1] To these three pillars should be added a fourth, which is sometimes viewed as prolegomenon to the others: anatomy.

Anatomy was still the queen of the medical sciences, the subject around which much medical education revolved, but it was also a source of considerable conflict between doctors and the public. The former argued that knowledge of anatomy was necessary to understand the functions of the body in health and disease, but the public viewed dissection as unsavory, associated with the fates of condemned criminals and encouraging ribaldry and loose morals among medical students. To the crowds who witnessed public executions in Georgian London, surgeons were as unpopular as the hangmen and riots against them were not uncommon. Persistent difficulties in supply led to the lucrative business of body snatching and grave robbing, linking anatomy teachers directly to the criminal underworld. The poor knew that, under normal circumstances, it was their bodies that were dissected, but solid citizens feared that no fresh grave was inviolate from ruffians who could sell the valuables to pawnbrokers and the body to anatomists. The French resolved the legal if not the emotional aspects of bodies for dissection in the 1790s, but in Britain and America problems persisted, fanned by revelations from the 1820s that Burke and Hare in Edinburgh and the Williams gang in London were actually generating their own corpses by murder. There were serious riots against doctors and medical students in New York in 1788 and in New Haven in 1824.

Knowledge of gross human anatomy was extensive enough and general works produced in the first half of the century by William Cheselden (1688–1752), Lorenz Heister (1683–1758), and Jacques Winslow (1669–1760) went through multiple editions in several languages long after their authors' deaths. The thirteenth edition (1792) of Cheselden's *Anatomy of the Human Body* was virtually unchanged from the fourth (1730), suggesting a stable – even a dead – science. Specific anatomical investigations occasionally paid direct surgical dividends, as in the development of new approaches in operating for bladder stones, repairing hernias, or removing tuberculous joints. But pre-Listerian surgeons avoided the abdominal, thoracic, and cranial cavities, whose opening almost invariably led to fatal infection, and the absence of anesthesia placed a premium on speed. This in turn left no time to consider during operations the finer anatomical details of the area. Amputations of an arm or a leg took only a minute or two and debates about amputation concerned timing, whether to cover the surgical wound with a skin flap

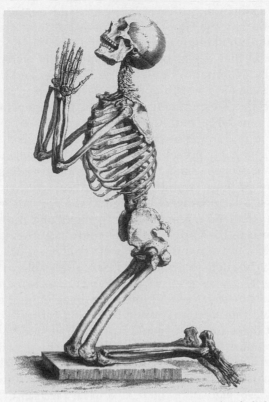

Figure 2. Despite the fact that anatomy was popularly considered slightly disreputable, many anatomical books had expensive and elaborate engravings with artistic pretensions, as in this skeleton saying its prayers, from William Cheselden's Osteographia *or the anatomy of the bones (London: W. Boyer, 1733), Plate xxxvi.*

and postoperative care rather than matters for which sophisticated anatomical knowledge was relevant.

Rather, much innovative anatomical investigation had been aimed at elucidation of function. Injection techniques were applied to the small blood vessels, lungs, glands, and lymphatics, the latter being the subject of a priority dispute between William Hunter and Monro *secundus*. Anatomy thus provided the backdrop for physiological experimentation or speculation: for what Albrecht von Haller called *anatomia animata* (living anatomy). In conjunction with anatomy, or under the rubric of the "Institutes of Medicine," physiological function was expounded as the theoretical foundation of medicine. Traditionally, of course, the humors, or fluids, had been emphasized as the active agents in both normal and abnormal function. The Hippocratic doctrine of four humors – blood, black bile, yellow bile, and phlegm – provided a framework and a vobulary for maintaining individual health and explaining disease. In 1790, admiration for the Hippocratics was still ardent, but humoralism's hold on medical thinking was being eroded. Early in the century, Boerhaave had held that the blood and blood vessels were the culprits in many diseases. Hoffmann, however, had emphasized the centrality of the nervous system in health and disease, a position subsequently reinforced by Haller's experimental work on the distinction between irritability and sensibility, and Robert Whytt's (1714–66) investigations of the spinal cord and involuntary bodily actions. From the 1750s, a new aesthetics of sensibility preached the association between delicate, "sensitive" nervous systems and refinement, good breeding, and culture. Cullen integrated these strands into his medical writings. Two-thirds of his physiological lectures were devoted to the nervous system, and his discussion of circulation, respiration, digestion, and nutrition made frequent reference to the body's ultimate control by the nervous system. The functions of the nervous system were *vital* ones, observable in their manifestations but not, according to Cullen, explicable without reference to an immaterial soul as a source of nervous power or energy. He used the traditional categories of will, memory, imagination, and perception in approaching the functions of the brain and central nervous system, insisting that these functions could not be understood mechanically.

At the same time, the peripheral nerves were being subjected to a lot of experimental analysis. Haller had exploited the fact that mechanical stimulation causes nerves to produce their effects, and from 1780, Luigi Galvani (1737–98) had investigated "animal electricity." Galvani's researches reinforced earlier speculation on the possibility that the *vis nervosa* (nervous power) was analogous to electricity. His major work, published in 1791, came too late for Cullen, but fascination with the physiological and therapeutic potentials of electricity was part of the Enlightenment's "discovery" of the nervous system. Only since the eighteenth century have people suffered from "nerves": earlier, they had been affected with things such as "spleen," "vapours," or "melancholia" (black bile).

The blood was the only real rival to the nervous system as the primary custodian of the life force in late eighteenth-century physiology. John Hunter's researches on blood kept that ancient, emotionally laden humor to the fore. The ubiquity of bloodletting for treating a wide range of disorders provided doctors with frequent opportunities to examine the substance, and chemically inclined medical men applied subtle reasoning to relate the appearance and behavior of shed blood to both physiology and pathology. For Hunter, blood was the essence of life itself (the *materia vitae*), and a whole range of diseases, including fevers, gout, and tumors was explained by reference to it. Secretion, by both the glands and the kidneys, was linked to the different substances comprising blood and the notion of "acrimony" was often cited as the reason blood turned bad and caused disease. Inflammation occupied a key position, as doctors debated whether it was a salutary or pathological process. Its cardinal features – heat, redness, swelling, and pain (*calor, rubor, tumor,* and *dolor*) – had been noted by Celsus (fl. A.D. 25), but its precise mechanism and purposes still preoccupied many. Hunter insisted that inflammation was defensive rather than pathological; for Cullen it was disease in itself, grouped, like fevers, within the class Pyrexia (from the Greek word for *fire*).

The hematological and nervous systems occupied such prominent places in physiological inquiries because they seemed most relevant to the second part of the Institutes of Medicine: pathology. Boerhaave, Hoffmann, and Hieronymous David Gaub (1705–80) published standard Enlightenment expositions of the subject, and the latter two directly influenced Cullen's major treatise on disease: *First Lines of the Practice of Physic* (1778–84). This multivolume text continued to be widely used – particularly in America – well into the nineteenth century, although it was usually modified by later editors. It was not a pathological work in the style of Gaub's *Institutiones pathologiae medicinalis* (The institutes of medical pathology, 1758), which treated general pathological issues, such as the nature, causes, and consequences of disease. Instead, Cullen organized his work nosologically: around a classification of specific diseases. His concern with disease classification was widely shared by many eighteenth-century physicians who built on the prestige of Carl Linnaeus's (1707–78) vast taxonomic enterprise.

Linnaeus had set himself the ambitious task of precisely naming (and hence classifying) the objects of the natural world: to name is to know. Most successful in botany, he also extended his taxonomic gaze to the other two kingdoms of nature, the animal and the mineral. A physician himself, Linnaeus also attempted a classification of diseases, a formal intellectual justification for which can be found a famous passage of Thomas Sydenham (1624–89) asserting that the symptoms produced by a particular disease are so constant that the physician can identify and classify disease in exactly the same way as a botanist classifies plants.

In addition to Linnaeus, a number of doctors – notably Boissier de Sauvages (1706–67), David Macbride (1726–78), and Cullen – produced systematic nosological treatises, based on symptoms. Boissier had insisted that only symptoms provided an adequate guide for the classifying doctor, postmortem lesions being too variable and unreliable. Cullen allowed gross pathological changes as one source of information, but he too, relied more on the sequence of symptoms as his principal guide. These symptoms he related to his physiological ideas, particularly to the primacy of the nervous system. One of his four classes of disease was the "neuroses," a term he coined, although one whose meaning has

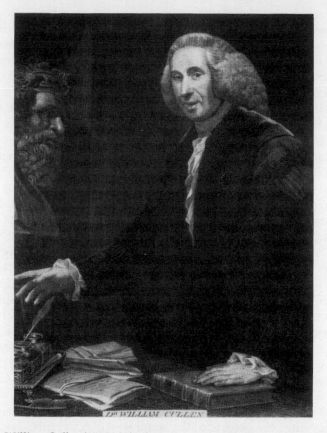

Figure 3. William Cullen (1710–90), shown here as a cultured man of letters. Engraving in Jesse Foot – extra illustrated copy of Life of John Hunter *(London: T. Becket, 1794), Vol. 2, p. 248.*

since changed. For Cullen, neuroses were primary diseases of the nervous system, without fever, affecting the senses or movement. They included apoplexy, palsies, fainting, and epilepsy (obvious neurological disorders) as well as diarrhea, asthma, indigestion, and colic, disorders in which the internal or "natural" motions were deranged.

Three points need to be made about Cullen's nosological scheme. First, based as it was primarily on symptoms, it thus embodied a holistic approach to disease. Although Cullen admitted that disease sometimes could be local (one of his classes of disease was *locales*), he conceived the human body as an integrated whole, so that individuals, not organs or body parts, were the actual loci of disease. His pathology was clinical, not anatomical, in its orientation. Second, this clinical orientation was directly based on his physiology, for he explained the sequences of symptoms in a disease on the basis of their physiological causes. Like most doctors of his day, Cullen sometimes spoke of disease causation in terms of contrasting pairs: remote and proximal, external and internal, predisposing and exciting. But for both nosological and therapeutic purposes, he stressed the more immediate of the pairs: proximal, internal, and exciting. Remote causes were relevant for prevention; proximate causes for treatment. What happened to the patient during the course of the illness seemed of more urgency than background issues such as inheritance, temperament, or constitution. He made no attempt to establish a classification based on *etiology*, as the germ theory was later to encourage doctors to do. Consequently, even while elaborating a nosology of specific disease entities, his discussions often harked back to his physiological principles, particularly the role of the nervous system: "In a certain view," he wrote, "almost the whole of diseases of the human body might be called NERVOUS."[2]

In this endeavor, Cullen shared a third characteristic with many of his contemporaries: the simultaneous concern with nosological splitting and the ardent search for basic pathophysiological principles uniting virtually all disease into an integral whole. Cullen's sense of the contingent protected him from the excesses of many systematists, but his own advocacy of nervous debility as an ubiquitous pathological symptom was carried further by two of his pupils who claimed to have discovered laws of Newtonian grandeur for medicine: John Brown (1735–88) and Benjamin Rush (1746–1813). Brown accepted the necessity of various nosological tags but believed that all disease was caused by excess or deficiency of a single biological property that he called "excitability": the capacity to react to external stimuli. A proper balance of excitability was healthy, but deviations could occur in either direction, too much yielding *sthenic* diseases, too little, *asthenic* ones. In practice, most diseases became asthenic, as exhaustion supervened after initial excessive excitability. Treatment was aimed at the underlying cause. For sthenic conditions, depletive or lowering measures, such as bloodletting, emetics and cathartics were appropriate, whereas asthenic diseases required stimulants, of which opium and alcohol were Brown's favorites. In Britain, Brown's system, wonderfully simple yet argued with considerable force, never made much headway, but in Germany and Italy it found many willing disciples. Brown himself did not live to enjoy his Continental fame. He died prematurely, worn out by gout and his personal fondness for his beloved remedies, opium and alcohol.

Rush also had the courage of his therapeutic convictions, permitting himself to be treated by the dictates of his own system, which was a monolithic one: all disease, he insisted, was caused by a preternatural tension in the arteries, thus combining the nervous and hematological systems into a pathophysiological unity. Massive bloodletting was his treatment of choice, although he also valued other depletive measures such as calomel, a mercury compound used as a purgative. Rush's most sweeping systematic pronouncements made only limited impact on the medical community, although vigorous depletive therapy could be pursued from other theoretical standpoints. But the pressure felt by eighteenth-century doctors to produce a Newton of medicine sustained the search for grand laws and wholesale generalizations. Unfortunately, there was nothing quite like gravity around in the medical sphere.

As can be seen, Cullen, Brown, Rush, and other late eighteenth-century physicians incorporated definite therapeutic implications into their pathological theories. The relations among the three parts of the Institutions of Medicine were close, because both pathology and therapeutics were approached physiologically. There is a great deal of historical continuity in therapeutics, much more so than in theories of disease. Much of Cullen's therapeutic armamentarium was available to the Hippocratics. Bloodletting, cathartics, and emetics; sudorifics for inducing sweating and febrifuges for combating fever: these were all described in the Hippocratic corpus but were still vital to Cullen's world. There had, of course, been numerous additions and modifications to the pharmacopoeia: New World imports like Jesuit's bark (or Peruvian bark, the active principle of which is quinine) for intermittent fevers, guaiacum for syphilis, and ipecacuanha for inducing vomiting; a variety of metallic preparations of arsenic, mercury, and antimony unavailable to the Hippocratics were popular; and always there was exploitation of local botanical preparations. Having lectured on materia medica, Cullen was sensitive to the range of medicinal possibilities. Further, unlike Brown or Rush, whose therapeutic systems can hardly be called subtle, Cullen insisted that therapeutics was an extremely delicate art. The timing, sequence, and dosage of the recommended agents could make the difference between success and failure, between cure and death. There was consequently much room for therapeutic debate, but the terms of these debates were Hippocratic in spirit: of correcting imbalance, lowering the overactive system, stimulating the debilitated one. In that sense, therapeutics was still geared to the peculiarities of the individual patient. Diet continued to play a large role in medical thinking and in this area Hippocratic precepts loomed large until the nineteenth century was well advanced.

Despite what to the modern eye is a sterility of much eighteenth-century therapeutic discussion, the subject was of considerable moment. Chairs in the practice of medicine were prized over those in the theory of medicine or in the medical sciences. Therapeutics was often the object of attempted medical reform, particularly from mid-century, as the practice gradually developed of reporting multiple therapeutic trials. James Lind had used twelve sailors with scurvy in his demonstration of the value of citrus fruit, and military doctors and hospital staff sometimes turned their enlarged medical arenas to the service of numerical reporting of therapeutic results. William Withering's *Treatise on the Purple Foxglove* (1785), in which digitalis was shown to be useful in many cases of dropsy (fluid accumulation), was a model of clinical pharmacology, reporting failures as well as successes, and laying down guidelines for use and signs of toxicity. Like many drugs, however, digitalis subsequently became a panacea, employed for diseases as far apart as phthisis and insanity, before late nineteenth-century clinicians began finally to limit its use along the lines originally suggested by Withering.

For Cullen, therapeutics meant not simply curing diseases; it also involved preventing them through understanding and acting on their remote causes. He duly discussed the remote causes of most diseases, for instance, the class Pyrexia, which included the fevers. These causes were traditional environmental factors, such as damp and cold, plus miasmata. The last, which Cullen conceived as poisons spread through the atmosphere, were necessary to explain epidemic outbreaks. For diseases such as smallpox, the intermediate vector was a contagion of unknown nature but communicable from person to person. As we shall see in Chapter 3, various Enlightenment doctors examined more general aspects of disease within the community, but Cullen himself was not a sophisticated social thinker. He knew it was difficult to identify remote causes of diseases, so he spent more time on their immediate causes within the individual patient. For him, prevention more usually involved the regulation of the individual life, but his remarks on prevention were scattered and do not add up to a systematic philosophy of health.

For someone like Cullen, then, medical knowledge could be integrated within the framework of the Institutions of Medicine. Pathology and therapeutics were grounded in physiology, which in turn was often inferred from observations made at the bedside. Cullen made virtually no direct use of experimental physiology. General symptoms were more important than local lesions for both nosology and therapeutics. He most commonly conceptualized symptoms in terms of the nervous, cardiovascular, and digestive systems. Nosology was a prestigious enterprise, but it jostled uneasily with the search for common underlying causes of all disease. The same cluster of proximate "causes" – cold, heat, spasm, debility – tend to recur throughout Cullen's expansive nosological scheme and he never satisfactorily resolved the question why similar causes can produce such diverse pathological effects. His therapeutics, like that of many of his contemporaries, tended to be optimistically aggressive: doctors spoke of cures and they meant it. Some laymen doubted medicine's capacity to intervene effectively and many books, like John Wesley's *Primitive Physick* (1747), Simon Tissot's *Avis au peuple sur sa santé* (Advice to the people on their health, 1761), and William Buchan's *Domestic Medicine* (1769) discounted doctors' claims to esoteric knowledge and instead offered laymen all they needed to know about coping with disease. But not much suggests that medicine and its institutions were under serious threat in 1790, even if the French Revolution was briefly to experiment with a kind of laissez-faire medical populism. Indeed, the fact that medical knowledge was not so remote from that of the educated layman, that doctors approached disease in terms of the symptoms the patient experienced, and that medical language had wide cultural resonances, may have weakened medicine's claims to professional status; but these very factors helped secure medicine's niche within late Enlightenment society.

III. PLACING DISEASES

Much morbidity and mortality in 1790 were the result of infections by microorganisms. Plague had disappeared more than a century before, but fevers, smallpox, dysentery, pulmonary consumption and the communicable diseases of childhood were widespread. Venereal disease was a leading cause of morbidity in the military and a common reason for outpatient visits among civilians. Convulsions, the most frequent recorded cause of death among small children, were usually the outcome of some acute communicable disease with high fever and body fluid disturbances.

The impact of these and kindred disorders on late eighteenth- and early nineteenth-century society will be considered in Chapter 3. Here, we can only sketch how Cullen perceived, diagnosed, and treated four selected diseases: smallpox, "typhus," pulmonary consumption, and "heart disease." This group will recur in later chapters as we look at the changing nosological, diagnostic, pathological, therapeutic, and prophylactic issues that they raised during the course of the nineteenth century.

Smallpox was virtually universal in Enlightenment Europe and America. Its distinctive rash made diagnosis easy and there was general agreement that its proximate cause was a specific contagion spread from person to person. Smallpox also attracted widespread attention during the period as the one disease for which a kind of specific preventive was available: inoculation. Introduced into England earlier in the century largely through the efforts of Lady Mary Wortley Montagu (1689–1762), inoculation was a folk-practice of ancient origin in Asia and the Near East, and Lady Mary had learned of it in Constantinople. Inoculation involved taking some material from a pustule of a person suffering from smallpox and introducing it through a break in the skin of someone who had not had the disease. The result was smallpox, but usually milder than ordinarily acquired through natural infection. Lasting immunity followed and given the almost certain chance of suffering from the disease sooner or later, inoculation made good sense. It became safer, cheaper, and more commonly practiced after mid-century, when the Sutton family introduced in England a simpler, quicker, and more effective procedure that avoided the esoteric and dangerous trappings with which the medical profession had earlier invested it. By 1790, inoculation was widely practiced in France, Russia, and elsewhere in Europe. It may even have produced a demographically significant diminution in mortality, particularly in the countryside where mass inoculations were often carried out in the wake of threatened smallpox epidemics. Such possibilities are intriguing but reliable data are scarce and in cities like London smallpox continued to account for about 5 percent of mortality into the nineteenth century.

As befitting a disease of such consequence, Cullen discussed it fully. He classified it as an eruptive fever, along with measles, scarlet fever, plague, and erysipelas. These exanthemata were united as an order of the class Pyrexia by virtue of their acute onset, skin and lymphatic involvement, and the presence of fever. Although, as we shall see, Cullen related the febrile symptoms to the nervous system, the associated rash (leading to the formation of pustules), salivation, lymphatic enlargement, and bleeding disorder (leading to bloody urine and to petechiae – red spots – under the skin) were discussed in humoral terms. The pustular rash seemed to be the body's attempt to get rid of the putrescent matter of the contagion. Accordingly, he recommended remedies to assist the body's natural defenses: cool air, cooling drinks, and gentle purging to counter the inflammatory state, tonics and wine if the putrescence led to debility, and blisters in serious cases with a confluent rash. Although generally an acute, specific disorder leading to death or recovery, smallpox could, Cullen believed, occasionally yield a more chronic inflammatory condition, including tubercles in the lungs. Although the Hippocratics did not describe smallpox, they would have understood most of Cullen's discussion and would have approved of the reasoning that underlay his treatment of the disease.

More complicated, however, was "typhus" fever. The fevers, another order of the class Pyrexia, were distinguished from the exanthemata by the absence of specific topical or local manifestations. For us, fever is a sign of underlying disease; for Cullen, it was a disease itself, of which excess body heat was only one part. Rather, Cullen taught that the disease *fever* consists of an invariable sequence of symptoms whereby debility or nervous weakness is followed by a chill that in turn produces a hot stage. Because both the chill and the hot stage were part of the process initiated by the debility, fevers were for Cullen disorders of the nervous system.

In 1790, "fever" was a common diagnostic tag, accounting for almost a quarter of the mortality between 1774 and 1793 in some London parishes. These bills of mortality did not distinguish among various kinds of fever, but Cullen and his contemporaries were much concerned with their detailed classification. Cullen's main division was between the intermittent and the continued fevers. He further differentiated the latter into other categories such as typhus, remittent, synochus, simple, and so forth. Cullen used the word "typhus" to describe the disease that John Huxham (1692–1768) had called a "nervous fever." With its features of headache, disturbance of consciousness sometimes leading to coma, and great prostration, Cullen's typhus shares some characteristics with the condition we now call "typhus." But the fit is hardly precise and the disease variously called typhus, nervous, jail, camp, or ship fever cannot be placed in a single modern diagnostic mold. Because Cullen believed fevers to be without specific local pathological manifestations, he did not expect to find any useful postmortem changes. Consequently, his diagnostic criteria were gathered at the bedside: in observing the condition of the patient's skin and tongue, state of the bowels, the pulse rate and its relation to body heat, the pattern of chill and heat, and the patient's reported feelings. He occasionally used a thermometer but believed it less helpful than noting these clinical phenomena.

At one level, Cullen's criteria for differentiating fevers into genera and species were precise, but he also recognized that the course of a fever in an individual patient did not always conform to a precise, idealized type. A typhus, for instance, might change into a synochus or simple fever, and a fever epidemic might change its character in the course of spreading through a locality. Thus, although he believed that typhus was remotely caused by a specific contagion, its precise nature was elusive. Further, under appropriate circumstances, other factors – miasmata, heat, cold, venery, fear, dirt, putrefaction, or bad air – could cause a fever. This difficulty in identifying precise and invariable remote "causes" of "typhus" reinforced Cullen's tendency to concentrate on the immediate, physiological "causes" of the particular patient's fever. Therapy was aimed at counteracting them: at correcting the debility, loosening the spasm of the cold stage, and reducing the excessive heat of the hot stage.

Many of the difficulties Cullen faced in categorizing acute disorders like fevers were compounded for chronic diseases such as consumption. As a diagnosis, consumption referred to almost any wasting disease with a pulmonary component; many but not all would now be diagnosed as pulmonary tuberculosis. Cullen, who preferred the phrase phthisis pulmonalis, defined the condition as "an expectoration of pus or purulent matter from the lungs, attended with a hectic fever,"[3] a definition that could include almost any chronic lung disease. Indeed, Cullen recognized this, for this purulent expectoration could result from ulceration of the lung (the consequences of tubercles), but also sometimes from pneumonias, asthma, hemoptysis (spitting up blood), or catarrh. Accordingly, although tubercles were "the most frequent cause of phthisis," they were only one of a cluster. Further, he observed that measles, smallpox, and syphilis could produce an acrimony (i.e., sharp, corrosive quality) in the blood that might yield – particularly in those of a phthisical "disposition" – full-blown pulmonary phthisis. The ancient observation that phthisis often ran in families underlay the belief that its remote cause was generally an inherited diathesis (predisposition). The phthisical habit or temperament was found in people with florid complexions, narrow chests, long necks, and prominent shoulders. Cullen denied that phthisis was contagious; rather its proximate cause was most commonly an episode of catarrh, pneumonia, or measles, leading to ulceration and tubercle formation. Dusty occupations – stone cutting, milling, flax-dressing – seemed to increase its incidence. The accompanying hectic fever occurred twice daily, morning and evening, the latter being more serious and producing night sweats.

Unlike smallpox or typhus, phthisis was a condition for which postmortem data were of relevance. Even so, Cullen was far more concerned with establishing clinical guidelines than precise pathological categories. For one thing, tubercles could often be found at autopsy in patients with few or none of the symptoms of phthisis. And since phthisis could occur in patients without tubercles, their presence guided prognosis rather than defined diagnosis. One of Cullen's aphorisms summarized this: "A phthisis from tubercle has, I think, been recovered; but it is of all the others the most dangerous; and when arising from a hereditary taint, is almost certainly fatal."[4] The onset of hectic fever, with debility, emaciation, sweating, and diarrhea, heralded the end. While noting the common association of pulmonary tubercles and scrofula, and the existence of tubercles in the lymphatic glands in the latter condition, Cullen denied that phthisis and scrofula were different manifestations of a single process. Rather, he grouped scrofula with syphilis, jaundice, and scurvy among what he called the cachexies or wasting diseases.

Cullen was honestly pessimistic about the effects of his therapy. Most of his measures were aimed at minimizing the lung's inflammatory response to the tubercle, since he believed that the uninflamed tubercle sometimes spontaneously disappeared. Thus, what was called an antiphlogistic regimen – low diet, avoidance of animal food and wine, occasional bloodlettings – was in order. Intense cold, violent exercise, and emotional excesses were to be avoided. Cullen found most of the favorite drug remedies of his day – mercury, quinine, myrrh – of no use and often positively harmful. Our art, he wrote, "can do so little towards the cure of this disease."[5]

In contrast to these other conditions, "heart disease" occupied an insignificant niche in Cullen's thinking. He briefly discussed inflammation of the heart ("carditis"), as well as palpitations (irregular heart-beats) and mentioned inadequate action of the heart as one cause of syncope (fainting). But these topics filled only a dozen or so pages in Cullen's four-volume work, and for the rest, he was not interested in this topic, which has become so central to modern medicine. Valvular heart disease was too local for Cullen's holistic orientation; his discussion of "rheumatism" included joint and muscle complications but he was silent on "rheumatic heart disease," and atherosclerosis went unnoticed. These and various other conditions affecting the heart had been de-scribed by earlier authors, but Cullen's vast "system of the Doctrines and Rules proper for directing the Practice of Physic" was too physio-logical, too holistic, and too symptom-oriented to pay much attention to heart disease.

Cullen's *First Lines of the Practice of Physic* continued to be edited by others well into the nineteenth century and it deserved its fame and influence. But it was also a book that, in its nosological organization and symptomatic approach, survived its author's death more as a mon-ument to his authority and wisdom in practical bedside situations than as a continued theoretical force. Cullen's clinical teaching at the Edin-burgh Infirmary was governed by different precepts from those who, especially in Paris, were soon to make the hospital into the central pillar of medical education.

2

Medicine in the hospital

Medicine must be taught in the hospitals.
> Philippe Pinel, *The Clinical Training of Doctors* (1793), trans.
> D. Weiner (1980), p. 67

THE Enlightenment had erected hospitals in considerable numbers and doctors were aware of their value both for education and for providing more concentrated fields of experience about disease. But the eighteenth-century hospital could reflect local pride, Christian philanthropy, or benevolent despotism as much as the aspirations of medical men. It was generally controlled by boards of governors or religious orders, in whose hands lay the power to decide which patients were fit objects of charity and to whom the discharged patient owed gratitude. Further, particularly in France and Italy, hospitals had more general custodial and coercive functions, for in many of them the sick were herded together with petty criminals, beggars, the infirm, orphans, prostitutes, the unemployed, and the mad. Much effort had already been made by 1790 to segregate the functions of the *Hôtel Dieu* (for the sick) from the *hôpitaux généraux*, which housed an eclectic variety of social deviants and unfortunates. But some of the associations with the earlier, more undifferentiated perceptions of illness, dependency, and deviancy persisted. At best, hospitals still conferred the stigma of poverty and social inadequacy on their inmates, for those who could afford it received formal medical treatment in their own homes or consulted with the doctor in his rooms.

Much of this was to change in the early nineteenth century with the emergence of "hospital medicine," or the "birth of the clinic." During the half-century following 1794, hospitals moved toward the center of medical education and research; they became sanctuaries of medical knowledge, crucial institutions within medicine's career structure, bastions of medical power. Whether this constitutes a "revolution" is almost a question of semantics. Ideas have long pedigrees and institutions are not created in social vacuums. Hospital-based medical education, hospital-focused medical practices, and systematic record keeping were not unknown in the Enlightenment. Many of the reforms effected during the French Revolution had been set into motion or at least called for in the previous decades. Many of the high priests of the new hospital medicine – Pinel, Corvisart, Cabanis – had practiced for years in the ancien régime. Nevertheless, in France as nowhere else, the Revolution made social and educational experimentation possible on a vast scale, and it was the sheer magnitude of an enterprise affecting thousands of students and tens of thousands of patients that set France apart and make 1794 an *annus mirabilis* in the history of medicine. In that year, the chemist Antoine Fourcroy (1755–1809), with the assistance of François Chaussier (1746–1828), a Dijon anatomist and physician, prepared for the National Convention a report that became the basis of a law, passed in early December 1794, instituting three new "health" schools (*Ecoles de santé*) in Paris, Montpellier, and Strasbourg. Shortly to be called Schools of Medicine, additional ones were established in 1796, primarily for training military doctors. By the end of the Napoleonic Wars (1815), Paris was universally recognized as the Mecca of medicine. Yet, like many laws (or events) seen in retrospect as turning points, the immediate concern of the 1794 law was more limited, in this case to the chaos in hospital finance, patient care, and medical education, institutions, and licensing created by the Revolution.

I. NEW SCHOOLS FOR NEW TIMES

Reports and surveys commissioned before the Revolution had already quantified many problems in and proposed various solutions to existing medical services in France. Most famous is Jacques Tenon's *Mémoires sur les hôpitaux de Paris* (Memoirs on the hospitals of Paris, 1788), in which the distinguished surgeon drew attention to the appalling sanitary conditions, overcrowding, inadequate facilities, and high mortality rates of the Paris hospitals. The *Hôtel Dieu*, the oldest, largest (1,200 beds) and most famous of them, had a mortality rate of almost 25 percent (most English hospitals reported rates of much less than 10 percent), making it, in Tenon's words, "the most unhealthy and uncomfortable of all hospitals."[1] Many beds held three or more patients, there was little attempt to segregate patients with contagious diseases, most surgery was performed on the wards, and women gave birth in beds shared with others in various stages of labor. Conditions in other hospitals, though not so bad, were far from ideal. There were more hospitals in Paris than in London, a city twice the size of its French rival. In 1801, there were only an estimated 3,000 hospital beds in the whole of England; Tenon found 6,236 persons in twenty-eight hospitals in Paris, with another 14,105 people housed in hospicelike accommodations. This con-

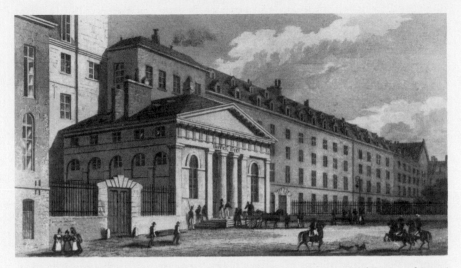

Figure 4. Hôtel Dieu, *close to Notre Dame Cathedral in the center of Paris, where so many of the leaders of French medicine trained and worked. Anonymous engraving, early nineteenth century.*

centration of patients contributed to the distinctiveness of the Paris school after 1794.

But the French hospitals suffered precarious existences in the early 1790s. Most of them, owned and run by the Catholic Church, were nationalized by the secular Revolution. Some monasteries were also turned into hospitals. With their financial and administrative bases disrupted, the hospitals were badly in debt, being rescued by periodic allocations of money from central coffers. In addition, the ethos of equality and individual rights fostered by the Revolution encouraged the hope that hospitals could be abolished, to be replaced by domiciliary care for a people made healthy by the new social order. "No more indigents, no more hospitals," rang one Revolutionary slogan. Doctors, too, came under fire as representatives of the old hierarchical order, and the medical schools, along with medical institutions like the Faculty, the Royal Society of Medicine, and the Academy of Surgery were closed in the early days of the Revolution. Medical licensing fell from favor as a symbol of the old inequality and, despite protests from some doctors, a medical laissez-faire developed.

There was pressure from some quarters, however, to improve (from above) the quality of medical services instead of letting them find their "natural" level. In particular, military authorities discovered they needed adequately trained doctors to care for French troops, which by 1792 were fighting against Austria, Prussia, and the Netherlands. Heavy losses of doctors (600 in 18 months) and a growing army required constant medical replacements. Military needs also encouraged the reform of the whole educational system, with the establishment of new technological, mining, military, and scientific schools whose pupils were selected by competitive examination from youths all over France. It was in this context, with Britain also joined in the war against France, that Fourcroy, a member of the Convention, turned his attention to problems of medical education. His report, with its famous dictum that, in the new medical schools, students were to "read little, see much, do much,"[2] established the framework for hospital medicine. The new law contained several features that encouraged this policy.

First, the law integrated French medical education into a single system. Gone was the old diversity of faculties, academies, colleges, schools, and universities vying for patronage and jealously guarding privilege. The three large schools that it created were instead much more uniform and subject to central bureaucratic control, with the national system of licensing (1803) soon further extending centralization. This latter law introduced a new hierarchy into the profession with the creation of a "second class" doctor (*officier de santé*) for rural areas and primary practice. These "health officers" went through a shorter, less rigorous period of training and, although never very popular with medical élites, the system survived until 1892. Before this new division of medicine, however, the Law of 1794 had established a second integrating principle: that of physicians and surgeons. "Medicine and surgery are two branches of the same science," Fourcroy had proclaimed, and the new law made physicians and surgeons equal within the hospitals, and the new schools taught both medicine and surgery to all students. This was important for the army, which needed doctors who were able to deal with wounds and injuries as well as diseases like fevers. It had even more important consequences for medical thought, for it taught generations of students to conceptualize disease as surgeons would: in terms of anatomic structures, the solid parts, local lesions. This systematic integration created the ambience for the emphasis on pathology, physical diagnosis, and clinicopathological correlation, which are the hallmarks of hospital medicine. Fittingly, the surgeon Desault is often cited as the father figure for the new medicine.

In other ways, too, the new medical schools were demarcated from older medical institutions. The law provided an adequate supply of bodies for anatomy teaching from those dying within the hospitals, where, from the first day of his education, the medical student began to learn about disease at the bedside. "Practising the art, observing at the bedside, all that was missing [in the old medical education] will now be the principal part of instruction."[3] The old medicine had been too much concerned with theory; the new medicine, like the old surgery, would be devoted to practice. Behind this empiricism stood the figures of Francis Bacon (1561–1626) and John Locke (1632–1704), particularly as the latter's writings had been modified in France by the Abbé de Condillac (1714–80). For Locke and Condillac, the senses were the ultimate source of human knowledge. It was fruitless to waste time speculating on the hidden causes of things. Rather, the mastery of nature, and the understanding and cure of disease would come through the careful observation, classification, and analysis of events, objects, or diseases. The "method of analysis" lay at the heart of P. J. G. Cabanis's (1757–1808) philosophy of "ideology" (the science of ideas). Knowledge, Cabanis insisted, comes from experience; it is of facts, not primary causes. These facts can be analyzed into useful generalizations and analogies, and then applied in the service of humanity. For the physician Cabanis, medicine was central to a comprehensive science of human beings that had as its task the understanding of both moral and physical aspects of human existence. An admirer of Hippocrates, Stahl, and the Montpellier vitalists, he viewed the history of medicine as a series of revolutions and regressions culminating in the Paris *Ecole de Santé*, where he was professor of hygiene and, later, internal medicine and medical history. Cabanis was also deeply committed to the value of hospitals for teaching, practical research, and patient care. He regretted the intrusion into medicine of chemistry and physics, which only encouraged sterile speculation. His political influence was considerable, as was his role in the transformation of Paris hospitals, but he remained in many ways a traditional figure, as close in his medical thinking to Hippocrates as to the apostles of localism and solidism. He analyzed symptoms, not lesions.

Other provisions of the Law of 1794 and later extensions also reinforced the move toward the hospital. The provision of full-time, salaried teachers meant that the professors and assistants no longer had to divide their time in private practice outside the hospital. Students, too, received state scholarships, on the basis of national competitive examinations, enabling poor boys from the provinces to study in Paris. The examination, or *concours*, system was soon extended beyond the entrance level, particularly after the creation, in 1802, of externships and internships in Paris hospitals for outstanding advanced students and recent graduates. An internship became a sine qua non for a subsequent hospital career; the prestige attached to hospital and teaching posts encouraged intensive competitiveness. After 1803, all medical practitioners of any sort had to pass formal examinations.

In just under a decade, then, French medical education acquired a structure that, with minor modifications, remained intact throughout the nineteenth century and whose essential features are still visible today. Rooted in the hospitals, the Paris medical school systematically imported surgical thinking into medicine. Its achievements are best examined under three heads: the localism of pathological anatomy, the development of appropriate diagnostic techniques, and the numerical approach to disease and therapeutics.

II. THE ANATOMY OF DISEASE

Eighteenth-century medicine was primarily one of symptoms, not lesions, of patients, not their organs. Even the erosion of Hippocratic humoralism by the cardiovascular or neurological systems of Boerhaave, Hoffmann, and Cullen had left almost intact much of the Hippocratic orientation of classical medicine. Nevertheless it is possible to overstate the neglect of pathological anatomy by nosologically inclined doctors. Cullen noted that even Sauvages – arch-exponent of the primacy of the symptom – had tacitly employed autopsy findings "in an hundred instances." "Dissection of morbid bodies is one of the best means of improving us in the distinction of diseases,"[4] Cullen insisted, echoing a theme easy enough to find in eighteenth-century medical writings.

The focus of this earlier pathological medicine was often the organ. Typical of this tradition was Jean-Baptiste de Senac's (1693–1770) treatise on the heart (1749), a work that owed much to Senac's own dissections as well as to the earlier monograph on the heart by the Italian doctor G. M. Lancisi (1654–1720). More broadly based were the works of Joseph Lieutaud (1703–80), particularly his *Anatomica medica* (1767), which collected autopsies over the previous three centuries in an attempt to correlate symptoms and pathological lesions, sometimes in parallel columns as an aid for students. Cullen pronounced this work confused, useful perhaps for a system of pathology but hopeless as the basis of medical practice.

In fact, Lieutaud's work had already been rendered virtually obsolete by a more successful pathological masterpiece, *De sedibus et causis morborum* (On the seats and causes of disease, 1761) by Giovanni Battista Morgagni (1682–1771). Morgagni's volumes, based on more than half a century's reading and experience, contained hundreds of case histories, presented in reasonably full detail and buttressed with autopsy findings. He hoped thereby to elucidate what Bacon had called the "footsteps of disease," to correlate symptoms with their structural manifestations. Accordingly, Morgagni eschewed any attempts to classify diseases into a nosological order, organizing his work instead topographically, starting with the head and brain and working his way leisurely to diseases of the lower extremities (*a capite ad calcem*). The resulting discursiveness was supplemented by analytical indexes, one arranged according to diseases and their symptoms, another listing the organs and their preternatural appearances in dead bodies:

so that if any physician observe a singular, or any other symptom in a patient, and desire to know what internal injury is wont to correspond to that symptom; or if any anatomist find any particular morbid appearance in the dissection of a body, and should wish to know what symptom has preceded an injury of this kind in other bodies; the physician, by inspecting the first of these indexes, the anatomist by inspecting the second, will immediately find the observation which contains both (if both have been observed by us).[5]

Morgagni's treatise systematized and extended anatomically based pathology, which had long been vigorously pursued in Italy, where the professional distinctions between physicians and surgeons were not so sharp. He left clear case histories and pathological descriptions of many conditions, including apoplexy (stroke), cirrhosis of the liver, pneumonia, valvular disease of the heart, and arterial aneurysms. His work quickly established itself as standard, rapidly going through several editions (in its original Latin) and, in 1769, a translation into English. Yet its immediate impact was particular rather than sweeping. Its monumental size discouraged wide circulation and Morgagni's prolixity diffused his central message. His discussions of etiology were eclectic and unsystematic, difficult to fit into more rigid schemes of disease causation. Cullen admired the work but made little use of it, for the organ-based approach could not be easily integrated into his nosological system. Further, doctors were acutely aware of the difficulty of correlating with any consistency symptoms with their underlying organic causes. This problem led Matthew Baillie to concentrate exclusively on the structural changes caused by disease in the first edition of his *Morbid Anatomy* (1794). He hoped thereby to alert doctors to the importance of routine postmortem examinations in delineating diseases. The symptomatic approach was less reliable, for:

the same symptoms are not uniformly connected with the same morbid changes of structure in the body. In many cases too the symptoms are nearly the same, where the morbid changes are very different. This is particularly exemplified in diseases of the brain, and of the heart.[6]

Baillie clearly distinguished between the symptoms and the disease *per se*, and, although both were part of what he called the "whole disease," the morbid changes yielded the most certain guidelines for categorizing disease entities and eventually formulating effective therapeutics.

These strands in eighteenth-century medicine are part of the conceptual background to the pathology of the French School. But the organ-based pathology of Morgagni and Baillie was further refined by the young and tragic genius of Xavier Bichat (1771–1802). His whole life seems foreshortened. By his early twenties he had trained as a surgeon, had a brief stint as a medical officer in the French army and had established himself in the capital, where he quickly became Desault's favorite student. He absorbed the localism of surgery but by 1799 he was physician to the *Hôtel Dieu*, where he continued a frenetic pace of physiological experimentation, patient care, postmortem dissections, writing, and lecturing, which ended only with his death. He was not yet thirty-one.

For Bichat, physiology and pathology were part of the same science of living bodies. Organisms have their own unique properties, irreducible to physics and chemistry. He divided living functions into two components, "organic" and "animal." Organic functions are involuntary and automatic, like digestion, secretion, absorption, and exhalation. Plants and animals share these functions. Further, human beings and other animals have additional, essentially voluntary functions such as movement, sensation, and voice. In this sense, Bichat sharply distinguished the living organism from inert matter (vitalism), but he was less concerned philosophically with the distinctions between humans and other animals. He held that both organic and animal functions, although irreducible to physical laws, are dependent on the particular organizational properties of the parts in which they reside. For him the functional unit of analysis was not the organ, however; it was the *tissues*. The heart, for instance, is not a single homogeneous organ. Instead, it is composed of different kinds of tissue, such as the pericardium (a serous membrane), the muscle itself, and the endocardium, which includes both fibrous and serous tissue. It was at the tissue level that Bichat sought to locate both physiology and pathology, normal and abnormal function. Bichat derived his tissue concept, he tells us, from a passage in Pinel's *Nosographie Philosophique*, in which the latter noted that the arachnoid, pleura, and peritoneum (the serous membranes lining the cranial, thoracic, and abdominal cavities), although located in different sites of the body, are subject to the same pathological afflictions.

Bichat distinguished twenty-one kinds of tissues. His list hardly stood the test of time. Some ("venous," "arterial," "absorbent") were subsequently recognized as conglomerates. Others ("medullary" – the substance of such organs as liver and spleen) would be utterly reconceived by cellular theory. Still others ("fibrous," "cartilaginous," "serous") were more homogeneous. But, despite the irony that this "father of histology" was a naked-eye anatomist who mistrusted the microscope, Bichat provided medicine with a new concept of "elemental unit," which transformed pathology. The "lesion" took on a more precise meaning; pathological analysis could go beyond the organ in the attempt to correlate lesion and symptom. "Pericarditis," "myocarditis," or "endocarditis" replaced "inflammation of the heart." Further, although Bichat recognized the importance of the blood and other bodily fluids, the tissues were solid; it was there that the vital properties – and the objects of pathology – were located. With pathological anatomy, medicine could hope to become an exact science:

> What is the value of observation, if one does not know the seat of the disease? You can take notes for twenty years from morning to evening at the sickbed on the diseases of the heart, lung, and stomach, and you will reap nothing but confusion. The symptoms, corresponding to nothing, will offer but incoherent phenomena. Open a few corpses, and immediately this obscurity, which observation alone would never have removed, will disappear.[7]

Bichat admitted that certain diseases – some fevers and nervous diseases – were beyond the ken of his localist, solidist pathology. But he firmly believed he had shown the way forward.

Certainly he had provided his successors with a hero. Men as different as Laennec and Broussais claimed him as their teacher. Even Jean Cruveilhier (1791–1874), whose beautifully illustrated works on pathological anatomy were not finished until 1864, worked squarely within Bichat's tradition of tissue pathology sans microscope. It was a tradition that never could have developed without hospitals, with their clusters of seriously ill patients and their dissection rooms where a final diagnosis could be made. Pinel had urged his colleagues to "paint disease," in Pinel's case in the service of classification. In the event, fascination with the minutiae of nosology barely survived Pinel as general classification gave way to monographic consideration of smaller groups of diseases. But the new pathological anatomy permitted more authoritative portraits of diseases, based on their lesions, but correlated by the symptoms and signs the lesions produced. We shall look below at French portraits of phthisis and typhus, after considering the other half of clinicopathological correlation: the diagnosis of disease during life.

III. DIAGNOSING DISEASES

Every medical student today learns that the four cardinal arts of the good bedside diagnostician are inspection, palpation, percussion, and auscultation: looking, feeling, thumping, and listening. The doctor primarily uses hands, eyes, and ears, occasionally supplemented by the senses of smell and taste. Before the nineteenth century, doctors also employed their five senses, but often in ways different from those dominating after the French canonized the ritual of modern physical examination. Earlier, ears were used principally for hearing the patient's own description of his or her symptoms, eyes for looking at the tongue and (perhaps) a specimen of the urine, hands for feeling the pulse and the condition of the skin. Notions of class, delicacy, and modesty reinforced a doctor–patient relationship in which (especially for those in

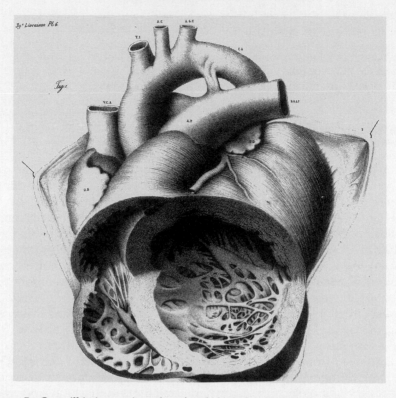

Figure 5. Cruveilhier's massive atlas of pathological anatomy offered both descriptions and engravings of diseased organs and systems. This engraving of the heart shows dilation of the chambers and growth of the heart muscle, typically found in patients with chronic severe high blood pressure. J. Cruveilhier, Anatomie pathologique du corps humain, *3 vols. (Paris: J. B. Ballière, 1829–42), Vol. 3, 39ᵉ Livraison Plate 6, Fig. 1.*

the upper part of the social scale) undressing was not part of a visit from the doctor. (For these patients, it was always a visit *from*, rather than to, a doctor.) Queen Caroline (1683–1737), wife of George II, suffered for three days with acute abdominal symptoms, including intense pain, vomiting, and diarrhea. She was blistered, bled, purged, and cupped. None of her physicians or surgeons actually examined her abdomen until virtually ordered to by the King. Once they had looked and felt, it was obvious that Caroline had a strangulated umbilical hernia. Unsurprisingly, the operation was unsuccessful, merely filling her last seven days with more agony.

In this instance, inspection and palpation might have permitted manual reduction of the hernia before gangrene set in, thus saving the Queen's life. Nor were the medical injunctions to look and feel all that novel, for the Hippocratics record many instances of careful inspection of parts of the body and they palpated enlarged spleens and livers in living patients. But the conventions of eighteenth-century medicine did not dictate the routine visualization or touching of parts of the body ordinarily covered from public view. The exceptions were largely surgical conditions such as abscesses or superficial tumors, where the patient's complaint focused attention on a local lesion. Within this context, it is hardly surprising that the introduction of percussion as a diagnostic procedure made only a minor ripple in the medical world.

Percussion was the brainchild of an Austrian physician, Leopold Auenbrugger (1727–1809). A successful physician in the Vienna of Maria Teresa and Mozart, Auenbrugger published little save a libretto for one of Antonio Salieri's operas and his short medical classic, *Inventum novum*, which appeared in the same year (1761) as Morgagni's masterpiece of pathology. Percussion consists of striking sharply the body with slightly curved fingers. The quality and pitch of the sound vary according to whether the region beneath the percussing finger is hollow or solid, and if the latter, whether densely solid or fluid. Auenbrugger learned the technique when, as a small boy, he could determine the fluid level in wine casks in his father's inn by tapping on the side of the cask. At the transition from hollow to fluid, the sound changed. As a diagnostic tool, percussion was of particular value in conditions involving the thorax, such as enlargement of the heart, consolidation of parts of the lung from pneumonia, or collections of fluid in the lungs or around the heart. In conjunction with other features of the patient's history, symptoms, and signs, percussion could be useful. Yet, it went largely unnoticed by Auenbrugger's contemporaries, partly perhaps because Auenbrugger never pressed his technique in later publications, but more pointedly because it yielded little significant information for doctors who still thought primarily about prognosis and general disease categories. Cullen mentioned percussion only to dismiss it. A couple of eighteenth-century surgeons extolled it, and it was taught in some German medical schools, but even in Vienna its routine employment seems to have lapsed with the early death of Maximillian Stoll (1742–87), one of Auenbrugger's early converts.

Auenbrugger himself resigned his hospital appointment in 1762 to devote his time to private practice. He had assumed that, for modesty's sake, a layer of cloth would separate the patient's chest from the percussing fingers. In the French hospitals, however, where patients were expected to be cooperative, and where local manifestations of disease were closely scrutinized, percussion took on a new significance. There, J. N. Corvisart (1755–1821), physician to *La Charité* and professor of clinical medicine in the medical school until 1804 (when he became Napoleon's personal physician), perceived the value of Auenbrugger's method, practiced and taught it, and translated the *Inventum novum* into

French (1808), with commentary four times the length of the original terse text. Two years earlier, Corvisart had published a monograph that demonstrated the diagnostic value of percussion: *Essai sur les maladies et les lésions organiques du coeur et des gros vaisseaux* (An essay on the organic diseases and lesions of the heart and great vessels). In it, Corvisart extolled the virtues of careful physical diagnosis and postmortem examination, the systematic practice of which would corroborate his belief that, save for pulmonary phthisis, the most common organic diseases were those of the heart. The operative word was *organic* – those with structural changes – for Corvisart's scalpel and keen eye detected lesions of heart disease that others might miss. He was ever conscious that different diseases could produce similar signs and symptoms. The doctor's task was to be aware of them all, and to approach diagnosis in a differential fashion, detectivelike, using his skills to arrive at the most probable disease.

Many of the characteristics of the French school were already maturely present in Corvisart's great work: the emphasis on differential diagnosis; sharp, economical case histories; the hospital orientation; the routine autopsy correlating signs, symptoms, and lesions. It is a quietly pessimistic book, permeated with Corvisart's personal melancholic stoicism. The diseases he wrote about were beyond the power of medicine to cure; his patients – many of them in their twenties and thirties – were admitted into hospital to die: "The prognosis was that the patient must die soon." "On the day he entered the hospital, I announced both the kind of disease, inefficacy of medicine, and the proximity of the patient's death." "The prognosis was hopeless." "The child, admitted April 22nd, died the 26th of the same month, after agonies of ten or twelve hours, during which his whole body was covered with a cold sweat, and a yellowish froth flowed from his mouth."[8] Little wonder that Corvisart's pupil and editor C. E. Horeau (who prepared the book, based on Corvisart's lectures and notes, for publication) suggested that the *Essay* could be looked upon as a meditation on death: organic heart disease could sometimes be prevented but never cured. The occupations of Corvisart's doomed patients reflect the ordinary clientele of the Paris hospitals: a washer woman, a cook, a wheelwright, a tailor.

Corvisart valued earlier work on the heart by Senac, Lancisi, and Morgagni, but dismissed Cullen's nosological descriptions of cardiac and thoracic disease. Above all, he appreciated the new orientation that the "celebrated Bichat" (twenty years his junior) had provided. Not simply heart disease, but diseases of the pericardium, heart muscle, endocardium, and heart valves attracted his separate gaze. "The heart, like all the other organs, is formed by the assemblage of several different tissues."[9] This provided him with a much richer sensitivity to the variety of cardiac afflictions and their relationship to more general signs and symptoms, such as difficulty in breathing and even apoplexy. He recognized the latter as a common consequence of diseases of the heart's valves, and his cases include what we describe as clear instances of subacute bacterial endocarditis, pericarditis, valvular incompetence, rheumatic heart disease, congestive heart failure, congenital abnormalities, aortic aneurysms, and atherosclerosis. Percussion helped him identify cardiac enlargement, collections of fluid around the heart, and effusions in the lungs secondary to heart failure. The consequences of organic heart disease were of course *physiological:* disturbances of respiration and circulation, pain, and loss of appetite. But Corvisart's physiology was clinical, not experimental; human, not animal; bedside, not laboratory. He opposed Fourcroy's desire to have a laboratory in every clinic, preferring to base his medical practice on the observations that could be made at the bedside. Only then could medicine rid itself of the pernicious speculative elements that had too long impeded it.

Corvisart was aware that cardiac diseases occasionally produce sounds that can be heard some distance from the patient and he was not adverse to placing his ear sometimes directly on the patient's chest (*immediate* auscultation). But sound was not an important diagnostic clue for him, as it became for R. T. H. Laennec (1781–1826), inventor of the stethoscope and probably the greatest clinician of the French school. The well-known story of Laennec's invention of the stethoscope, whence *mediate* auscultation derives, is best told by him:

> In 1816, I was consulted by a young woman labouring under general symptoms of diseased heart, and in whose case percussion and the application of the hand were of little avail on account of the great degree of fatness. The other method just mentioned [immediate auscultation] being rendered inadmissible by the age and sex of the patient, I happened to recollect a simple and well-known fact in acoustics, and fancied, at the same time, that it might be turned to some use on the present occasion. The fact I allude to is the augmented impression of sound when conveyed through certain solid bodies, as when we hear the scratch of a pin at one end of a piece of wood, on applying our ear to the other. Immediately, on this suggestion, I rolled a quire of paper into a sort of cylinder and applied one end of it to the region of the heart and the other to my ear, and was not a little surprised and pleased, to find that I could thereby perceive the action of the heart in a manner much more clear and distinct than I had even been able to do by the immediate application of the ear. From this moment I imagined that the circumstance might furnish means for enabling us to ascertain the character, not only of the action of the heart, but of every species of sound produced by the motion of all the thoracic viscera.[10]

Between 1816 and 1819, when Laennec published his two-volume masterpiece, *De l'auscultation médiate, ou Traité du diagnostic des maladies des*

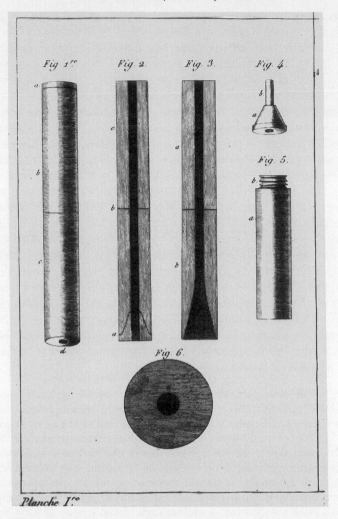

Figure 6. The depiction of Laennec's monaural stethoscope, a wooden tube with the bell and diaphragm adaptations at the bottom to assist in hearing high and low pitched sounds. The "binaural" stethoscopes, with flexible rubber tubing going to both ears, began to appear around the middle of the nineteenth century. R. T. H. Laennec, De L'auscultation médiate (Paris: J. A. Brosson and J. S. Chaudé, 1819), Plate 1.

poumons et du coeur (Mediate auscultation, or treatise on the diagnosis of disease of the lungs and heart), he perfected his diagnostic innovation and conclusively demonstrated its pragmatic value. He had been well prepared to exploit the stethoscope's potential, having absorbed the surgical orientation of pathological anatomy as a young military surgeon and as a student of Dupuytren, the surgeon and pathologist, and, above all, of Bichat. He had in addition assimilated Corvisart's message, even if the pious, politically conservative royalist Laennec had little personal regard for Napoleon's agnostic physician.

During the Napoleonic period Laennec had devoted himself to private practice, intermixed with medical journalism, intermittent military duties, and periodic residence in Brittany, where the air was better for his weakened lungs. The Restoration brought him the post of physician at the Necker Hospital, where he introduced the stethoscope. His Catholic royalism, more than his great book, eventually secured him a chair at the *Collège de France* and one at the *Charité*, where Corvisart had worked. With Laennec, the last of the routine bedside diagnostic procedures emerged, and, unlike Auenbrugger's advocacy of percussion, auscultation was quickly adopted, particularly among hospital and military doctors. This was partly due to the authority with which Laennec stamped his new technique, for auscultation of the lungs (the heart sounds still largely baffled him) appeared maturely dressed in 1819: that medical students today still learn the terms râles, rhonchi, pectoriloquy, and crepitations derives from the original French vocabulary that Laennec's musically gifted ear created.

As its title suggested, his treatise was actually two books, one on stethoscopy, the other on lung and heart diseases as diagnosed in life and confirmed at autopsy. His stethoscope, illustrated in the most famous plate from the work, was a simple wooden cylinder that could be unscrewed in the middle for carrying in the pocket. Although somewhat less convenient to use than the binaural stethoscopes with flexible rubber tubing introduced from mid-century, Laennec's stethoscope conveyed sound perfectly adequately and was the most important diagnostic innovation until the introduction of x-rays in the 1890s. His knowledge of the different kinds of normal and abnormal breath sounds, systematically discussed in the first part of his book, permitted him to diagnose a variety of pulmonary afflictions: bronchitis, pneumothorax, effusions, pneumonia and, above all, pulmonary phthisis. Sensible of the value of his friend G. L. Bayle's 1810 monograph on phthisis (itself based on some 900 dissected cases), Laennec did not hesitate to extend and modify Bayle's framework. He even insisted that a patient (still living) whom both had treated had been misdiagnosed by the stethoscope-less Bayle. Bayle had been concerned above all with nosological issues, distinguishing six distinct species of pulmonary phthisis. Laennec had little interest in nosology *per se*; rather, he unified all varieties of tuberculosis into a single disease, whose hallmark was the tubercle. This lesion Laennec minutely described (without the microscope, of which he shared his teacher Bichat's suspicions), in both its pulmonary and extrapulmonary manifestations. Scrofula (glandular tuberculosis) was merely another form of this same disease, as were tuberculous lesions in the gut, brain, liver, or prostate. But its most common manifestation was pulmonary, where it usually began in the upper part of the lungs and yielded a series of changing breath sounds that Laennec insisted were unique to the disease, thus making it diagnosable during life. Although his case histories sometimes referred to clinical aspects of earlier definitions of pulmonary phthisis, such as the hectic fever, Laennec put more stock in its anatomical manifestations and the specific signs and symptoms that they yielded. For him, the disease had an essential anatomical, rather than symptomatic, character.

The relevance of the hospital to his work was obvious; so was the relevance of the work to the hospital, where, Bayle had reported, of 696 deaths, 244 were from phthisis. Percussion ("one of the most valuable discoveries ever made in medicine")[11] and auscultation went together hand in glove, for as Laennec's English translator John Forbes noted, symptoms:

> for the most part, have only a remote connexion with the morbid lesion, and are, indeed, frequently present in other and very different diseases. M. Laennec's diagnostics, on the contrary, are the immediate and almost physical result of the individual derangement of parts. . . . In short (if his new diagnostics are as certain as he affirms) he may be said to have realized the wish of the ancient philosopher, and to have placed a window in the breast through which we can see the precise state of things within.[12]

Being able to hear and interpret breath sounds gave Laennec an insight into the whole course of the diseases under his ken. It convinced him that pulmonary phthisis was sometimes (though not often) compatible with survival, although he suspected that this had little to do with doctors' ministrations. He was accused (perhaps correctly) of concentrating more on diagnosis than on therapy, but this was probably from his awareness of therapeutic limitations rather than lack of sympathy for his patients. "I live in the midst of the dead and the dying," he once wrote in despair. He hoped that the careful description of disease would eventually lead to a more effective therapy, but he believed that medicine should always be based on the observable and that the causes of disease would probably always remain hidden. There was certainly not much to be gained by chemical speculation or by magnifying disease processes through the microscope.

Contemporary reviews of Laennec's book were mixed, partly for political and personal reasons, but stethoscopy took hold, and by 1825 the medical shops of Paris were displaying stethoscopes prominently in their windows. Translations of his book into English, German, and Italian helped spread the technique, as did a steady stream of foreign students during Laennec's last years. Simply owning a stethoscope did not make an expert, and penetration of the skill beyond the few hospital elites was slow, but at least the instrument was rapidly available. By 1832, the year in which George Eliot set her great novel, *Middlemarch*, the stethoscope symbolized the progressive forces in medicine; Tertius Lydgate, the doctor she created in her novel, upsets his conservative colleagues by preaching the value of this new French instrument. By mid-century the stethoscope had come near to its present symbolization of the profession itself.

By the former date, too, a generation of post-Revolutionary doctors had grown up taking the newest diagnostic attitudes for granted. This can be seen clearly in the work of men like Andral, Chomel, Bretonneau, and Piorry, and above all in Pierre Louis (1787–1872). Louis's career and writings embody many of hospital medicine's main features. Graduating in Paris in 1813, he spent seven years practicing in Russia before a diphtheria epidemic there convinced him of the relative powerlessness of his knowledge. Returning to Paris, he immersed himself in the wards of the *Pitié* for some five years before publishing the fruits of his experience. In 1825 his massive book on phthisis appeared, followed four years later by one on fever. Both relied on his broad diagnostic and postmortem experience available only in the hospital. His idea of pulmonary phthisis was essentially Laennec's, diagnosed stethoscopically and confirmed in hundreds of cases by autopsy. Likewise, his work on fevers made diagnosis, clinical course, and pathological examination the basis of delineating typhoid fever, with its abdominal, lymphatic, and splenic involvement. Foreigners – particularly the Americans – flocked to his wards and lectures and read his books.

His little *Essay on Clinical Instruction* (1834) is a clear statement of his own attitudes and catches the essences of French hospital medicine. Four features stand out. First, he preached not simply the value of bedside diagnosis, but of the systematic investigation of the patient's background, history, and general health. The "Other Illnesses," "Family History," and "Review of Systems," which are part of the routine admission record of a patient today, were also part of Louis's world:

> Before commencing the study of the symptoms, [the doctor] will inform himself of the age and profession of the subject; of his habitual state of embonpoint or of emaciation, of strength or of weakness, of health or of disease; of the affections under which he has labored previously to the present, of his good or bad natural conformation.[13]

Second, the value of the patient's symptoms (i.e., what the patient experiences and which he called "secondary") lies in their pointing toward signs (i.e., what the doctor detects on examination), whence the lesions of the involved organs may be determined. These lesions, determined by physical diagnosis and confirmed by pathological anatomy, are the most consistent guides to naming the diseases, planning the therapy, and assessing prognosis.

It followed from this that clinical medicine was to Louis an observational rather than an experimental science: "particular observations are to the physician, what experiments are to the natural philosopher." It was learned at the bedside and in the morgue by observing and correctly interpreting facts. The purpose of medical education was to teach the student how to interpret the sights, sounds, feel, and smell of disease: to train his senses. Clinical judgment or tact consists simply of proper interpretation of what is presented to the active senses, with one final step, the placement of these observations within the systematic laws of medicine. These latter laws are accumulated by *counting*, by employing what Louis fondly called his *méthode numérique*, the numerical method. Medical facts must be quantitatively expressed. Here, as in much else, Louis consolidated previous thinking, and, as always, needed the hospital in which to base his activities.

IV. THE NUMERICAL METHOD

Numbers had never been of more than intermittent use to doctors. William Harvey had made a crucial calculation of the amount of blood ejected from the heart during each systole; iatromechanists like Giovanni Borelli (1608–79) had been intrigued by the force generated by muscle contractions; Sanctorius (1561–1636) had measured various physiological phenomena such as insensible perspiration and temperature. But these were isolated examples, of more physiological than clinical relevance, and even the thermometer was but rarely used by Enlightenment doctors. At the same time, the "political arithmetic" of seventeenth-century thinkers like John Graunt (1620–74) and William Petty (1623–87) introduced a quantitative element into the public domain, with their attempts to estimate population, occupational distribution, mortality rates, and trade and commerce statistics. The London Bills of Mortality had been published regularly since the early sixteenth century, and, although recognized even at the time as not entirely reliable, they represent a continued concern with broader, quantitative parameters of disease and death.

Mathematics, then, might be used to study either the individual – the heartrate or force of muscle contraction – or collections of individuals – deathrates or relative frequency of different diseases. Neither approach required mathematical expertise, merely the right frame of mind and industry sufficient for the task. Social or vital statistics became important for public health (see Chapter 3), but, in a modified form, numerical thinking also influenced clinical medicine and therapeutics. From the mid-eighteenth century, multiple case reporting became more common. Earlier doctors often reported only single instances of disease and therapies, and only "cures." James Lind's famous experiment (1747) in treating twelve patients with scurvy with the same basic diet supplemented by six different possible remedies for scurvy (including citrus fruit) was a well-designed attempt to evaluate rival therapies rather than simply "prove" a particular favorite one. Lind and other British military doctors advocated systematic record keeping, a procedure that Gilbert Blane (1749–1834), James McGrigor (1771–1858), and other high-ranking medical officers had succeeded in making widespread by the time of the Napoleonic Wars. These summaries – of hospitals, campaigns, and ships' sick bays – helped quantify the cost of sickness and injury to the military, and initiated doctors into the importance of multiple-case evaluation. "Detached cases, however numerous and well attested, are insufficient to support general conclusions . . . The test of arithmetical calculation [ought not to be] evaded," wrote John Millar in 1777.[14] The numbers game was central to various late eighteenth-century nosological and therapeutic debates, and civilian hospital doctors increasingly published yearly tabulations of their hospital experience.

It could be (and was) argued that a hundred ill-diagnosed and variously treated cases merely quantified chaos and confusion, and that, in any event, the individual sick person had to be treated as an individual, taking into account his or her peculiar symptoms, temperament, nourishment, and personal circumstances. The Hippocratic tradition, still strong among late eighteenth- and early nineteenth-century British and French doctors, encouraged this individual approach. Nevertheless, hospitals provided dense concentrations of diseased humanity, and lesions proved more constant than symptoms. Pinel had stressed the greater objectivity of multiple observations, and the monographs of Corvisart, Bayle, and Laennec were infused with a confidence wrested from thousands of patients and hundreds of autopsies. At the same time, the work of Condorcet, Laplace, and others on probability theory suggested to various doctors that the surest foundations of clinical science lay in the rigorous quantification of experience. Against the charge that idiosyncrasies in each patient made precise prediction impossible (unlike many instances in the physical sciences), Pinel, Chomel, and Louis replied that probabilistic thinking must still guide medical decisions.

Louis was the most ardent spokesman for numerical methods in medicine. His claims are those of the proselytizer rather than innovator, for he was actually the culmination of an outlook with Enlightenment derivations rather than a blazer of new trails. His mathematics was simple, his methods straightforward. They consisted in no more than quantitatively basing symptom, lesion, and disease categorizations, and (more significantly) in applying similar techniques in evaluating his therapies. This he had been doing since the 1820s but his systematic examination of the problem was in his pioneering monograph, *Recherches sur les Effets de la Saignée* (Researches on the effects of bloodletting, 1835). In it, Louis compared patients matched for diagnosis, age, general condition, and other variables receiving several traditional therapies varied in their timing and strength. Bloodletting in pneumonia and other inflammatory conditions was his most controversial clinical experiment, but he also examined the use of antimony (tartar emetic) in pneumonitis. He did not, as is sometimes claimed, advocate abandoning bloodletting; indeed, he did not even consider withholding phlebotomy completely. What he showed was that it made little or no difference to the course of pneumonia whether bloodletting was performed early or late in the disease, or whether a small or large quantity of blood was taken. Similarly tartar emetic had little influence on the mortality or duration of pneumonitis, although Louis felt his figures showed it to be of some value.

To the modern eye, Louis simply recorded the natural histories of these diseases, unhampered by any therapeutic intervention with power to change their courses. Louis's contemporaries did not see it quite so starkly, but his treatise was an indictment, not so much on therapeutics *per se*, as on the claims made by doctors for their remedies. His chief target was F. J. V. Broussais, who had extolled the virtues of letting blood through leeching for virtually all diseases. (For a discussion of Broussais, see Section V.) On balance, Louis was no more skeptical about his armamentarium than were Corvisart, Laennec, or Andral, the latter of whom had countered the classic therapeutic epigram of "Better something doubtful than nothing" with his own version: "Better nothing than something doubtful."[15] But Louis, by making therapeutics a particular study, brought into the open the apparent inefficacy of some commonplace remedies, when subjected to scrutiny by his numerical method. It was consistent with his empiricism that he hardly speculated *why* these therapies might or might not work: he merely devised clinical trials to see *whether* they did. Only through the accumulation of numerous instances could doctors hope to formulate general laws. No wonder one of his American pupils called him the "Bacon of Medicine."

The French hospital doctors, then, were not aggressive therapists. Laennec compensated for his relative unconcern with therapy by occasionally extolling the old Hippocratic notion of the healing power of nature: the capacity of the body, unaided by the ministrations of doctors, to restore itself to health. Nature, he wrote, could sometimes cure pulmonary phthisis; medicine could not. Corvisart, who doubted both nature and medicine, was even more pessimistic. At its core, the whole issue was fused with cynicism: Louis was cynical about Broussais, who claimed too much for his simple-minded therapeutics; Broussais was cynical about Louis and Laennec, whom he accused of neglecting their patients. But one thing is certain: in the French school, therapeutics remained the poor relation of diagnosis and pathological anatomy.

V. THE NORMAL AND THE PATHOLOGICAL

The greater precision with which men like Corvisart, Laennec, and Louis described disease reinforced the nosological ideal of diseases as discrete, separate entities. The shift from diagnostic dependence on variable symptom to much more constant lesion gave credence to the notion that diseased states are qualitatively different from normal ones. If lesions (gross structural changes) define diseases, then the absence of the lesion testifies to the absence of the disease. Pathologically inclined physicians like Laennec were of course aware of the dynamics of structural (and functional) change, for instance in the development of tubercles in pulmonary phthisis. But the thrust of pathological anatomy was toward a static view of disease.

It was possible, however, to start from the same principles of localism, tissues, solidism, and lesions, and arrive at alternative conclusions about the relation between the normal and the pathological. F. J. V. Broussais (1772–1838) did just this in a series of polemical works that rent apart the medical world of post-Napoleonic Paris. A pupil of Bichat and Pinel, he believed that Laennec, Bayle, and Louis were leading medicine astray with their pathological anatomy, ontological obsessions, and therapeutic pessimism. The true legacy of Bichat rather lay in his recognition of the primacy of physiology, and of the continuity between the normal and the pathological. Disease, Broussais asserted, occurred when normal functions went awry. The dynamics of pathophysiology rather than the statics of pathological anatomy were his concern. This principle, subsequently to assume such significance with the young Rudolf Virchow and Claude Bernard, hit at one of the weaknesses of the anatomical school. But Broussais diluted his lasting impact in developing the details of his pathophysiology. First, he turned it into a monolithic system. Always interested in the relation between inflammation and disease, he turned localism and pathological anatomy on their heads by suggesting that virtually all diseases are caused by gastrointestinal inflammations. It is "the destiny of the stomach always to be irritated."[16] Local lesions in other parts of the body were the result of sympathetic reactions to this primary seat and cause of disease. Second, Broussais based this system on a theory of life similar to that of John Brown some half-century earlier. Organisms live only by virtue of stimulation or irritation, and oxygen was the most potent of these external stimuli. Inflammation being the consequence of excessive stimulation, it followed that depletive or antiphlogistic remedies were required. Broussais's favorite was phlebotomy through leeches, a procedure that enjoyed a considerable vogue in France in the 1820s and early 1830s, when his influence was at its peak. Like many another ardent medical reformer past and present, he made sweeping claims on behalf of his therapy: any disorder, from cancer to phthisis to syphilis would, under the right conditions, respond to leeching.

Even before the end of his life, Broussais's star had begun to wane. His lasting importance resided not so much in his system but in the critique he offered of the medicine of the hospitals. He stood for a busy optimistic therapeutics against the diagnostic pessimism of his contemporaries; for an approach to disease that abolished ontology and saw only individuals suffering physiologic abnormalities; and, ironically, for the universality of the lesion, even in the "essential" fevers (those without striking local manifestations). Casting himself as Newton to Louis's Bacon, he saw that a medicine without theories was vacuous. Unfortunately his physiology was hypothetical, deduced at the bedside and in the autopsy room. But, like his professional rivals Laennec and Louis, he reckoned that "basic" sciences like physics, chemistry, and experimental physiology were not essential foundations of clinical medicine. In that sense, at least, he was a true son of French hospital medicine.

VI. HOSPITAL MEDICINE ABROAD

The acrimonious polemics that Broussais and Louis exchanged remind us that even the "Paris school" did not espouse a single cohesive philosophy of medicine. Nor did the clinicians who came to maturity in the 1830s and 40s simply recapitulate the values and attitudes of their teachers. Nevertheless, even foreign contemporaries knew there was something distinctive about Paris medicine, and for the three or four decades after the close of the Napoleonic Wars, students flocked to Paris from all over Europe and North America. "Thither came almost all the youth of the medical world. Nowhere are conditions more splendid, more multifarious than in Paris,"[17] wrote the German physician Carl Wunderlich in 1841. Laennec had as many as 300 foreign pupils, and Louis, Chomel, and Andral (among others) drew many more to their lectures, clinics, and wards. Foreign students even founded their own medical societies to provide assistance in practical aspects of living and working in a transplanted environment, and a forum to discuss what they had learned there. Translations of the major works produced by the Paris school made the findings of hospital medicine easily available to others who had not the time, inclination, or resources to experience Paris first hand.

So many young men who studied in Paris between 1815 and 1850 for periods varying from a few weeks to several years subsequently became eminent in their native countries that it is tempting to picture enclaves of disciples at work in places like London, Geneva, Vienna, Philadelphia, Dublin, and Edinburgh. At an individual level, this may be valid, for many students retained intense affection and admiration for their Paris teachers, often dedicating their books to them: books that in content and approach were sometimes *à la mode Parisien*. But the notion of a kind of intellectual apostolic succession is too simple, for foreign students brought to Paris a vast array of cultural backgrounds, and went back to local settings with indigenous traditions, values, and medical institutions. While they were there, some were put off by the moral laxness of the Parisians, the callousness with which patients were often treated, the filth of the hospitals and streets, the casualness about therapeutics, the size of the classes, and the difficulties of the language. Ideally, they would be expected to carry away with them an appreciation of, and skills in, physical diagnosis and clinicopathological correlation and would have seen for themselves the importance of the hospital setting for the French educational enterprise. Curiously, they often also took back with them knowledge and skills in "basic sciences" like chemistry and microscopy, disciplines not routinely valued by the leading teachers in the Paris medical school. For foreign students also often attended lectures and demonstrations in the Collège de France, Sorbonne, and other institutions not directly connected with the medical school. The bedside–morgue axis was rarely duplicated so purely outside of Paris.

Paris hospital medicine did provide a model, though, and one that certainly had a significant impact on medical thinking and education abroad. Three localities – London, Philadelphia, Vienna – can serve for the much larger number of places where students returning from Paris adapted what they had acquired there to indigenous situations. English pupils were swift to forget that England and France had been at war for two decades ("the sciences were never at war," one historian has insisted), and after 1815 they went to Paris in force. Several early English stethoscopists, including Thomas Hodgkin (1798–1866) and Charles Williams (1805–89), learned the technique directly from Laennec himself. James Hope (1801–41) arrived in Paris just after Laennec's death, but he still consolidated there his appreciation of the stethoscope's value in diagnostics. Other Paris-trained doctors who subsequently succeeded in the London hospital scene included W. H. Walshe (1812–92) in medicine, Robert Carswell (1793–1857) in pathology, and Astley Cooper (1768–1841) and William Bowman (1816–92) in surgery. The individual contributions of these men were firmly based on their hospital work: on the daily round of ward and morgue, of physical diagnosis and postmortem correlation of symptom and lesion, of the press of medical students "walking the wards," eager to absorb practical medicine and surgery. But the London scene remained far more eclectic than Paris. It is true that the major voluntary hospitals in London developed their

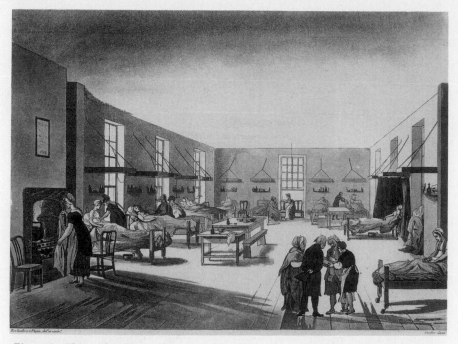

Figure 7. This early nineteenth-century interior from the Middlesex Hospital in London still looks rather domestic, save for the consultation of two doctors with the nurse and apothecary in the foreground. Aquatint, 1808, by Stadler after T. Rowlandson and A. C. Pugin.

own formal medical schools about this time, but their timing and organization belie any simple transplantation of French hospital medicine into a rival capital city.

Most of the London medical schools grew up gradually and had had both physicians' and surgeons' pupils since at least the mid-eighteenth century. In 1820, (Sir) Robert Christison (1797–1882) remarked that St. Bartholomew's Hospital had only three medical [i.e., physicians'] students, but several hundred surgical students, who learned no medicine save "the few crumbs they might pick up now and then during the medical treatment of surgical cases." Several hospitals claim foundation dates for their medical schools well before 1794 (e.g., Guy's, 1769; the London, 1785) and those started during the "Paris era" (e.g., Middlesex, 1835; Westminster, 1841) did not differ noticeably in organization from sister institutions in London. Teaching staffs made some money from student fees, but they also maintained private practices, and it was there that fame and fortune lay. Hospital governors sometimes looked on the medical school as a necessary evil and suspected that the presence of too many students deflected attention away from the hospital's primary aims of philanthropy and patient care. Autopsies were never so common in English hospitals as in French ones and English hospital patients were less likely to be subjected to repeated physical examinations or intimate surgical operations in front of a crowd of students. Some British doctors objected to the French habit of discussing details of the case in front of the patient and believed either that Latin should be used or diagnosis and prognosis talked over away from the bedside.

Differences such as these should not hide the fact that, in London as in Paris, a significant restructuring of medical teaching and clinical research around the hospital occurred during the early decades of the nineteenth century. Partly it was the result of simple market forces, for the 1815 Apothecaries Act specified that all apothecaries must henceforth be licensed by the Society of Apothecaries, and in addition to passing the examination of the Society, candidates needed to present certificates proving attendance of lectures on anatomy, chemistry, botany, materia medica, and the theory and practice of physic. But, in addition, the candidate had to spend six months in clinical work in a hospital, infirmary, or dispensary. By the 1830s more than 400 students per year were taking the Licentiate of the Society, and the demand for clinical opportunities had increased accordingly. The Act further encouraged the hospitals to expand teaching facilities, for the private medical schools had never been able to provide much bedside instruction, and the private educational sector began to wilt after this intrusion of the State into medical education. On the other hand, it must be remembered that the six months' clinical stint need not have been full-time, so apothecary students (still for the most part indentured apprentices) would often spend a year or so of their apprenticeship in London, simultaneously attending several lecture courses and discharging their clinical training.

But if hospitals in London were hardly arranged along pure Parisian lines, at least the doctrines of localism, clinicopathological correlation, and hospital-based statistics were often embraced by London hospital élites. A good example of this tendency is that of James Hope himself, a medical graduate of Edinburgh, student of Paris, and physician at St. George's Hospital in London. His *Treatise on the Diseases of the Heart and Great Vessels* (1832) shows how utterly changed was the concept of heart disease since the work of Cullen, or even Corvisart, and how much stethoscopy itself had developed even in the few years following Laennec's death.

Hope subscribed perfectly to the Parisian notion that symptoms should be explained in terms of structure: "I am satisfied [he wrote] that ... the process of thought which passes through the mind at the bed side and in the post-mortem theatre is from symptom to lesion."[18] Being convinced that the doctor's task was to translate the one into the other, Hope found the stethoscope of immense value, for the heart sounds gave clues to the structural basis of the functional impairment. The nature of these sounds, Hope insisted, had first been elucidated by him, for Laennec had believed that the heart sounds were muscular in origin, whereas he had determined (by experiment as well as clinicopathological observation) that the heart's valves were actually the origin of the famous "lub-dub" of the normal heartbeat as well as most of the variety of murmurs audible to the trained stethoscopist. Cardiac palpitations, so central to Cullen's "cardiology," were of minor consequence to Hope, and Cullen's vague notion of "carditis" was transformed in Hope's treatise into a detailed discussion of inflammatory heart disease. But, above all, valvular disease intrigued Hope, and his stethoscopy allowed him to understand it clinically. He described a number of murmurs, including what we would now call hemodynamic murmurs of anemia and pregnancy, and recognized the difference between "cardiac asthma" (pulmonary edema, in modern parlance) and asthma from other causes.

Much of Hope's work on the origin of cardiac sounds was controversial in his own time, and certainly did not lay to rest speculation in the area: in 1878 one commentator wryly noted that, since Laennec's time, no fewer than thirty-five theories had attempted to account for these sounds. Nevertheless, Hope's career does illustrate an English version of hospital medicine: "hospital" because of the fact that his own records of more than 1,000 instances of organic disease of the heart were drawn from the 15,000 in- and outpatients he examined during the 1830s (he explicitly excluded his private patients from his account); "hospital" because Hope valued his public dispensary and hospital appointments above his private practice, returning to London in 1840 from a rural retirement (brought on by declining health) so that he could try to do justice to the appointment he had so long desired: physician (as opposed to assistant physician) to St. George's Hospital. He died, less than a year later, aged forty, of pulmonary consumption.

By the time Hope died, St. George's had 200 pupils, St. Bartholomew's Hospital had 300, and besides the hundreds of students in other London hospital schools, London also boasted a teaching university, with two colleges, King's and University, each of which had medical faculties and purpose-built hospitals to provide clinical instruction. It is likely that much the same phenomenon would have occurred in London, even without the Paris model and the steady influx of Paris-trained doctors onto the London scene. Nevertheless, so many monographs by London doctors made such explicit use of diagnostic and postmortem strategies similar to French ones, that it would be parochial to deny an important Parisian dimension to London hospital-based education and research. The existence in London before 1794 of numerous hospitals and medical students simply made the transition easier, and the Parisian catalyst more potent.

The American situation was different: less organized so that the Parisian educational impact on individual doctors was often more striking, but at the same time, less able ultimately to change medical structures in the New World. Not surprisingly, the links with the Old World were closest among doctors on the East Coast, and Boston, Philadelphia, and (to a lesser extent) New York City provided the majority of the recent medical graduates who crossed the Atlantic. As a group, the American students have been closely scrutinized, and it was they who through translations of French works and dedications of their own productions made their debts most explicit. Boston (and Harvard) medicine probably felt the impact most strongly, but the realities facing American doctors returning from Paris can be seen particularly well in Philadelphia, home of the oldest hospital (the Pennsylvania Hospital, 1751) and oldest medical school (now called the University of Pennsylvania, 1765) in the United States. From the beginning the Medical College had used the hospitals, students being required to attend the practice of the hospital for one year before being eligible for the M.D. degree. Benjamin Rush had added his own particular luster to both institutions for more than forty years.

During the middle third of the century, three key individuals in hospital and medical college – Alfred Stillé (1813–1900), W. W. Gerhard (1809–72), and S. G. Morton (1799–1851) – had been trained in Paris. Morton produced (1834) the first systematic American monograph on consumption. Gerhard studied the symptoms and postmortem lesions of tuberculous meningitis and of typhus and typhoid fevers (1837), and Stillé also contributed to the latter enterprise (1838). These were works of permanent value, clearly bearing the stamp of Paris. Gerhard also published books on physical diagnosis. But the history of medical education in nineteenth-century Philadelphia (much less many other parts of the country) was hardly one of easy triumph of the ideals of hospital medicine. The medical school managed to maintain reasonable standards throughout the period despite formidable problems caused during the Civil War (1861–5). But the university's medical school did not have its own hospital until after that war, so it was dependent on loose arrangements with the Pennsylvania Hospital and the Philadelphia Hospital (the old alms house at Blockley). Furthermore, the medical school found itself in competition with a steady stream of new medical schools founded at regular intervals through the century. Jefferson Medical College (1824) was the most successful of these rivals, and others, especially the Medical Department of Pennsylvania College (with which both Morton and Stillé were briefly associated), were serious enterprises with some attention paid to academic standards. But others were blatantly commercial in conception and execution, inadequately staffed but offering degrees at cut-rate investment of time and money. These proprietary schools were long to dot the American landscape, and though Philadelphia had perhaps sufficient medical traditions to discourage some educational sharks, the established medical institutions there were not immune from pressure from these newer establishments, including a Homeopathic Medical College (1848), and no fewer than three "eclectic" medical schools. In fact, returning Americans from Louis's wards in Paris discovered that many of their countrymen had turned to botanical, homeopathic, or eclectic medical systems. Well-educated allopathic doctors were thus faced with the dual problem of factory-mills from within their own ranks, and alternative therapeutic cosmologies from without. Besides, Parisian neglect of therapeutics had unsettled many American students, who perceived it as ethically callous and professionally disastrous. The formation of the American Medical Association in 1847 (with Stillé as one of its secretaries) gave the "regulars" an organized voice, but the middle third of the century was an uneasy period in American medicine. Although the Paris ideal provided an inspiration for some, the realities of Jacksonian America were not conducive to the sustained cultivation of hospital medicine.

At the University of Vienna, there were established traditions on which to build. There had been bedside teaching on the Boerhaavian model in the old medical school, but decay had set in toward the end of the eighteenth century. The curriculum was reformed from 1803, under a new Dean, J. A. Stifft (1760–1836). Although the final two years of the five-year course were to be primarily clinical, Stifft was intent on expunging all foreign medical theories (including Brunonianism and German *Naturphilosophie*), engineering appointments among colleagues who subscribed to his call for a return to a kind of Hippocratic humoralism. Curiously, a new brand of humoralism was introduced (albeit briefly) by one of two Paris-inspired doctors who, after Stifft's death, came to dominate the Viennese school. This was Carl von Rokitanski (1804–78), who had through independent study absorbed the message of the lesion before he visited Paris in the 1840s. During that decade pathological anatomy was made a compulsory subject in Vienna, with Rokitanski appointed professor in the department in which he had worked since his student days. By then he had already perfected postmortem protocol, completing his 30,000th autopsy by 1866. In many years he performed as many as 2,000, an average of more than five each day, Sundays and holidays included.

Rokitanski had a superb grasp of anatomy, normal and pathological, and left important studies of congenital malformations and memorable descriptions of a large number of conditions, such as peptic ulcer, acute yellow atrophy of the liver, pneumonia, and valvular heart disease. He left behind so many precise anatomical pictures of disease that it was no wonder his contemporaries sometimes called him the Linnaeus of pathology. Rokitanski was brilliant at the hospital-based portraiture of diseases and their lesions, but he was not just a slavish imitator of Paris. For one thing, he was enthusiastic about the value of science for medicine, using chemistry whenever he thought it could help him, introducing the microscope to Viennese pathology (and encouraging his assistants to develop histology) and, after he became an advisor to the Austrian Ministry of Education, overseeing the expansion of science teaching at all levels. He was also prepared to speculate about the cause of disease, and the first edition of his great multivolume *Handbuch der pathologischen Anatomie* (Handbook of pathological anatomy, 1842–6) contained an ambitious, and ultimately unsuccessful, attempt to explain all disease in terms of what he called a "crasis" of the blood. The blood being an ubiquitous fluid, Rokitanski believed that the general cause of disease resided in disturbances – probably chemical – in this primary humor. His theory bore some structural similarities with Broussais's slightly earlier attempt to yoke the general condition and specific lesion into a single interacting whole. The notion of the crasis was elastic, fitting whatever was required of it in individual situations, but Rokitanski had made a serious attempt to marry humoralism and solidism, the new chemistry and the new pathological anatomy. It was, however, a sterile union, which found no favor among contemporaries and was quietly dropped in later editions of his *Handbuch*.

Rokitanski's main colleague was Josef Skoda (1805–81), who worked closely with him on the clinical half of clinicopathological correlation. Stethoscopy was Skoda's forte and he spent long hours working with sick and healthy people, with animals, corpses, and models, seeking to elucidate the physical conditions that produce breath and heart sounds. He was more cautious than Laennec had been about pathognomonic auscultatory patterns for disease like tuberculosis. He went beyond Hope in elucidating the nature of heart sounds, and attempted to clarify and standardize further the vocabulary of auscultation (which unlike the demonstrable lesion of the pathologist always had an element of subjectivity). His *Abhandlung der Perkussion und Auskultation* (Treatise on percussion and auscultation, 1839) passed through multiple editions and translations, and, though he sometimes complained that his French contemporaries failed to appreciate the nuances of his researches on auscultation, his work was in the Paris mold, certainly in the premium he placed on diagnosis. Skoda could be openly contemptuous of medicine's therapeutic capacities and it was rumored that the medicine he put most stock in was cherry brandy.

It should be recalled that, although Rokitanski and Skoda worked within the *Allgemeines Krankenhaus* (General Hospital), it was affiliated with the University of Vienna, which provided a broader educational context than the Paris hospitals. By 1841, when Wunderlich compared

Paris and Vienna, he hinted that the center of medical excellence was shifting northward and eastward. Certainly, in the decades following, Americans went to Vienna in far larger numbers (as many as 20,000 before World War I): although by then they were going not just for the opportunities of the bedside and autopsy room, but the specialty clinic and the scientific and diagnostic laboratory. We shall look at this phenomenon later. But before then, in the first half of the century, the assumptions and techniques underlying hospital medicine – localism, solidism, physical diagnosis, and clinicopathological correlation – transformed the map of disease. Pathological anatomy provided the basis for many "new" descriptions, even in the absence of much etiological understanding, or enhanced therapeutic power. Many of the same phenomena – population increase, urbanization, industrialization – that made the hospital such a prominent feature of modern medicine, also had a significant impact on corporate health, and the critical realization of therapeutic impotence made the prevention of disease seem more urgent.

3

Medicine in the community

The cholera is the best of all sanitary reformers, it overlooks no mistake and pardons no oversight.

The Times (London), 5 September 1848

B Y the mid-nineteenth century, the hospital had become a permanent feature of the medical landscape, a pillar of medical services and a crucial site of medical education. But its limitations were recognized even as its value was defended. Hospitals catered to individuals only after they were taken ill, were usually available only for the acute phase of the illness, and in any case were often limited to persons with certain diagnoses and from particular socioeconomic groups. Their ideal was curative rather than preventive, their constituency the individual and only incidentally society as a whole. Hospitals were material monuments to the failure of the preventive ideal.

That it was better to prevent disease than afterward to cure it (no matter how spectacular the method) was a medical commonplace older than Hippocrates. Doctors after all should be constantly trying to make their curative roles unnecessary, as people learned how to prevent disease through healthy living. In practice, of course, preventive regimens have been imperfectly conceived, even less rigidly followed and in any case required a level of self-consciousness and economic security obtainable by only a fraction of society. It has always been easy enough to explain away medical failure (doctors can bury their mistakes) and if one lived long enough, "old age" or "natural causes" could still be invoked at the end. Disease may be preventable; death is not.

Historically the thrust of most preventive medical writing has been toward the individual. Galen's *Hygiene*, the twelfth-century *Regimen sanitatis* ('Regimen of health') and Luigi Cornaro's (1467–1566) *Sure methods of attaining a long and healthful life* (1558, translated and reprinted many times throughout the nineteenth century) were all guides for people concerned with preserving or restoring their health. The economics of this kind of personal hygiene could be fitted into the mold of curative practice. Doctors can always dispense advice along with their prescriptions.

55

There are communal health issues, however, that are inadequately tackled by the ordinary method of individual doctors seeing patients one at a time. Questions of water supply, sewage disposal, housing and work conditions, and food adulteration are not best left to the uncontrolled forces of the marketplace. Epidemic diseases create situations whereby the health of a society is more than a simple summation of multiple individual healths. Ancient societies tackled these issues in a variety of ways ranging from the employment of town or state doctors devoting themselves to communal health matters to the use of tax money to provide water and sewage facilities (generally in proportion to one's wealth or social standing). From the Middle Ages, especially, there has been an increasing recognition of the interdependence of human beings in society ("Never send to know for whom the bell tolls . . . "), and, with the regular return of plague following the devastating Black Death of the fourteenth century, a variety of measures, including quarantine, surveillance, and isolation hospitals were employed in an attempt to contain plague and other epidemic diseases.

From the seventeenth century, an explicit political philosophy began to equate populous nations with wealthy, strong ones. The premium placed by the New Philosophy of the Scientific Revolution on the mathematization of truth – even social truth – encouraged the attempts of John Graunt and William Petty to examine the phenomena of health, wealth, and population quantitatively (as discussed in Chapter 2). From the eighteenth century, the right of each human being to health (as well as to liberty and the pursuit of happiness) was increasingly articulated, although the relation between these individual rights and the responsibilities and privileges of the State was not always clear. The doctrine of economic laissez-faire of Adam Smith (1723–90) cast doubt on the wisdom of state interference in the market forces of supply and demand.

This philosophy of laissez-faire was strongest in English-speaking countries, where relatively weak central governments, minimal bureaucracy, and individualism went hand in hand. On the Continent, more absolutist states (sometimes acquiring the epithet "benevolent despotisms") enshrined different values. Two Continental enterprises were particularly important as background to nineteenth-century public health and community medicine: Johann Peter Frank's elaboration of the idea of medical police, and the *Société Royale de Médecine's* collaborative study of epidemic disease.

I. FRANK AND THE MEDICAL POLICE

Johann Peter Frank (1745–1821) was an internationalist who faithfully served, during a peripatetic career, the governments of Germany, Italy, Lithuania, Russia, and Austria. Only Napoleon he declined to follow, turning down the offer to become his personal physician. For it was Austria, with its Viennese capital and (all-too-briefly) its genial Emperor Joseph II (1741–90), which commanded his deepest affections. Frank was a favorite of the reformist-minded Joseph, and, had the Emperor lived, Frank might well have been able to put into operation many of his ideas on social medicine. As it was, they remained only partially realized, although classically stated in his *System einer vollstandigen medicinischen Polizey* (System of complete medical police), published in six volumes and three supplements between 1779 and 1826.

Polizey and *Polizei* are usually translated "police," but with the now archaic meaning of "regulating or administering a state." Chairs in *Polizeiwissenschaft* ('police science') were created at various Continental universities from the early eighteenth century. Lectures in the subject would be aimed at future civil servants, lawyers, and administrators. The Emperor Joseph's mother, Maria Teresa, had established a chair in "police science" at the University of Vienna in 1765 for Frank's friend and colleague Joseph von Sonnenfels (1732–1817). Inevitably, Sonnenfels was forced to deal with medical issues in his writings on the regulation, financing, and administration of the enlightened state. Frank made medicine the core of his own vision of the humane society.

Frank drew from his wide experience as a physician and medical educator. His *System* dealt with virtually every aspect of health and medical care, from hospitals and medical licensing to marriage, abortion, and infant feeding. It followed the individual from the womb to the tomb, examining every stage of life and the factors that influenced the people's health. The title of one of his famous lectures, delivered in 1790, already indicated the broad sweep of his vision: *The People's Misery: Mother of Diseases*. The police in his ideal state were to ensure that neither the social conditions nor individual habits obtained if these were detrimental to health. There were, he recognized, potential conflicts between the wishes of the individual and the needs of the state: but most of the unhealthy things human beings wished to do – like eating too much, dancing during late pregnancy, or frequenting brothels – were not really conducive to lasting happiness. Our intemperance and the strength of our passions have overpowered the instinct of natural, simple self-preservation originally implanted in the species by the Creator.

Three themes permeated Frank's work from beginning to end. One was the paternalism that characterized the relationship between medical police and people. He was not afraid to recommend legislation and other positive measures to ensure that individual acts of folly could not be easily committed. Thus, sex outside of marriage was to be closely regulated but foundling hospitals rather than abortions were the solution to indiscretions resulting in pregnancy. The same paternalism made it incumbent on the State to ensure that food and beverages were not adulterated, so the consumer could be guaranteed decent standards of quality.

The justification for the paternalism ultimately lay in the *System's* second major theme: Frank's equation of communal health and prosperity with a large population. The motto to the first volume stated this in no uncertain terms: *Servandis et augendis civibus* ('For the preservation and increase of the population'). Both police and people were to dedicate themselves to this collective good, for a healthy, populous nation was, in the end, a happy one. Curative and preventive measures worked hand in hand, but Frank saw clearly the suffering caused by disease and so placed the higher premium on the creation of social conditions compatible with health, fecundity, and long life. Foundling hospital statistics showed that illegitimate children had far higher mortality rates than legitimate ones, so the sanctions surrounding marriage could be justified on the same grounds as those requiring employers to provide salubrious workplaces and reasonable working hours. The more people the better for all.

But (third) Frank also recognized certain paradoxes of prosperity previously glimpsed by one of his major inspirations: Jean Jacques Rousseau (1712–78). Rousseau was the great Enlightenment apostle of the "natural" life, with its emphasis on fresh air, simple food, comfortable clothes, breast-feeding and uncomplicated, direct human relationships. Sometimes called "primitivism," Rousseau's message had important medical ramifications, for both he and Frank attributed many of the diseases of civilization to the rigid and artificial constraints placed on people in pursuit of beauty, social esteem, or wealth. Powdered wigs, corsets, make-up, and closed windows were equally anathema to Rousseau and Frank. But the problem did not end simply with the temptations and pitfalls that modern life placed in the way of the unwary. Frank's ideal state also created its inherent difficulties, for its very populousness inevitably led to large towns, which by their nature, were unhealthy. The powerful state with so many subjects generated its own pollution, its own smoke and dust, its own overcrowded and insanitary dwellings.

The full statistical realization that people living in densely populated areas had – other things being equal – higher mortality rates than those who inhabited the countryside or more spacious parts of towns was a powerful nineteenth-century discovery. At one level, Frank himself recognized it, but his *System* never really came to grips with the health problems created by the twin forces of industrialization and urbanization. Rather, his medical police would have operated within what was essentially a preindustrial world, where land was plentiful, cities only larger villages without unique social or hygienic problems, and population increases an inherently good thing. Ironically, even as Frank was visualizing a state with vigorous, sustained population increases, T. R.

Malthus (1766–1834) in England was drawing attention to the problems created by too many people chasing too few resources. "Malthusianism" is still part of the modern worldview.

Frank's ideas naturally had greater impact in German-speaking countries, Eastern Europe, and Italy, where individualism was less valued than collective strength, although in practice no government was prepared to invest the money to implement Frank's idealized welfare state. There was a brief flirtation with medical police in early nineteenth-century Scotland, but the mixture of individual and communal regulation contained in the *System* was alien to dominant Anglo-American philosophies. In these countries, as in France, most organized medical pressure came to be exerted in areas more directly touching the generation and spread of what were called "filth diseases." A systematic attempt to understand why such diseases occurred was made by the *Société Royale de Médecine*.

II. THE SOCIAL ECOLOGY OF DISEASE

Epidemics had long been a major disruptive feature of human life, a particular threat in times of war and famine, but seemingly always lurking behind the regularities of seasons, harvest time, and festival. Some outbreaks could be expected: jaundice, fevers, and infantile diarrhea in hot weather; catarrhal fevers in cold, wet conditions; malarial fevers ("ague") in marshy areas. Plague, common in Europe from the Black Death of 1348–50 to the mid-seventeenth century, usually began in the spring, peaked by late summer, and abated with the coming of cold weather. Smallpox could erupt at any time.

The "causes" of these epidemic disorders were variously explained, but two different elements – the one environmental and secular, the other personal and essentially religious – reflect the mingling of Greek and Judeo-Christian strands in the Western medical tradition. The *locus classicus* of environmentalism was the Hippocratic treatise *Airs, Waters, Places*. Although partially concerned with the nature of the physical and cultural differences among human groups, the Hippocratic authors of this work (there were undoubtedly at least two) yoked together medicine, physical geography, and ethnology so persuasively that subsequent medical speculations on why epidemics occurred, and why certain diseases were prevalent in particular regions, made frequent reference to features such as wind, climate, temperature, soil, and humidity. At the same time, both individual and collective sickness could be rationalized in terms of moral or religious failings. Epidemics, for instance, could be the result of the wrath of God, who sent them to chasten and punish a wicked people. Aspects of both these explanatory schemes can be seen in words like "infectious" and "contagious," both originally carrying implications of pollution, taint, and defilement, moral as well as physical. "Miasma," too, was derived from the Greek word for stain or pollution, although with the stipulation that miasmatic diseases were spread through the air.

Moral and physical, supernatural and natural explanatory schemes need not be incompatible or mutually exclusive ("Praise the Lord, but keep your powder dry"). Gradually, however, most of the supernatural dimension to explaining epidemics was shorn, and discussion centered on the physical causes of disease. The continuing legacy of Hippocratic environmentalism can be seen in late eighteenth-century projects like that of the *Société Royale de Médecine*. The *Société* sponsored a questionnaire sent to physicians and surgeons throughout France. The aim was to establish a central, empirical body of evidence that would relate local variations in temperature, rainfall, wind speeds and direction, atmospheric pressure, quality of available food, prices, and hygienic conditions, to the local prevailing diseases. Inspired by Vicq d'Azyr, the project continued for two decades from the 1770s, and was to provide a massive, numerically expressed and observationally based guide to the total environment and its causal relationship to health and diseases (of both human beings and their livestock). Month after month, year after year, dozens of local doctors completed their questionnaires, providing standard environmental information and correlating it with the prevalent diseases in their towns and regions. In the event, Vicq d'Azyr's death and the Revolution supervened before the massive cache of facts and figures was molded into publishable shape and the *Société* archives lay in obscurity until this century. But the project itself is indicative of the increasing concern of late eighteenth-century doctors in the environmental causes of disease, and in the augmented medical role in affairs touching the common health.

What could be called the *Société*'s ecological approach to disease can also be seen in the activities – more famous in their own day – of John Pringle (1707–82) and James Lind (1716–94) aimed at improving the health in the British armed forces. Lind is associated today primarily with scurvy, but both he and Pringle had broad medical interests. Lind's *Essay on diseases incidental to Europeans in hot climates* (1768) was a product of his medical experience in the West Indies and other parts of the world where indigenous diseases were particularly virulent for Europeans. Yellow fever, malaria, and other acute fevers took a heavy toll in garrisons and settlements, and seriously hampered imperial enterprises. Climate (in its widest meaning) was the most striking difference between Europe and the tropical countries and naturally it played a prominent explanatory role in Lind's analysis of why the tropics were so often the white man's grave. Likewise, his perception of disease aboard ship led him to single out the close living quarters, foul air, spoiled food, and lack of personal hygiene as leading to the high incidence of fevers, scurvy, and other diseases on long sea voyages. Pringle's *Observations on the diseases of the army* (1752) took a similar ecological approach, placing particular emphasis on good sanitation and ventilation in the prevention and treatment of the common diseases of the army.

The contexts of the *Société*'s cooperative surveys and the more personal, individual observations of Lind and Pringle were different: the first one French, civilian, and never completed, the other British, military, and producing some changes in medical policies. But the differences are less significant than the similarities, for all this late eighteenth-century activity reflected broad environmental approaches to diseases within the community and formed a matrix continuous with the heroic decades of public health agitation in the 1840s and 50s. Certain themes and problems had permanent relevance in the whole of this period.

First, there was the ongoing concern with dependent groups, especially the poor and the common soldier or sailor. It was they who suffered the brunt of epidemic diseases, premature death, and appalling living conditions. Since the late sixteenth century the English Poor Laws had sought to provide a net to catch the deserving poor who through misfortune, death of a breadwinner, sickness, unemployment, or inadequate wages were unable to secure the bare necessities of life. Even the concept (and certainly the reality) of the Welfare State was well in the future, but the Poor Law embodied a rudimentary acceptance of public responsibility for those fallen on hard times. The level of maintenance thus available was of course meager, to receive it sometimes required removal to a poorhouse or workhouse ("indoor relief"), where the able bodied were expected to work for their keep, and always the stigma of dependence followed. Poor Law support had to be essentially disagreeable, a last resort, for otherwise the will to work might be sapped. Furthermore, as originally conceived, Poor Law provision was expected merely to supplement the occasional breakdown of private, Christian philanthropy, but the latter was to be the primary means whereby the well-to-do helped their brethren down the socioeconomic scale. Medical services were only a fraction of this survival kit for the unfortunate, but many Poor Law Guardians hired the part-time services of a local doctor to care for the sick and injured poor whose resources were inadequate to buy these services or who were unable to obtain them through voluntary hospitals, dispensaries, and other private medical charities. It took no great leap of the medical imagination to perceive that prevention might be cheaper than cure, particularly because the illness or death of the breadwinner might have ramifications beyond his own case. The military was a particularly obvious instance of the economics of health,

since as Pringle and Lind both pointed out, sickness usually took a
heavier toll than battle, and an army unfit for fighting still had to be
maintained.

Certain post-Keynesian economists like to point out that there is no
such thing as a free lunch, and past philanthropy was often two-edged,
not only by its ultimate harshness but by the deference and gratitude it
was designed to engender. Philanthropy is commonly written about
nowadays in terms of social control, but an important category of earlier
concern was its relation to the economic system. Many of the debates
about the role of medicine in the community were permeated with worry
about its effects on the principles of laissez-faire economics, and on the
paradoxes of philanthropy articulated by Malthus. Labor and goods were
worth precisely what the free market determined, and to interrupt the
system whereby both workers and capitalists were permitted to buy
cheaply and sell dearly (if possible) was to court disaster and inhibit the
general good. Quarantine laws during epidemics inhibited the free flow
of goods and services (and were consequently resisted on economic
grounds), and the repair of substandard housing might have the un-
desirable effect of forcing up rents and driving out the very individuals
who were supposed to be helped. Malthus further analyzed poverty in
terms of the differential growth of population and the means of subsis-
tence, pointing out that saving lives might merely increase the poor's
misery, as more people competed for scarce resources.

All these matters were thrown into even sharper relief by the third
phenomenon of continuing relevance for nineteenth-century public
health activity, the spreading impact of industrialization. The relationship between industrialization and general living standards is still a
matter of historical debate; some groups benefited whereas others,
whose skills or cottage-based industries were no longer viable in the
marketplace, clearly did not. The total quantity of manufactured goods
– cottons, cooking utensils, pottery – increased, but so did the population
and data on these parameters are often insufficient to permit conclusions
about standards of living commanding general assent. What is more
certain is that the factory system imposed great demands on workers
who were compelled to slog long hours at monotonous jobs in unhy-
gienic surroundings. The system also imposed considerable demands
on women and children (who of course had not been exempt from the
rigors of farm labor or cottage industry), and it certainly intensified the
processes of urbanization.

In terms of population distribution, Britain remained a rural society
until the mid-nineteenth century, and France and Germany even longer,
but it was the Industrial Revolution that caused former towns and villages such as Manchester, Sheffield, Glasgow, Birmingham, and Liverpool to grow into the cities of the 1830s, and that fueled the largest

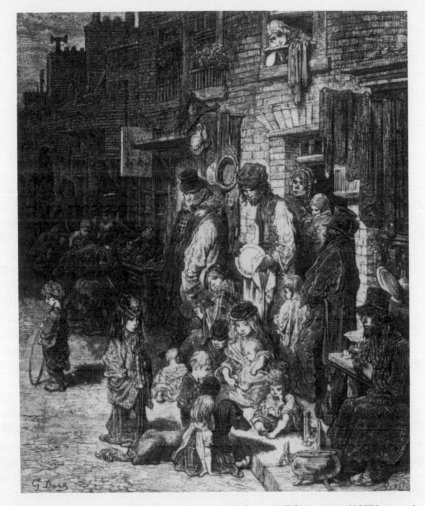

Figure 8. The images from Gustave Doré's London: A Pilgrimage *(1872) were impressive reminders of the association of poverty and overcrowding in London and other European and American cities. G. Doré and Blanchard Jerrold,* London: A Pilgrimage *(London: Grant, 1872), f. p. 124.*

industrial center of all, London, where a population of about 675,000 in 1750 had doubled to almost one and a half million in 1831. Manchester's population increased more than sixfold between 1770 and 1831, from about 27,000 to 183,000. Liverpool grew almost as rapidly (from about 34,000 to 165,000 during the same period), and Birmingham, Sheffield, Leeds, and other industrial cities experienced similar population explosions. The pattern was somewhat different in France, where both industrialization and population increases were delayed until the nineteenth century and where the largest cities (Paris, Marseilles, Lyons, Bordeaux, Rouen) were less dependent on factory-based industry. Nevertheless, Paris almost doubled its population between 1801 and 1846 (from 548,000 to 1,054,000) and other cities underwent similar or even greater rates of growth, even if Paris dwarfed its French rivals in size and complexity as did London its British ones.

It had long been known that cities and large towns were less healthy than the countryside. The London Bills of Mortality had shown in the seventeenth and eighteenth centuries a general excess of deaths over births in the capital (whose ever-increasing population was thus achieved only through sustained immigration from the surrounding countryside). Rousseau's gospel of rural simplicity had wide vogue from the 1750s, and few doctors would have denied the contrast between the dirty, unhealthy, insanitary cities and the rustic, glowing countryside. The reality of course did not always fit the image, but the worst effects of rural poverty could be buffered through poaching, a garden, and the produce of the forests and lanes. Urban poverty was more brutal, as mushrooming cities spawned jerry-built houses, which were densely packed and without gardens or sanitary facilities. The rough and tumble of the marketplace produced a disturbing new element, the trade cycle, which in turn led to seasonal unemployment. Successful entrepreneurs could make fortunes but bankruptcies were also common and had wide repercussions. Government spending on the Napoleonic Wars created price inflation and the close of the Wars unfortunately coincided with several years of bad harvests, high prices, and little employment for returning veterans. In Britain, corn laws imposed high duties on foreign imports of grain, thereby protecting agriculture at the expense of low-paid workers for whom the cost of bread was crucial. Trade unions were still illegal and workers responded by machine breaking, industrial sabotage, and food riots. Although there was little direct starvation in Britain, demands on the poor rates soared and serious outbreaks of fever occurred between 1816 and 1819 in London, Leeds, Glasgow, and many other cities. The Glasgow Infirmary, which had admitted 90 cases of fever in 1814, had 1,371 cases in 1818. Workhouses in London in 1818 were reported overflowing with paupers suffering from fever; the London Fever Hospital treated 80 patients in 1804, and 760 in 1817. Despite the social turmoil and widespread hardship, the Government of the day was in no conciliatory mood; it imposed censorship and prosecuted the authors and publishers of seditious or blasphemous works (such as those of Tom Paine). The turbulent decade ended with the Peterloo Massacre (16 August 1819), when the militia charged a peaceful meeting in Manchester, which was calling for repeal of the corn laws and parliamentary reform, killing 11 people and injuring 400.

The Peterloo Massacre may be thought to have little to do with medical history, but the issues at stake – the right to work, freedom from want, responsible government – were precisely those that Rudolf Virchow identified three decades later as central to the healthy society. It had become apparent by the 1820s that factories had come to stay and that urban growth was one consequence: they were two hallmarks of the modern, rational society. The extent to which such phenomena were affecting society was more clearly seen because of another common characteristic of industrial rationality: the rise of quantification. We have already noticed seventeenth-century attempts at counting heads and estimating social structure, and examined the use of large numbers of cases in early nineteenth-century hospitals. The accumulation of hospital statistics merely reflected a more general reliance on numbers, and a widespread belief that numbers yield objectivity and reliability.

Between 1750 and 1810 many countries started collecting national censuses and during the nineteenth century these became more reliable and began to provide information on household size, age structure, occupation, marital state, religion, and so forth. In 1837, civil registration of births, marriages, and deaths was initiated in Britain. Trade statistics and other economic indices became more commonly and reliably available. By the 1830s, interested individuals began to establish statistical societies, which held regular meetings, encouraged members to investigate vital, social, and economic events numerically, and sometimes published proceedings. The Manchester Statistical Society dates from 1833, a year before the one in London and coincident with the Statistical Section of the British Association for the Advancement of Science. There was an official Bureau of Statistics in Germany as early as 1805, France had various temporary national and provincial statistical bureaus during the Revolution and Empire, and a permanent one by 1833. Paris moreover had its own statistical bureau by 1818, and the *Académie des sciences morales et politiques* provided from 1795 a semiofficial forum for investigating and discussing sociomedical and statistical matters.

These and other expressions of what was predominantly a middle-class desire for objective "facts" were facets of the social and economic rationality assumed to underpin the new industrial order. Membership in British statistical societies was heavily weighted toward the established professions – medicine, law, church – with generous representation from the new industrial entrepreneurs and a reasonable sprinkling of improving landowners, gentry, and aristocrats. By the 1840s Queen Victoria's husband Prince Albert graced the statistical movement with his own interest and patronage.

If figures were required to validate the images just mentioned – the greater healthiness of countryside over city, of rich over poor, of legitimate children over illegitimate ones – the widespread passion for statistics amply supplied them. "There are," the British Prime Minister

Benjamin Disraeli was reported as saying, "three kinds of lies: lies, damned lies and statistics." It was, ironically, those very statistics that brought home to Disraeli's novel-reading public the stark reality of his own insistence that the rich and poor of England constituted two nations, ignorant of each other's habits, thoughts, and feelings, "formed by a different breeding, . . . fed by a different food, . . . ordered by different manners, . . . and not governed by the same laws."[1] Early statistical social investigators rarely examined the familiar; instead they sought the exotic within their own countries – the criminal and the vagabond, the unemployed and the unemployable, the destitute and the prostitute, the Great Unwashed. Disraeli was undoubtedly correct to insist that a barrier existed between rich and poor, for just as the ethnographic literature of the 1830s and 40s often betrayed travelers and missionaries recoiling from the cannibalism or puberty rites they witnessed in savages, the early statisticians were often repelled by the sloth, drunkenness, sexual promiscuity, and fiscal irresponsibility of the unwashed. Yet it was these very segments of society for which much of the early public health agitation was voiced. Whether reformers were motivated by a fear of the Other, by Christian benevolence, humanity, a grandiose sense of paternalism, or revulsion at the way the irrational and inefficient poor did not blend into a rational, industrial society, is not always apparent: but in most European countries and in the United States, from about the 1820s the poor were discovered en masse, were described as an irreducible residuum of society, and were perceived to be suffering needlessly from the excessive debility and premature death of filth diseases.

III. THE FIRST INDUSTRIAL NATION

The initial "statistical" discovery of the health problems of the poor varied, of course, from country to country, as did the timing, pace, and consequences of industrialization. The two phenomena – industrialization and public health concerns – were closely related, though not in ways that can be completely understood by a crude economic determinism. Britain provides a particularly illuminating example, as the first nation to industrialize and as one that by the 1870s had a set of public health legislation more comprehensive than any other country in the world.

Some preventive dimension had been present even in the hospital movement, particularly the fever hospitals. Fever hospitals were inspired by the work of John Haygarth (1740–1827) in Chester, a small city in Northwest England. A physician to the Chester Infirmary, Haygarth became intrigued by the correlation between economic standing and the prevalence of diseases such as "fever." During an epidemic in the 1770s he surveyed the whole town, noting that the densely populated suburbs (where the poor lived) were more affected than the spacious and elegant center of the town. Surveys of individual households convinced him that the fever was contagious, spread from person to person through the atmosphere in which human effluvia had been generated to toxic levels by overcrowding, unwashed clothes and bodies, and insanitary habits. "If a regulation could be universally adopted of immediately removing out of the family such of the poor people as are seized with fevers," he wrote, control of its spread could be achieved. In 1783, during another epidemic of fever, the Governors of the Infirmary permitted him to turn an attic room of the Infirmary into a fever ward, where victims could be taken immediately when they fell ill, and nursed in circumstances in which a free flow of fresh air prevented spread to other patients or staff at the Infirmary.

Haygarth's success encouraged others in the 1790s and early 1800s to start fever hospitals ("Houses of Recovery" they were euphemistically called) in industrializing towns and cities like Manchester, Liverpool, Stockport, Newcastle, Leeds, and London. A fairly uniform set of nursing and medical procedures evolved for treating fever victims, including fresh air, clean bedclothes, cold water baths, special diet, and purgatives, but hospital concern was not just curative, but preventive. Early removal of the patient prevented his becoming a focus of spread, and clean clothes, soap, and whitewash for the walls were provided for his family. Advocates of the fever hospitals claimed good results, both in reducing mortality among those affected and in reducing incidence during times of epidemic. Any "contagious" fever (though not smallpox) qualified for admission, and most patients were diagnosed as suffering from "typhus," "low," "continued," or "spotted" fever or erysipelas. Patients did not have to pay anything, nor did they need to secure letters of recommendation from hospital governors, as was necessary for admission to the general voluntary hospitals.

Financial support for the fever hospitals came from middle- and upper-class individuals, many of them associated with the Society for the Betterment of the Condition of the Poor. This was one of hundreds of philanthropic societies started during the early Industrial Revolution. Like many others, the S.B.C.P. had strong medical interests, though it was also concerned with education, living and work conditions, and moral purity. Its dominant religious orientation was Evangelical Anglicanism, the branch of the Church of England that sought to make evangelical, salvational Christianity a potent force for religious, moral, and social reformation. William Wilberforce (1759–1833) was the key figure in the early Evangelical movement, Lord Shaftesbury (1801–85) in its high Victorian phase. In addition to their fervent, emotional religion, both men were keenly interested in social problems, knowing full well that it was difficult to save a man's soul if his stomach was empty, or to teach him to read his Bible if he worked fifteen hours a day in a factory or mine, and was illiterate to boot. The people's health concerned them both: Wilberforce was Vice-President of the London Fever Hospital (as well as many other medically oriented charities), Shaftesbury (as we shall see) an active member of the General Board of Health, created in 1848.

Evangelical solutions to social problems were generally paternalistic, offering reform from above of a kind that never challenged the legitimacy of deferential relationships between master and servant, governor and governed, capitalist and worker. The poor were expected to be grateful for the rich man's offering. Evangelicals hoped factory owners would take paternalistic interest in their workers' welfare, who in return would behave like obedient children. Many prominent Evangelicals (including Wilberforce and Shaftesbury) were active in Parliament and helped pass a good deal of early social legislation, beginning with the Factory Act of 1802, which dealt with child labor. Paternalism continued to hold sway among many (particularly the pious) throughout the century, though it was not always in accord with the new economic realities, where (according to the novelist Sir Walter Scott) the manufacturer could "assemble five hundred workmen one week and dismiss them next, without having any further connection with them than to receive a week's work for a week's wages, nor any further solicitude about their future fate than if they were so many old shuttles."[2]

The other major motive for social reform during the period was a desire to improve the nation's efficiency. This was a particularly common theme among those inspired by the social philosopher Jeremy Bentham (1748–1832), the apostle of utilitarianism. Essentially secular in its values, utilitarianism preached the gospel of "the greatest happiness of the greatest number," and Bentham believed that institutional and legal corruption and lethargy caused much needless suffering. Men and women were uncomplicated organisms who sought to increase pleasure or avoid pain, and given rationally planned institutions and environments, could be expected to behave appropriately. Bentham was most concerned with reforming the law and its associated penal institutions, busying himself with numerous projects, including the design of the ideal penitentiary where criminals (under constant surveillance) could be environmentally "reprogrammed" and turned into productive members of society.

Like many members of his generation, Bentham recognized that the Old Poor Laws were ineffective and inappropriate for the new economic circumstances of the age. Between 1780 and 1830 an increasing volume of books, pamphlets, and parliamentary debate offered comment on these Poor Laws, through which payments had increased fourfold during those decades. Their administration varied wildly in the 15,000 parishes in England and Wales (Scotland had its own separate procedure), each responsible for collecting and distributing the Poor Rate (tax) to eligible paupers. The Law tried to distinguish between the "worthy" (orphans, widows, the injured, or ill) and the "unworthy" (beggars, vagabonds, the willfully unemployed) poor, and to deal with each according to his or her deserts. Paupers had the right to relief only in the parish of their birth, and from the mid-seventeenth century one line of thought had advocated that most paupers should be made to go into a poorhouse (or workhouse) to be eligible for support. There authorities could keep closer check on their charges, putting the able-bodied to work and teaching the unskilled a trade. This form of relief ("indoor," as opposed to "outdoor," which permitted the pauper to stay in his residence) was never very common, since most parishes were too small to afford to build and maintain a workhouse, and parishes were often unwilling to cooperate with neighboring parishes for fear that they would be saddled with the cost of keeping paupers who were not actually their legal responsibility. Because much poverty was health-related, many parishes hired the part-time services of a local doctor to provide medical care for their dependant population.

Many middle-class commentators decried the way in which the very existence of the Poor Laws sapped the energy and spirit of the English workman, who knew that the Parish would not let him or his family actually starve, even if his troubles were due to idleness, drunkenness, or debauchery. Economic rationality dictated that those who do not work should not eat, and Malthusianism preached the potential hopelessness of even well-meaning philanthropy since it might merely permit more hungry wretches to survive: "Industry and subordination [should] once more be restored," insisted Malthus, by firmness if necessary. Further, Christian moralists could argue that the Poor Laws made Christians forget to do their duty through individual, private acts of charity and mercy.

After several decades of debate, Parliament in 1832 finally ratified an official inquiry into the operation of the Poor Laws, against a backdrop of increasing social and industrial unrest. There were nine Commissioners, including three clergymen with Evangelical leanings and two lawyers who represented the newer economic thinking. Of these, Edwin Chadwick (1800–90) was ultimately the most important. Chadwick, one of the lawyers, had been Jeremy Bentham's last Secretary (Bentham died in that eventful year 1832) and had imbibed from the old philosopher a passion for rational reform. He proved to be the most energetic of the Commissioners, personally visiting many parishes to inspect the Old Poor Laws in operation, and playing the most important part in writing the Commissioners' *Report* (1834), detailing their findings and recommendations for change. Their "fact-finding" mission (published in

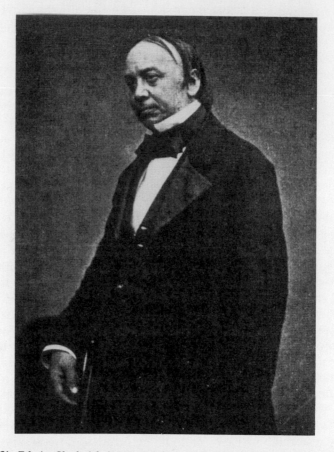

Figure 9. Sir Edwin Chadwick (1800–90) became the dominant figure in the attempt, from the 1830s, to impose an economic rationality on the relief of poverty and the control of paupers. His concern with public health developed gradually. From J. A. Delmege, Towards National Health *(London: W. Heinemann, 1931).*

twenty-two volumes), on which the *Report* was based, was a pioneering attempt, using questionnaires and site visits to conduct a social survey. The Commissioners were particularly concerned to show that the Old Poor Laws made relief for an able-bodied individual too easy to acquire, thereby sapping his independence to his own detriment and that of society as a whole. Poverty they felt to be fundamentally a moral problem, caused by laziness, vice, and moral decay: its worst features could be solved if the nation – rich and poor – adopted simple Christian virtues. What should be eradicated was the belief that the able-bodied had a right to relief. For the "impotent" poor (the sick, injured, children), they had somewhat more sympathy and expressed general satisfaction with the provision of medical services under the old system.

The Commissioners' attitudes thus mixed the older paternalism and the newer economic rationality. Their recommendations (encoded in the New Poor Law of 1834) were more aggressively rigorous. In order to standardize proceedings, the old Parish system was abolished, to be replaced by larger geographical units – the Union – each of which was to build a workhouse to accommodate the deliberate emphasis on indoor relief, since the harsh conditions and public stigma of pauperism associated with workhouses would discourage abuse. The general principle of "less eligibility" (that the level of support under the Poor Law should be less than the minimum that could be made by working) would further encourage the lower orders to use the system as nothing but a desperate appeal of last resort. Workhouses were to have infirmaries associated with them, and each Union was required to employ a Poor Law Medical Officer. To ensure that the New Poor Law was uniformly administered throughout the country, permanent Poor Law Commissioners were appointed. Chadwick was disappointed not to be one of them, having to content himself with becoming their Secretary.

Nevertheless, the inferior social status of his position did not stop him from throwing himself wholeheartedly into his work, and between 1834 and 1842 his intense – almost obsessive – concern with the daily operation of the New Poor Law changed his ideas about the relationship between social class, ill health, and poverty. He not only discovered, but he went a long way toward quantifying, the extent to which poverty and disease operated in tandem. We might almost say that the conclusion was forced on him by the sheer weight of the evidence, for it represented a significant departure from the moral analysis of poverty embedded in the 1834 *Report*, and, in any case, the lawyer Chadwick had little faith in the capacity of doctors to diagnose and cure disease. The annual reports on the operation of the New Poor Law that Chadwick had to prepare on behalf of the Commissioners show the gradual evolution of his thinking, a process aided by cooperation with several equally concerned doctors, including Thomas Southwood Smith (1788–1861) and James Kay Shuttleworth (1804–1877), who carried out systematic surveys on the relationship between poverty, bad living conditions, and disease in the slums of London, Manchester, Glasgow, and other cities. These surveys and those of Chadwick himself made abundantly clear the extent of class- and income-specific mortality in early Victorian Britain. In Whitechapel (a working-class district in east London), middle-class individuals were on average 45 years old when they died; tradesmen (and their families) were on average dead by the time they were 27; laborers, servants, and others in the working class were 22. In Liverpool (with a large unskilled Irish population and vast areas of slums) the figures were even worse: 35, 22, and 15. In the rural shire of Rutland they were 52, 41, and 38. Inevitably, much of this wastage was among those under five years old, but even among adults, mortality rates were significantly higher among working-class individuals than those of the middle class, and among urban dwellers when compared with those living in the countryside or small villages.

That there existed a direct correlation between poverty and disease was not unfamiliar to those of Chadwick's generation. But Chadwick went further in exploring the dynamics between the two categories, arguing not just the common theme that poverty causes disease, but the more radical proposal that disease causes poverty. Individuals were being forced onto the poor rates because illness had destroyed their capacity to work, or had killed the family breadwinner. It was of course a vicious circle, for depressed earning capacity reduced the poor's ability to support a physical environment (including food, clothing, and shelter) conducive to health. Chadwick's analysis shifted the emphasis from moral causes of poverty (laziness, dissipation) to environmental ones, since the relevant diseases of poverty (fevers, cholera, phthisis, infantile diarrhea) were deemed to be caused by environmental factors, in particular miasmata. Chadwick believed these miasmata were generated by squalor, dirt, and excrement and were above all associated with the putrid smells of insanitary conditions: "All smell" (he wrote) "is, if it be intense, immediate acute disease."[3] On strictly utilitarian grounds, health had become for him a national priority and economic desideratum. It was an investment that paid dividends.

Chadwick's thinking along these lines culminated in his *Report on the Sanitary Condition of the Labouring Population of Great Britain* (1842), a stout volume that Chadwick had widely distributed to peers, Members of Parliament, key clergymen and doctors, and others in positions of power. For Chadwick was no armchair philosopher, but a political being whose *Report* contained not simply analyses of the economic and social costs of disease, but a program for action. His attitude toward medicine is apparent in the details of his program. Socially consequential diseases are easy to diagnose, and are all caused by the same cluster of environmental pollutants. In fact, these "filth diseases" were (Chadwick thought) simply variants of the same disease that under different conditions could produce different symptoms. In any case, diagnostic quibbling was much less appropriate than preventive action.

For a book that was fundamentally about health and disease, there was (it could be argued) surprisingly little about doctors, hospitals, or therapies. This was not because Chadwick believed that doctors could be entirely dispensed with, but because he held that sufficient knowledge and technology already existed to prevent the most important diseases. The solution was not so much medical as social and (above all) engineering, and the operative word in his preventive program was cleanliness. Clean was virtually synonymous with healthy, dirty with unhealthy, and one need only improve ventilation (clean air), washing, drinking, and cooking facilities (clean water), waste disposal (clean privies), and housing (clean walls) to prevent disease among the laboring population. Although not a notably pious man, Chadwick undoubtedly pondered much on the scriptural injunction: "Wash and be clean." Much of Chadwick's recipe for health revolved around his proposal of an "arterio-venous" system of water supply: clean water was to be piped under pressure into houses, and human and household waste were to be removed suspended in water through sewers made of impervious glazed pipes. This would prevent seepage of decomposing excrement and animal matter (the single most common cause of disease) into the soil as was then common from individual cesspits or enormous sewers made of porous substances. As a brilliant bureaucratic coda, Chadwick proposed that the refuse be taken (under high pressure) to great vats in the countryside, where the water could evaporate, leaving rich manure that, when sold to farmers, would raise revenue to fund the scheme. There was "gold to be won from muck." The farmers, with pure fertilizer, could produce more food, which further enhanced economic output. With this single bold stroke, he believed an average of thirteen years could be added to each laborer's life, and the poor rates correspondingly reduced.

Chadwick's *Report* appeared in a decade of intense political and social unrest, sometimes known as the "hungry forties." During this decade a series of bad food harvests, including the potato famine in Ireland, compounded by the continuation of the "Corn Laws" (which taxed imported grain, thereby keeping bread and other staple food expensive) led to widespread hardship among the poor. The anti-Corn Law League and Chartism (a working-class movement aimed at securing the legal right to form trade unions) occupied more public attention than did the public health movement. Nevertheless, there was growing concern about the continued deterioration of living conditions in the industrial cities (the deathrate in the five largest English cities rose from twenty per thousand to thirty per thousand between 1831 and 1841), and the cholera epidemic of 1832 had seemed to many like a return of the plague.

Cholera made an impact on British (as well as European and American) consciousness beyond its actual mortality, although even that was significant enough. The 1832 epidemic caused some 23,000 deaths in England and Wales, a large number but one that should be seen in context. It represented only about 6 percent of the total deaths during the year, putting cholera no higher than third in the table of leading causes of death, behind "consumption" (pulmonary phthisis), and "convulsions," and not far ahead of typhus, pneumonia, smallpox, dropsy, and "debility." Since cholera virtually disappeared in 1833, over the quinquennium surrounding the epidemic, it was not one of the top ten causes of death. Why then do we still recognize the middle third of the century as "the cholera years"?

IV. CHOLERA AND OTHER SPECIFIC DISEASES

In the 1830s, cholera was a new disease, without precedent in Europe, thus giving it a status not unlike Legionnaire's disease or AIDS in our own time. Doctors since antiquity had used the word "cholera" to describe a condition characterized by vomiting, intense diarrhea, and gripping abdominal pain, and many cases of infantile summer diarrhea were called "cholera infantum." But, as European doctors with Asian experience well knew, another acute disorder with the same general signs and symptoms was endemic in India and the Far East, and it was this "Asiatic cholera" which, for no apparent reason, broke out of its traditional confines in 1817, and began slowly creeping westward. By 1823 it had reached the Caspian Sea, in 1829 it turned northwestward, to Moscow, Poland, and the Baltic ports. By then, nations in Western Europe were thoroughly alarmed, and several delegations of doctors had been dispatched to study the disease and try to answer basic questions: Was Asiatic cholera contagious? What caused it? How should it be treated? Could anything be done to prevent its further spread into Western Europe? Public confidence was hardly helped by the fact that there was no consensus on any of these matters, and, though much ink was spilled, and some preparations mooted, a kind of hypnotic paralysis took hold, as the epidemic gradually crept closer. Some ships were quarantined, but although cholera's contagiousness was accepted by some medical opinion, everyone knew that quarantine disrupted trade and transport, and so hurt economically. As cholera moved closer, a central Board of Health, consisting of six doctors and five public servants, was established in June 1831, but it had only advisory powers, and most of its members had no experience with the disease they were supposed to turn back from Britain's shores. The Board sponsored various experiments (was chlorine an effective disinfectant against cholera?) and made various proclamations but nothing it did or said stopped cholera from reaching Britain in October 1831. Like the old bubonic plague, cholera entered through a port – Sunderland, in Northeast England. It took four months to reach London, 300 miles away, in a pattern that suggested to contagionists that it was contagious, and to anticontagionists that it was not.

Its novelty made it more awful, and so did the way it worked, for it killed quickly and nastily. Victims would be well in the morning and dead by nightfall, dying after a few hours of intense vomiting, diarrhea (called "rice and water," since the stools were mostly liquid with a few solid particles), cramps, clamminess, and shrunken features. The *facies*

Hippocratica (the facial features presaging death described in the Hippocratic Corpus) had not been so common for centuries. Only a minority of victims lingered beyond a day or two, and most who survived the first forty-eight hours pulled through. The dramatic dehydration gave the skin an ominous bluish tint and the new corpses seemed to decompose more rapidly than normal. All this endowed cholera with a surreal character, and gave force to many a sermon suggesting that the epidemic was a divine chastisement.

Certainly the helplessness of the medical profession to do anything about it reinforced notions of a visitation. "It is passing strange that our *Pharmacopoeia* should always be behind the progress of science," lamented one medical journal in 1832, and despite competing claims among practitioners pushing their own favorite remedies (mostly traditional ones like bloodletting and purging – as if the disease did not purge enough!) doctors recognized that their therapeutic armamentarium was far from adequate. The public responded with a fair amount of antimedical hostility, and the hospitals came under particularly virulent criticism, because most of them were reluctant to admit cholera patients and stories circulated of victims being carted from hospital to hospital and finally being left to die in the streets. In London the Royal Free Hospital was converted from an outpatient dispensary to an inpatient facility during the crisis, to provide a place where even cholera patients could go, but with more than 11,000 cases and 5,000 deaths in the capital, this one small medical establishment (which treated 500 cases) could hardly make a major impact – its founder William Marsden (1790–1867) had no better treatment for cholera than his fellow doctors. Throughout Britain, medical services were regularly shown to be helpless in dealing with the new disease despite the establishment of temporary cholera hospitals in many places. Riots against doctors, hospitals, and hospital attendants in a dozen cities attest to the fear the disease engendered, and to the widespread belief among the working classes that those in authority *could* have done more, had they wished to. That 1832 also witnessed the passage of the Anatomy Act, providing for the use of dead paupers for anatomical dissection by medical students, also fueled public sentiment against the doctors. This further made the poor less willing to receive treatment in hospitals, for fear they would be experimented on and dissected. Statistics from seven towns and cities suggest a hospital mortality almost twice as high as cholera victims receiving treatment at home, although it is not always clear whether or not those going into hospitals were, on average, more seriously ill, and Marsden in London believed that the Royal Free Hospital had reduced mortality from about 50 percent to about 20 percent.

As always, it seems, the poor suffered most and working-class slums were often hit the hardest. Largely working class Glasgow (population

202,000) recorded 6,208 cases of cholera (about 1 in 32) whereas more genteel Edinburgh (population 136,000) had 1,886 cases (about 1 in 72). Mortality in both places was about 50 percent. But cholera never acquired so class-specific an image as typhus, and certainly all economic groups were affected, thus augmenting its impact among the powerful. In addition, the impression it made on contemporaries was increased by the almost perverse way it hit some areas hard, and others not at all. Some counties, such as Leicestershire and Dorset, almost completely escaped for reasons that seemed to defy analysis. The epidemic occurred just as the taste for statistical information was becoming well established, and although figures for the country as a whole are merely approximations (many areas never reported to the central Board of Health), the epidemic was followed more carefully by more people than any previous one, and many found it frustrating that its mode of spread did not fit into any easily understood pattern.

Nevertheless, the epidemic did leave its mark on early Victorian public health consciousness: cleanliness and good ventilation were the cornerstones of most of the prophylactic directives put out, and although the central and local boards of health had not been particularly effective (and in any case lapsed once the epidemic died down in 1833), they did give the nation experience with such bodies and probably paved the way for more permanent establishments in the following couple of decades. Cholera was a significant backdrop to the inquiries of the Poor Law Commissioners, the Anatomy Act, and to the Reform Bill of 1832, the first of a series of Parliamentary reforms that began to extend the franchise and to redraw boundaries for Parliamentary representation in greater harmony with the urban realities of industrial Britain.

By 1842, the year of Chadwick's *Report*, memory of the epidemic was receding, although "cholera" (much of it the earlier variety) figured modestly in the annual tally of national mortality after 1837, when the civil registration of births, deaths, and marriages was introduced. The compiler of these statistics was William Farr (1807–83), another doctor in the Chadwick circle, and one of the most creative minds in the public health movement. From 1837 until he finally retired in 1879, he supplied not just the tabulated raw data of the nation's biological indices, but thoughtful commentary on the geographical, class, age, sex, and occupational distribution of fatal disease. In his quietly professional way, Farr provided the framework for much epidemiological speculation about the causes of infectious diseases (he coined the term "zymotic" to describe diseases that he believed were caused by a process analogous to fermentation). He also developed a series of nosologies to guide those signing death certificates. Many Victorian disease categories do not conform to modern ones, of course, but Farr was acutely aware that many of his labels were imprecise. "The term *convulsions*" (he wrote in 1840) "is vague; and is applied too indiscriminately to the affections of infants under six months of age. It is often merely a symptom – a shadow of the disease, which escapes observation."[4] Some of Farr's most sophisticated epidemiological work related to cholera, wherein he devised mathematical formulas relating the incidence of the disease in any particular area to its height above the water table. High, well-drained areas were safest.

There was a widespread assumption during the century that with the availability of reliable information about any social condition, whether it concerned child labor, prostitution, or needless working-class mortality, appropriate remedies would follow. Certainly the annual reports on the nation's health that Farr prepared kept the brute facts of urban poverty and disease to the front, as of course had Chadwick's magnum opus. But if Chadwick expected immediate legislative action, he was disappointed. What he got instead was another commission – the Health of Towns Commission – that collected yet more opinion and facts about the deteriorating conditions in British cities, published in several massive volumes from 1844. At the same time, a private pressure group, the Health of Towns Association (1844), began campaigning for something to be done. Chadwick declined to be too closely associated with it, since this might compromise his effectiveness in government circles, but he certainly approved its plan of pamphlets, publicity, and petitions and agreed with its proposition that "the heaviest municipal tax is the fever tax," that is, the cost of caring for and burying those felled by fever.

Some of the momentum of 1842 was lost in the years immediately following, since nothing formal could be done while the Commission sat ("a bad substitute for action," one irate reformer called it) and the anti-Corn Law legislation preoccupied the government. A trial public health bill was debated briefly in Parliament in 1845, but not until 1848, with widespread political revolution in Europe, and cholera again approaching from the East, was a bill introduced that went some way toward satisfying Chadwick's ambitions for the public's health. Already, several local authorities had successfully experimented with his "arterial system," using small-bore glazed sewage pipes. The Public Health Act of 1848 set up a centralized General Board of Health, with Chadwick and Shaftesbury as two of its original three members. The Board had the power to require the formation of local boards of health (which reported to them) if petitioned by 10 percent of the local ratepayers or if the locality's death rate exceeded 23 per 1,000 (the national average was 21 per thousand). Liverpool had taken the lead by appointing a Medical Officer of Health (M.O.H.) in 1847 to oversee preventive arrangements, and the City of London and a number of other local authorities followed suit. For the most part the Board's powers were advisory rather than compulsory, but it did have the right to oversee the financing of sewers and water supplies to unhealthy districts. Chadwick, it will be recalled, believed he already had sufficient expertise to mastermind the eradication of most "filth disease," and his engineering approach underlay the Act. (Doctors complained that no member of the Board of Health was a medical man, although this was shortly remedied when Southwood Smith was added to it.)

In fact, the Board was largely a failure, but not for want of dedication and effort. The second cholera epidemic was a mixed blessing for Chadwick's plans, for, although it again focused the nation's attention on public health, it deflected to the crisis at hand what should have been the Board's long-term concerns with housing, sanitation, and poverty. It encouraged Chadwick to invoke emergency powers aimed at centralization and compulsion, two aspects of health policy that he felt were necessary. In 1848, he was correct in the sense that many local authorities would have done little or nothing had they not been forced. However, he misjudged the ferocity of opposition to his hope to centralize control of public health policy and activity. Local officials responsible for the many civic functions touching on health resented being told what they had to do, and even during the cholera epidemic the Board's work was often resented. Chadwick found it difficult to compromise and had little patience with the capricious, corrupt, and inefficient conglomeration of local government administration. He drove himself at a frenetic pace, but made many enemies and found few admirers. *The Times* (London) poured scorn on Chadwick, who was (it wrote) asking "for powers which a beleaguered community would hardly consider [giving] to a military dictator." The newspaper believed that, for all his trying, Chadwick and his Board had not made the nation healthier, but even had they done so, the price – compulsion and centralization – would have been too high. "The truth is, we do not like paternal governments . . . This is another reason why the CHADWICKIAN sanitary *regime* so signally failed."

Initially, the Board had been given a life of only five years and, despite the return of cholera in 1854, the nation decided that cholera was easier to tolerate than Chadwick. England would not be "bullied into health," and the Board was dissolved and Chadwick pensioned off to a long and frustrating retirement. There was, however, no returning to a pre-1848 amorphousness, and a new sanitary authority, with John Simon (1816–1904) as its chief medical officer, was established. Simon, a surgeon by training, had been appointed in 1848 Medical Officer of Health for the City of London, where he was independent of Chadwick's Board, since the City had been excluded from the Board's sphere of influence. His main attractions to the City Fathers, who hated Chadwick and wanted no interference, were good City connections (his father was a wealthy London businessman) and no exceptional involvement with the public health agitation of the mid-1840s. Simon subsequently showed himself to be everything that Chadwick was not: an elegant writer, a compromiser, a charming man, a persuader rather than a dictator. Simon was picked up by *The Times* and became the darling of the moderates, who wished to reform by suasion and local option. He was also eminently acceptable to the doctors, since he was more open-minded about the causes of epidemic diseases than Chadwick, and Simon's own evolving vision of health administration rested on a bedrock of medical knowledge. Even during the Chadwickian era, the nonspecific idea of miasmatic "filth disease" was being challenged through the work on cholera by John Snow (1813–58).

Snow experienced the 1832 cholera epidemic as a young surgical apprentice in the north of England, and the 1848 and 1854 epidemics as an established London practitioner. The '48 epidemic was the most devastating of all, claiming 53,000 victims in England and Wales, and Snow published several papers and a pamphlet (*On the mode of communication of cholera*, 1849) arguing that cholera is a specific, water-borne disease. During the 1854 epidemic he clinched his arguments by two separate epidemiological investigations, the one dramatic and famous, the other more mundane yet more brilliantly conclusive. In the first, he systematically mapped out the cases of cholera occurring in his own neighborhood in Soho (a district of central London), implicating a single contaminated well in Broad (now Broadwick) Street, where raw sewage was seeping back into the public well. He located several visitors who had drunk water from the well and subsequently come down with cholera, and suggested that workers in the local brewery were relatively immune from the disease because they could drink all the beer they wanted as a perquisite of their jobs, so there was no need to drink water. His carefully prepared analysis convinced local councilors that the well was the source of cholera and they removed the handle to the pump. The local epidemic soon subsided, although it had already been abating, so the gesture was more symbolic than directly effective. Nevertheless, there had been more than 500 fatal cases in a ten-day period within a 250-yard radius of the well.

Even more conclusive evidence for the water-borne spread of cholera came from Snow's analysis of the variable incidence of the disease in households throughout London that bought water from different water companies. (Although many London households were still dependent on drawing water from public wells like the one in Broad Street, an increasing number of them bought mains water supplied by several private, profit-making companies.) Snow was convinced that untreated sewage was the primary culprit for contaminating water, and thus companies that drew their water from downstream the Thames, into which many of the sewers of London emptied, should be more dangerous than

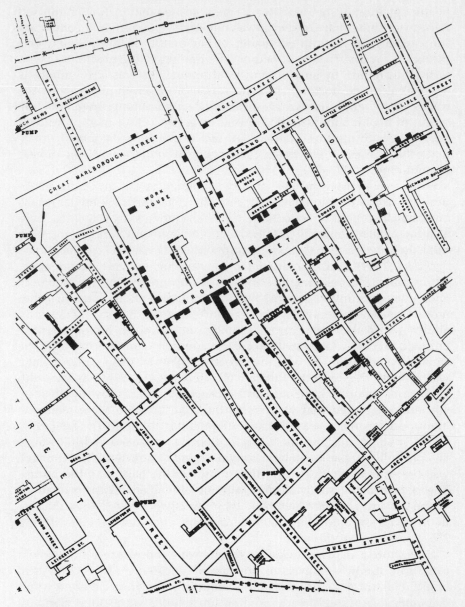

Figure 10. Snow plotted the cases of cholera in the area around the Broad Street pump during the 1854 epidemic in London. Modern epidemiologists would call this phenomenon "clustering." From John Snow, On the Mode of Communication of Cholera 2nd ed. *(London: Churchill, 1855).*

those that used Thames water upstream from London. There was no rigid geographical distribution to the areas supplied by the competing companies, and often houses in the same street would receive water from two or more different companies. Two companies supplied most of London south of the Thames, and Snow's massive survey showed that in one four-week period households receiving water from the Southwark company (with downstream pumps) suffered more than fourteen times the deathrate (71 per 10,000 houses) as the customers of the Lambeth company (upstream pumps and 5 deaths per 10,000 houses). The interdigitating nature of the supply ruled out air-borne, "miasmatic" spread. Snow examined the water microscopically and chemically and although the causative agent eluded him, he believed the *materies morbi*, whether living or simply chemical, was capable of procreation during the chain of infection. Boiling water before use was his advice, and he also advocated the employment of filters by the water companies, who should not be permitted to sell sewage-infested water from the Thames. Snow's data were useful for reformers campaigning for cleaner water and, though the private companies were reluctant to install expensive filtering plants (and municipal water supply was still in the future), a series of Parliamentary acts improved the quality of pumped water. The acceptance of Snow's message by public officials took some time, even if popular magazines began preaching the gospel of clean water in the 1850s. Nevertheless, neither Snow's investigations, nor the announcement, in 1854, that Filippo Pacini (1812–83), an Italian microscopist, had identified a unique microorganism in the feces of cholera victims, convinced many scientific élites. The issue of cholera's contagiousness and mode of spread was the main item on the agenda of seven successive International Sanitary Conferences held between 1851 and 1892, but the work of neither Snow nor Pacini figured in the deliberations.

An analogous piece of epidemiological work by William Budd (1811–80) in the west of England implicated contaminated water and feces-soiled linen in the spread of typhoid fever. A student of Pierre Louis, Budd could use his master's pathological criteria to define the disease he investigated epidemiologically, thus marrying hospital and community medicine. Although both Snow and Budd had no quarrel with Chadwick's plea for clean water and adequate sewage disposal (the sewer is "a direct continuation of the diseased intestine,'"[5] Budd wrote), their works were much more sophisticated medically in their rejection of the general notion of "filth disease" in favor of a series of specific noninterchangeable infectious diseases, spread through a variety of means, and each requiring separate study.

Their work was certainly appreciated by John Simon, who, during his twenty years as Chief Medical Officer successively to the reconstituted General Board of Health, to the Privy Council, and then to the Local

188 PUNCH, OR THE LONDON CHARIVARI

THE WONDERS OF A LONDON WATER DROP.

The freshest fruits of microscopical research are the wonders which have been revealed in a drop of London water through the Molecular Magnifier, illuminated by the Intellectual Electric Light. For the ability to behold these astounding marvels, a certain preparation is necessary, bearing, superficially considered, some resemblance to Mesmerism. The person intended to be the Seer is placed on a seat. Any competent individual then takes him in hand, and explains to him the composition of water, showing him how the pure fluid differs from the liquid constituting the Thames, and from that which exists in the metropolitan wells, when the former has received the contents of the sewers, and the latter the oozings of intramural graveyards. Some delicate subjects, even of the male sex, cannot endure this process, it affecting them with faintness and nausea.

Having been subjected to the above preliminaries, most people are in a sufficient state of enlightenment to discover, by the aid of the Molecular Magnifier, the curiosities contained in

A DROP OF LONDON WATER.

The drop to be magnified is taken from a mixture of the common well-water of London with that supplied by the various Companies. Mr. Hassell, it is already known, has enabled philosophers to discriminate between these waters, by the verminous and other peculiarities which he has demonstrated in each particular form of beverage.

The Molecular Magnifier differs from all other microscopes, in displaying the ultimate constitution of objects; a spectacle not only defying the naked eye, but all vision which is not in a measure psychical.

And wondrous indeed is the scene disclosed within the sphere of a little drop of water—of that water which Londoners drink, swallowing daily, myriads and myriads of worlds, whole universes instinct with life, or life in death! It transcends all that has hitherto been deemed astonishing. America herself will confess that it stumps the revelations of Andrew Jackson Davis.

Creatures—who shall name them? things in human shape—in all appearance London citizens—aldermen, deputies, common councilmen, —are seen disporting in the liquid dirt as in their native element. Behold them, fiercely hustling each other in competition for atomic garbage. What pushing, poking, fighting, kicking, scrambling! There goes an unfortunate wretch fast as if for dear life, with a hook-nosed homunculus—evidently a genuine water-bailiff—darting after him. Here a cheap slop-seller has caught a smaller individual of the same species by the head, and is trying to bolt him. There again, as plainly as possible, you see a funeral procession with an undertaker at the head

Figure 11. This Punch *cartoon, from 1850, shows that the general public was beginning to show concern about the quality of its water supply, even as Snow was implicating water in the spread of cholera.* Punch, 18 *(London: 1850).*

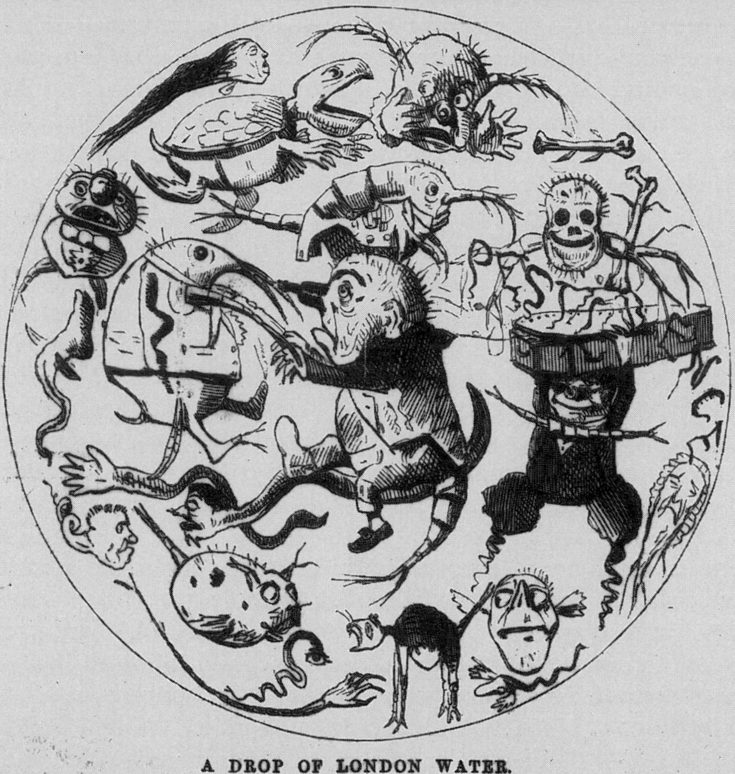

Government Board, managed to divert public money (often on an ad hoc, per diem basis) to fund epidemiological and even laboratory investigation of a number of communicable diseases, including diphtheria, typhoid, cattle plague, venereal disease, and smallpox. If 1834 to 1854 was the "Chadwickian era," 1855 to 1876 belonged to Simon, who was the key figure in the transition from sanitary reform to State medicine. Simon's style and values were always different than Chadwick's. His friends included high Victorian aesthetes like the art critic John Ruskin (1819–1900), and his prose, even in government reports, often exuded an impassioned, vivid, almost Dickensian quality. Behind the prose, however, was a mind that was far more open, far more subtle than Chadwick's, and, although Chadwick was a pioneer statistician, Simon was a true scientific epidemiologist. Significantly, Simon made the transition into the bacteriological age, whereas Chadwick remained to the end of his long life a miasmatist of the 1840s. Simon did some original work himself, but his forte was turning the investigations and statistics of men like Snow, Budd, Farr, and his own distinguished group of associates into blueprints for action.

Further, Simon knew how to gain the confidence of powerful politicians and so was able to influence a wide variety of important health legislation. These bills ranged from an 1855 Act requiring the appointment of Medical Officers of Health to each of the forty-nine sanitary districts of Metropolitan London to the 1875 Public Health Act, a comprehensive piece of legislation that consolidated and integrated the dozens of uncoordinated sanitary acts of the previous three decades. It touched housing, ventilation, sewage drainage, water supply, nuisances, dangerous trades, contagious diseases, and a host of other public issues in providing the backbone for what was the most efficient and extensive public health system in the world. The 1875 Act provided the basis of British sanitary administration until after World War I.

Ironies abound in the British public health movement, for the country that dismissed Chadwick for striving to create a central sanitary administration organized around compulsory legislation (stating what *must* be done rather than what might or should be done in matters touching the public health) actually permitted one to be assembled soon after his departure. Its principal architect was Simon, a man who began his public career believing that the dissemination of information and permissive legislation would lead local citizens and their elected officials to effect adequate sanitary reforms. His years in office gradually changed him and he became pragmatically if not ideologically a champion of a centrally administered and rigorous public health policy, which needed "the novel virtue of the imperative mood." Preventing disease was more humane and ultimately more efficient than attempting to cure it, and he came to view many of the medical and social payments made under

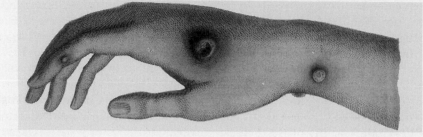

Figure 12. The lesions of cowpox on Sarah Nelmes's hand, as illustrated in Edward Jenner's An Inquiry into the Causes and Effects of the Variolae Vaccinae *(London: S. Low for the author, 1798), Plate 1, f. p. 32.*

the New Poor Law as a kind of arrears that could and should have been paid earlier in the form of decent wages, working conditions, and housing. He recognized, of course, that public health was as much a social as a medical issue, but he never wavered in his belief that those responsible for sanitary administration, such as the medical officers of health, should be medically trained and that medical research – in the community as well as in the hospital and laboratory – provided the underpinning for an evolving rational preventive program.

Although the details of the program that did evolve during Simon's tenure of office are beyond the scope of this volume, some indication of its complexity is provided by the case of smallpox, the one disease for which a specific prophylaxis existed in the mid-nineteenth century, *viz.* vaccination. Like smallpox inoculation (see Chapter 1), vaccination against the disease was an instance of folk knowledge turned into medical practice. Farmers in the west of England knew that a sporadic disease of cattle called cowpox could occasionally cause a mild, self-limited condition in human beings that seemed to protect against smallpox. The west-country surgeon-apothecary (i.e., general practitioner) Edward Jenner (1749–1823) put the possibility to experimental test in 1796. A pupil of John Hunter (who did not live to see his friend and correspondent achieve international fame), Jenner took some material from the hand of Sarah Nelmes, a milkmaid who had acquired cowpox from the udder of a diseased cow, and inoculated it into the arm of a young boy who had never had smallpox. The boy, James Phipps, developed a local scab and a mild fever. Six weeks later, Jenner challenged the boy with an inoculation of smallpox matter, in the manner of a Suttonian inoculation. No smallpox occurred, and Jenner called his procedure vaccination (from *vacca,* Latin for cow) to distinguish it from the older practice of inoculation, although the only difference was the nature of the matter being inoculated just under the skin.

By 1798, Jenner was able to publish in a slim volume the cases of twenty-three patients whom he believed had been protected from small-pox by vaccination. He was not a very clear writer, and his theoretical ideas about the nature of the animal disease that conferred immunity to smallpox were confused and badly presented. Nevertheless, within a few years, most people had become convinced of the superiority of vaccination over inoculation, and the British Parliament not only gen-erously rewarded Jenner financially, but set up in 1808 a National Vac-cine Establishment, publicly funded and empowered to investigate Jenner's claims and to provide free vaccination for smallpox. In fact, it conducted no research, but the Establishment, together with several philanthropic vaccine charities, did supply free vaccine lymph to vac-cinators throughout the country. Nevertheless, the simple availability of free vaccine did not prevent smallpox from remaining one of the leading half-dozen causes of death, nor did the more dangerous practice of inoculation die out completely. A serious epidemic in the late 1830s (between 1837 and 1840, the annual smallpox toll was 12,000) prompted a medical group (forerunner of the British Medical Association) to agitate for the prohibition of inoculation and the provision, by the State, of a universal and free vaccination service.

In 1841, Parliament responded with the first of a series of Bills that, by 1871, created what has been called a "Victorian National Health Service." The 1841 Act banned inoculation and made vaccination free and nonpauperizing (no means test was necessary to be eligible for it), even though it was actually administered through the Poor Law Boards. The system increased the frequency of vaccination in Britain and deaths from smallpox were almost halved in the following decade. However, the ratio of births to vaccinations varied widely from place to place and smallpox was still claiming some 5,000 victims a year in 1850. The Ep-idemiological Society of London took up the cause, investigated the system and called for compulsory infant vaccination with central med-ical supervision and registration. In 1853, just as Chadwick was being maneuvered out of office, Parliament agreed to this unprecedented infringement of individual liberty by making infant vaccination compulsory with penalties for failure to comply. The new legislation increased the level of vaccination, even without enforcement of the com-pulsion clause, but it alarmed various members of Parliament and fueled a nascent antivaccination campaign. When Simon became Chief Medical Officer to the new Board of Health, he became convinced that his office was a more appropriate authority than the Poor Law Boards to admin-ister the Act. Parliament deflected proposed legislation along these lines by appointing a Select Committee to examine the vaccination question, and, although this turned out to be another substitute for action, it gave Simon the excuse, in preparing his testimony, to examine smallpox and vaccination in its European context. This convinced him utterly that the value of vaccination far outweighed the minimal risks of reaction to the vaccine, secondary infection, or inadequate protection. It persuaded him that the State had a moral responsibility to control supplies of vaccine, to ensure that vaccinators were properly trained, and to require its citizens to participate in the program, which was for the common good.

Vaccination henceforth became one of the key issues in Simon's public health program, and during the 1860s he managed to secure funding for a systematic examination of the way the vaccination system operated, and to effect legislation aimed at training vaccinators, at improving the quality of the lymph, and at putting claws into the compulsion clause. Piecemeal legislation of the 1860s was consolidated and extended in 1871, passed as Britain (and Europe) were in the throes of the last smallpox pandemic. Deaths from smallpox in England in 1871 were as high (23,000) as from cholera during the 1832 epidemic, but to Simon and his colleagues the epidemic proved conclusively the value of vaccination and the necessity to extend the program. Most deaths occurred among the unprotected and they could point grimly to the Franco-Prussian War of the same year, where 300 German soldiers died of smallpox as compared to more than 20,000 French troops. Vaccination was compulsory among German soldiers, but not French, and, moreover, not among German civilians, where nearly 130,000 died in Prussia alone.

Compulsory vaccination was not without its problems, for many felt that the intrusion of the State into individual freedom of action was too high a price to pay for what could be viewed as a measure of dubious preventive worth. But the whole episode demonstrates how someone like Simon could gradually change his mind about the role of a strong, centralized health administration, once confronted with the complexities and possibilities of preventive medicine. His years in office were marked by notable administrative triumphs, and by his capacity to convince politicians of the value of medical science and epidemiology in understanding disease in the community. Despite individual successes, however, like vaccination, or the much better control of water-borne diseases like cholera and typhoid, the national deathrate hardly budged during the heroic years of the British public health movement. It was about 23 per thousand when Chadwick took office in 1846, about 21 per thousand when Simon left in 1876. These crude figures hide one important achievement, however: between 1850 and 1871, England's *urban* population rose from nine to fourteen million, whereas mean urban deathrates remained essentially constant (24.7 as compared with 24.8 per thousand). At least urban deterioration had been halted, and although England in 1871 was the most urbanized nation in Europe, only Sweden, Norway, Denmark, Ireland, and Greece had lower deathrates. London was the largest city in the world, but it had a significantly lower mortality than any other major European capital. How much would have been achieved along

Chadwickian sanitary engineering lines, and how much was added by Simon's cultivation of medical research and scientific epidemiology, are questions with no easy or entirely satisfactory answers, but are best understood within the context of medical science (see Chapters 4 and 5).

V. THE SANITARY ERA

During the middle third of the nineteenth century, investigators throughout Europe and North America affirmed the power of social statistics to elucidate the causes and correlates of disease within the community and to provide the factual basis for social action. "We are a statist – a dealer in facts," wrote Lemuel Shattuck in Massachusetts. "Statistics is the science of agreed upon and numerically expressed facts," insisted Louis René Villermé (1782–1863) in Paris. We are today more suspicious of claims that "facts" can be quite so unproblematical, or collected without reference to theories, hypotheses, or opinions. Facts are not the naked beings that early statisticians admired; they come arrayed in many garments.

Even at the time, agreement was not quite so universal as Villermé asserted. And if the facts themselves could be disputed, even more so could their interpretation or significance. The same facts could tell one inquirer that epidemic diseases were spread by person-to-person contact, and another that more general miasmatic influences were instrumental. Statistical facts could equally "prove" that laziness, indolence, and vice generated diseases, or that those diseases themselves engendered lethargy, fatalism, and disastrous social consequences. One reformer might believe that his facts illuminated a clear path of action, another that the path was in the opposite direction, or that standing still was the best course. There should therefore be no surprise to learn that conflict as much as conciliation marked this sanitary era, or that differing national, political, local, and individual circumstances dictated a multiplicity of reactions to the new statistical findings. No detailed examination of the circumstances surrounding the local or national implementation of sanitary ideas is possible here, but a brief examination of some ideological commitments of three key individuals will at least suggest the variety of religious, social, and scientific motivations behind sanitary reform in the period. Shattuck, Villermé, and Rudolf Virchow each worked in unique political and social circumstances and approached the burning question of differential deathrates – between urban and rural dwellers and between rich and poor – with his own special beliefs and solutions.

Like Chadwick, Lemuel Shattuck (1793–1859) came to sanitary reform from outside the medical profession. A sometime teacher, then bookseller and publisher by vocation, his avocations were statistical inquiry and sanitary improvement, activities he approached with a sense of religious mission. The factual certainty guaranteed by numerical methods made possible the discovery of the grand laws of human nature and human society, particularly the skeins that indissolubly linked the moral and the physical dimensions to man's being. A statistical orientation permeated his historical studies of Concord, Massachusetts (1835) and he called the meeting in 1839 that led to the foundation of the American Statistical Society. Improving the quality of the census data and the more systematic introduction of vital registration of births, marriages, and deaths were two areas of lasting concern to him. As a member of the Massachusetts Legislature he helped shape that state's Registration Act of 1842 and was an obvious member of the three-man commission appointed by the Governor in 1849 to conduct a Sanitary Survey of Massachusetts. The commission's 1850 *Report* was essentially Shattuck's. More wide-ranging than Chadwick's 1842 *Report* (whose value Shattuck acknowledged), this 1850 document proposed the establishment of a General Board of Health that would oversee a vast array of activities, touching home and workplace, public squares and bathhouses, cemeteries and lunatic asylums, vaccination and quarantine, smoke nuisances and adulterated foods, water supply and vital registration.

In the event, Massachusetts got a General Board of Health only in 1869, a decade after Shattuck's death. It would be easy to overestimate the immediate impact of the *Report*, despite its subsequent elevation to classic status. However, the attitudes reflected in Shattuck's work were typical of much mid-century sanitary writing, in their urgency and their optimism. Both were born of the certainty with which statistics endowed sanitary labors. The urgency was partially economic: preventable losses due to medical attendance on the sick poor, with consequent reduced productivity, losses to the workforce, and burial expenses for the dead. Shattuck quoted annual losses due to illness and premature death compiled for Britain of £20,000,000 and an economic mentality informed his *Report*. There was, however, also an urgency that was ultimately moral and religious. He divided the causes of disease into atmospheric, local, and personal. The first group included factors such as climate, seasonal variations, "malaria" and atmospheric "contagion" and was partially amenable to collective amelioration. Local causes were those found in neighborhoods or houses, including filth, damp, and animal effluvia. Personal causes were sometimes inherited, but more often acquired by bad habits, irregular living, and vice. Eradication of these latter two categories was possible, by slum clearance, clean water and moral, temperate behavior. The urgency – but also the optimism – was related to the failings of curative medicine, and to the power of preventive measures. As Shattuck announced, "We believe that the conditions of perfect health, either public or personal, are seldom or never attained, though attainable; ... and that measures for prevention will effect infinitely more, than remedies for the cure of disease."[6]

Despite Shattuck's lack of confidence in curative therapeutics, he did allow a substantial medical contribution to the preventive enterprise. His proposed Board of Health would have included two medical men, along with a lawyer, a chemist, a civil engineer, and two persons "of other professions or occupations." This diverse representation reflected the broad nature of prevention, with science, the law, and engineering not subservient to medicine. And, like Chadwick, Shattuck insisted that traditional medical education did little to prepare doctors, in experience and sometimes in sympathy, for prevention: "the constant direction of the [medical] faculties to the cure of actual disease, does not seem likely to leave much observation to devote to the study of its external causes." Until the medical profession took seriously the social and moral causes of disease within the community, and appreciated the statistical bedrock of facts needed to evaluate the community's collective health, disease prevention could not achieve its real potential.

Shattuck's ardent Protestantism and patriotism were reinforced by his own statistics, which showed that native-born Americans were on average healthier than immigrants and that in Boston, only about one-third of the Irish-Catholics reached a tenth birthday, whereas in affluent, Protestant Newton, Massachusetts, the figure was 78 percent. The interpretation might not have been so straightforward as Shattuck assumed, but similar statistics were easy enough to produce, as Shattuck and Chadwick's French counterpart, Louis René Villermé, discovered. His own inquiring eye turned often to prisoners, prostitutes, and the unruly proletariat (what the French called the "dangerous classes"), and his streams of papers, reports, and monographs established for France the same, familiar pattern of mortality correlates between those of varying social and economic status. He uncovered the appalling mortality in Parisian prisons (as many as one-quarter of the inmates in the Dépôt de Saint-Denis died each year between 1815 and 1818), showed dramatic variation in mortality of almost 100 percent between rich and poor *arrondissements* of Paris (fluctuations that could be pushed even higher if notoriously squalid streets and quarters were singled out for analysis), and calculated that the expectancy of life at birth among poor textile workers and their families was not much over a single year. Even those few who survived to age twenty could expect to be dead by the time they were thirty-five.

Villermé penned his medical thesis (1814) when Napoleon was in exile, just before Waterloo; his career subsequently spanned several fundamental changes in government, swings in the fortunes and influence of the Catholic Church (and of conservatism and liberalism in politics), and the gathering impact of industrialization in France. Although he lived until 1863, his work was virtually over by the time the Revolution of 1848 brought (however briefly) yet another experiment in government. Not notably religious, Villermé nevertheless brought to his studies a faith in the power of his social investigations to provide the factual bedrock on which to build a healthier and more prosperous nation. Science first, action second. He was, in fact, a bolder diagnostician than social prescriber: for all his trenchant criticism of the way in which low wages, insanitary housing, and the rigors of the factory system had produced a weakened and diseased working class, Villermé was true to his bourgeois origins and values, believing that men of good will would respond constructively to his findings. Philanthropic, benevolent entrepreneurs and a disciplined, prudent workforce epitomized his solution.

In the German-speaking lands, however, Rudolf Virchow (1821–1902) offered a more strident analysis of the health conditions associated with poverty and ignorance. Although actively concerned with the pathological investigations for which he is still remembered, the young Virchow was a thoroughly political creature. He was sent by the Prussian authorities in February 1848 to investigate a typhus epidemic in Upper Silesia. There had been serious food shortages during the winter and, not surprisingly, the disease had been more prevalent among the repressed Polish-speaking minority of the region. Virchow had read his Chadwick and his Villermé, so he would have been expecting associations between poverty and premature death. His report on the epidemic emphasized not just those (by 1848) commonplace liberal findings, but the much more politically sensitive one of the association between disease and social, religious, and political repression. His proposed solutions were not the obvious ones of more medical aid, or even more food to see the poor through the winter, but a fundamental, long-term social and political reorientation: democratic self-government, workers' cooperatives, progressive taxation, and individual freedom. The Prussian authorities were not too impressed at having responsibility for the epidemic laid on their plates.

Back in Berlin (the Prussian capital) in March 1848, Virchow was in time for the revolution, helping to build the barricades and caught up, for over a year, in the hopes and dreams of the revolutions of '48 that swept Europe. One outlet for his political energies was *Die medizinische Reform*, a weekly journal he coedited from July 1848 to June 1849. This journal gave him the opportunity to pen some of his most stirring rhetoric, claiming medicine as the queen of the social sciences ("medicine is a social science and politics nothing but medicine on a grand scale") and arguing that epidemic diseases always represent symptoms of social disturbance and that improvement of social conditions offered the quickest, most effective, and humane way of controlling disease such as tuberculosis, typhus, and cholera.

In the short run, the revolutions of 1848 did little to change the political and socioeconomic structures of European countries. The authorities pressured Virchow to leave Berlin in the early 1850s for the political backwater of Würzburg, and though he was to return to Berlin a decade later – and to play an important role in that city's public health program – his years in Würzburg were devoted primarily to medical research. By the late 1860s, when he was asked to oversee the overhauling of the Berlin sewage system, ideas of disease specificity and bacteriology were making themselves more explicitly felt, and he could draw on the experiences of those involved in the public health activities of other European cities.

Nevertheless, there can be no sharp demarcation between the sanitary era and the more technologically and conceptually sophisticated period that succeeded it. But the sanitarians had established a platform on which to build. With inspection, survey, and statistics, they had demonstrated the extent to which urban, industrial society created its own special health problems and had grappled with the tensions between the individualistic, laissez-faire ideology of early industrialization and the more communal issues of premature death and debility, the economic and human costs of their age.

4

Medicine in the laboratory

I consider hospitals only as the entrance to scientific medicine; they are the first field of observation which a physician enters; but the true sanctuary of medical science is a laboratory; only thus can he seek explanations of life in the normal and pathological states by means of experimental analysis.

Claude Bernard (1813–78), *An Introduction to the Study of Experimental Medicine* (1865; Eng. ed., 1957), p. 146

BY the middle of the nineteenth century, both the hospital and the community were claiming the energies of doctors and social investigators interested in understanding, diagnosing, treating, and preventing disease. Hospital and community were not mutually exclusive poles, for many public health activists (Southwood Smith, Simon, and Virchow, for instance) also had hospital appointments, and the quantitative mentality permeated the activities of many in both sites. There was, however, yet another location where work of importance for the medical enterprise could take place: the laboratory. By 1850, laboratories were just beginning to make an impact on medical education, although their direct relevance for medical practice was less clear.

Laboratories themselves were not new to the century. The word is derived from the same Latin root from which we get "labor": a laboratory is the place where one works. "Laboratory" was in English usage at least by the beginning of the seventeenth century, and a contemporary cognate word – "elaboratory" – points to an earlier existence of special rooms where one elaborated substances, that is, tried to produce through labor a finished product, especially gold from baser metals. Early laboratories were thus usually alchemical ones, but by the Enlightenment both the word and the place it described had become familiar, and not just for the study of chemistry but for investigating other dimensions of the natural world.

If laboratories were not new, neither was what Claude Bernard was to call experimental medicine. There was an actively experimental tradition in medicine going back at least to the Alexandrians of the third century B.C. and including such luminaries as Galen, William Harvey,

92

and John Hunter. It is easy to find many instances of animal investigation and of human and auto-experimentation in earlier generations aimed at elucidating physiological, pathological, or therapeutic questions. Experimental inquiry in medicine was hardly a unique product of the nineteenth century. Nor was the legitimate place of science in medicine problematical for many doctors who had worked long before Laennec or Simon were born. Medical science and medical knowledge had been affected by the Scientific Revolution of the sixteenth and seventeenth centuries, the general cry being more science, rather than less, for and in medicine. Furthermore, the practitioners of hospital medicine or the advocates of preventive medicine would never have dissociated themselves from science, with its resonances of objectivity, knowledge, and control. Few doctors since the early modern period would have embraced nonscience or would have rested claims to diagnostic acumen or therapeutic efficacy on explicitly unscientific grounds, or if they had, they would almost certainly have been branded as quacks. Notions of what constituted good science could, and did, vary, but the alliance between science (however perceived) and medicine was no nineteenth-century invention. Why, then, did certain mid-nineteenth-century practitioners of animal chemistry, or microscopy, or physiology, feel called upon to justify their activities, and why was physiology once called the "romance of medicine"?

Part of the answer is suggested by the word "romance": the correlations of pathology or social statistics seemed to many to be solidly scientific in ways that earlier explanations of function or disease causation were not. The old medical systems based on mechanical principles (iatromathematics or iatrophysics) or chemistry (iatrochemistry) symbolized the extent to which a putative scientific context within medicine had given rein to wide-ranging speculation, and nineteenth-century advocates of physiology or chemistry were conscious of this. They were conscious too, of a potential public distrust or even fear of too much fondness for science among those entrusted with their health, and with access to their bodies. William Harvey's complaint that his medical practice "fell off mightily" after he published *De motu cordis* (1628) may have been exaggerated, but, nearer to home, doctors in the 1830s would have been aware of public loathing of anatomical dissection, of the poor's fear of hospitals as places where they might be experimented upon (or treatment withheld in the interests of following the "natural history" of the disease), or of the assumption that animal vivisections engendered a callous attitude toward human suffering and so disqualified those who perpetrated ("practiced" being too weak a word) them from the personal characteristics necessary for the humane doctor. Humane or not, most doctors throughout the country were concerned primarily with earning a living – with the business of medicine – and so were caught between the demands of a professional identity that was increasingly allied to science, and the pressing realities of daily practice. This and the following chapters will examine aspects of this phenomenon. Here we shall be concerned with the broad framework within which medical science developed in Germany, France, Britain, and the United States.

I. THE PROFESSION OF SCIENCE AND THE PROFESSION OF MEDICINE

In Samuel Johnson's great *Dictionary of the English Language* (1755), a profession was defined as "calling; vocation; known employment." Vocation in turn could have the dual meaning of "calling by the will of God," or "trade; employment." In more recent times, the word profession has acquired additional connotations, though the definition of "known employment" would have served to identify medical practitioners of Johnson's day as members of a "profession," fragmented though it might have been.

By contrast, the pursuit of science would until sometime in the nineteenth century be qualified as a profession only in the inspirational aspect of Johnson's definition. Many who studied nature in earlier times professed to find inspiration and religious satisfaction therein, but most would have got their daily bread in other ways; as doctors, clergymen, teachers, or men of independent means. Within medical science, three of the most energetic experimentalists of the eighteenth century were Lazzaro Spallanzani, Albrecht von Haller, and John Hunter. The first was a clergyman, the second a university professor turned local civil servant, the third a practicing surgeon. They were never called "scientists," since that word was not coined by William Whewell until 1833 (on the analogy with "artist"). The suffix -ist now commonly denotes practitioners of many branches of science: chemist, physicist, physiologist, bacteriologist, and so forth.

Until the nineteenth century, then, few people earned a living from science. There were some exceptions, of course: members of the French Academy of Sciences in the eighteenth century were paid and thereby became civil servants, and professors in science subjects in universities often did research as well as teaching. The exceptions do not disprove the rule that the pursuit of science in earlier times was an amateur activity.

This changed during the nineteenth century, and those modest beginnings of "big science" had important implications for medical education, medical knowledge, and (eventually) medical practice. The growth of science within medicine was related to the more general phenomena of scientific development, though only those medical dimensions can be described here. The medical scientist can be defined as someone who earns at least part of his living from "doing" science; who is engaged in experimental (or sometimes only observational) work; who generally spends part of his time teaching the knowledge he and fellow scientists have discovered; who belongs to specialist societies of people with similar interests (or if they do not exist would like to create them); who usually works in a laboratory and uses scientific equipment; and who (increasingly) publishes in specialist journals papers that are often the result of collaborative research.

The emergence of groups of individuals who fulfilled these criteria occurred at different times in different countries. Most historians agree that the modern scientist first came into being in the German-speaking lands, before a unified Germany was created under Bismarck.

II. MEDICAL SCIENCE IN GERMANY

"There is no people which has given so much thought and pains to the development of its university system as the Germans have done – none which has profited so much by the services universities render – none where they play so large a part in the national life."[1] So wrote a British observer in 1885, at a time when the flow of foreign students to German universities was ample testimony to their reputations abroad. From little more than glorified high schools a century or so earlier, the universities in Germany – and above all their specialist *institutes* – had become prestigious centers of research in virtually all areas of scholarly inquiry.

The German word for science is *Wissenschaft* but it carries far broader connotations than its English equivalent. *Wissenschaft* means systematic knowledge and there was a science of history, or philology, or literature just as much as a science of chemistry, physics, or biology. To be sure, these latter were often distinguished as *Naturwissenschaften* (natural sciences), but all *systematic* inquiry marched under the common banner of *Wissenschaft*.

Even with the outpouring of resources into the universities, many of them remained poor and certainly could not expect to excel in all subjects. This mattered less because students were free to move easily from one university to another, absorbing what they wanted from each. This freedom of movement (*Lernfreiheit* – freedom to learn) was balanced by the freedom of their instructors to teach as they saw fit: *Lehrfreiheit* (freedom to teach). And what they taught was increasingly the methods and fruits of research, within institutes devoted to particular subjects. Although attached to the universities, these institutes were more autonomous and powerful than the departments of American or British universities: the professorial head of an institute could thus be a lord within his own kingdom and competition between the universities encouraged an entrepreneurial spirit among ambitious academic staff.

For many in the medical profession abroad, perhaps the first inkling of what German science was to come to mean would have been provided by Justus von Liebig's Institute of Chemistry at the University of Giessen. Liebig's career and those of several others accent some of the main features of the German system in operation.

Liebig (1803–73) developed an early interest in chemistry that led to a brief apprenticeship to an apothecary and then to the universities in Bonn and Erlangen, to study the subject. German chemical education in the 1820s lagged behind French, and Liebig thus spent two years in Paris, where he obtained instruction and laboratory experience from leading chemists, especially Gay-Lussac. In 1824 (at age twenty-one) he became professor of chemistry at the University of Giessen, where his Institute (in recently evacuated military barracks) began to attract students who valued the practical training in the newer methods of qualitative analysis. Sometimes acrimonious debates about chemical notation and some experimental results during the late 1820s and 30s, especially with French chemists, carried nationalistic overtones that were to continue to dog the gospel of internationalism in science, but Liebig was fêted as a kind of conquering hero when he attended the meetings of the British Association for the Advancement of Science in 1837. He had already trained several British students and another of his protégés, the German A. W. Hofmann (1818–92), was to spend many years at the Royal College of Chemistry in London.

Success bred success. Liebig's laboratories at Giessen were enlarged to accommodate more students and more research facilities, although the University of Munich lured him away in 1852 by building an even bigger Chemical Institute to his own specifications. By then his primary interests had already shifted through inorganic and organic chemistry to agricultural and what was called animal chemistry. Although Liebig came to recognize that the chemistry of living bodies was exceedingly complicated, his early notion was that an animal could be treated as a kind of black box. By measuring what went in (food, water, oxygen) and what came out in excretions and exhalations (urea, various salts and acids, water, carbon dioxide), much could be inferred about the chemical processes inside the animal (or human) organism. Respiration brought oxygen, which combined with starches to liberate energy, carbon dioxide, and water. Nitrogenous substances were digested and absorbed into muscle and other tissues; when their breakdown occurred, the urinary urea was the end product, along with phosphates and other simpler chemical by-products. Ultimately, he postulated, plants are the source of complex organic substances, as they use sunlight to provide energy to synthesize compounds out of simple nitrogenous compounds and carbon dioxide (releasing oxygen in the process). This was neatly symmetrical and, although it embodied some profound insights about the interrelationships between plants and animals, criticism from others and further investigations by Liebig and his colleagues convinced him that physiology and chemistry would need to be joined before the whole complexity of living processes could be revealed.

Nevertheless, the methods and concepts that Liebig advocated encouraged many to begin chemical analyses of animal tissues such as muscle or liver, or of fluids such as blood, sweat, tears, urine, and bile, and to measure the relationship between food and oxygen consumption and energy production in living organisms: in short, to investigate nutrition, metabolism, and what eventually was called biochemistry.

Several aspects of Liebig's career and scientific aspirations are worth noting: First, he worked in the laboratories of successive institutes, located within universities but with a good deal of autonomy and, after he went to Munich, built to his own specifications. He insisted on the latest scientific equipment and recognized the extent to which many scientific problems could be solved only through ever more sophisticated experimental design. Second, he trained many students in research methods and set them to work on problems related to his own broad concerns. Much of their work was reported in papers in the specialist journal that he edited for many years, the *Annalen der Pharmacie und Chemie*. In short, he created a research school in chemistry with outreaches in medicine, pharmacy, agriculture, and industry. Third, he stressed the importance of physical and chemical methods in understanding biological processes and, although he was no crude materialist, his research program had the reductionist aim of applying the laws and methods of the physical sciences to living organisms. As early as 1828 his lifelong friend Friedrich Wöhler (1800–1882) (from 1836 professor of chemistry at Göttingen) had synthesized the organic substance urea from inorganic substrates: proof that no absolute barrier separated "vital" compounds found in living animals from the ordinary chemicals of the laboratory.

Scientific materialists in mid-nineteenth-century Germany saw themselves as reacting against the speculative, idealistic and Romantic philosophy (*Naturphilosophie*) that, through the works of men like Goethe, Schelling, and Oken, had dominated German culture in the Napoleonic period and just after. Liebig was a sober experimentalist who seems to have been little touched by Romantic concerns. Johannes Müller (1800–58) never completely turned his back on the intellectual currents of his youth, although he and his students also cultivated a spirit of experimentation within medical science. Müller spent most of his academic career at the University of Berlin, as professor of anatomy and physiology. The University of Berlin was one of the newer ones, but its foundation in 1810 was a signal event in the history of higher education and research in the German-speaking lands and its rise to prominence mirrored that of Prussia and its capital, Berlin.

The development of physiology as an independent, experimental discipline was one of the main features of nineteenth-century medical science, and Müller's occupancy of a joint chair of anatomy and physiology was further symbolic evidence of the transitional character of his career and work. He was a gifted, sometimes brilliant, animal experimentalist whose neurophysiological research helped elucidate the reflex activities of the neuromuscular system and whose massive *Handbook of Physiology* (2 vols., 1833–40) was fundamental in the development of the discipline, despite its mixture of anatomy and physiology, its vitalism, and its long section on the soul. In later life he became ambivalent about the limits and justification of experiments on living animals, turning his attention to the observational sciences of morphology, embryology, and paleontology. Subject to serious bouts of depression (his death may have been suicide), he was nevertheless an inspiring teacher whose students – Theodor Schwann, Hermann von Helmholtz, Emil du Bois-Reymond, Ernst Brücke, Jacob Henle, Rudolf Virchow – became leaders in mid-century scientific and medical research.

Three of those students, Helmholtz, du Bois-Reymond, and Brücke, joined with Carl Ludwig in 1847 to publish a kind of manifesto announcing that the aim of physiology was to explain all vital phenomena through the laws of physics and chemistry. Before he turned to physics in the 1870s, Helmholtz devoted himself at a new physiological institute in Heidelberg to a series of physiological problems, such as the measurement of the production of animal heat and the velocity of nerve conduction, and the investigation of the physics of sight and hearing. His invention of the ophthalmoscope aided his work on vision. Ludwig – whose Institute of Physiology at Leipzig became an international training ground for experimental physiologists – experimented and directed research on a number of physiological problems, notably the elaboration of urine by the kidneys. When, on Müller's death, the chair of anatomy and physiology was divided, du Bois-Reymond became professor of physiology in Berlin, where he was eventually able to preside over a purpose-built physiology institute. His preoccupation was electrophysiology. Brücke went to Vienna, where his interests spanned many areas of physiological chemistry, histology, and neuromuscular physiology.

The thrust of this experimental physiology was the attempt, in Ludwig's words, to understand functions "from the elementary conditions inherent in the organism itself." It required the use of animals (made much easier after the introduction of anesthetics in the 1840s) but, equally characteristically, German physiologists developed many new instruments to record and analyze data. In 1847, Ludwig introduced the

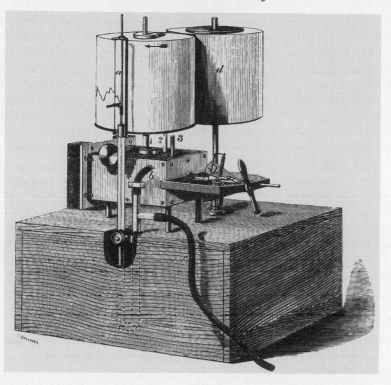

Figure 13. The kymograph, as it had been modified by the 1870s. The rotating drum (a in figure) allowed for the continuous recording of various physiological actions, such as arterial or venous pressure, respiration, and muscle contractions. J. Burdon-Sanderson, ed., Handbook for the Physiological Laboratory, *2 vols. (London: J. and A. Churchill, 1873), Vol. 2, Plate lxxiv, Fig. 202.*

recording device that more than any other can be identified with nine-teenth-century physiology: the kymograph. It allowed for the graphic recording of a variety of physiological phenomena, such as blood pressure fluctuations or muscle contractions. Ludwig also devised an instrument for measuring blood flow, and Helmholtz and Brücke used a good deal of newly developed equipment in their own researches. This increasing reliance on technology is another hallmark of modern science, and the machinery of research not only increased its cost, but it also began to make the private laboratory a thing of the past.

Amid the panoply of equipment that began to surround the medical scientist, one rather more familiar piece should not be forgotten: the microscope. Although these instruments had been around since the seventeenth century, technical improvements from the late 1820s corrected two sources of distortion and brought the microscope from the periphery to the center of medical and biological research. Histology always served as a kind of halfway house between anatomy and physiology (even after these latter two disciplines were administratively separate, histology was sometimes taught by anatomists, sometimes by physiologists), and in the long run, the microscope was Müller's principal scientific tool. "Learn to see microscopically," Virchow liked to say, crystallizing the message that Müller drilled into all his pupils. Virchow's *Cellular Pathology* (1858) did for the cell what Morgagni's *Seats and Causes of Disease* (1761) had done for the organ, or Bichat's *Treatise on the Membranes* (1800) had for the tissues: established a new, essential unit for thinking about function and disease.

Virchow's microscopical work in the 1840s and 50s had much broader biological significance: *Omnis cellula e cellula* (All cells from cells) was his ringing motto, a phrase extending the cellular theory that another Müller pupil, Theodor Schwann (1810–82), had enunciated in 1839. Schwann's model for cell formation was a reductionist one: cells, he believed, were the fundamental units of zoological and botanical activity. They consisted of a nucleus and an outer membrane and could be formed – in a process he explicitly likened to a crystal growing within a solution – out of an amorphous organic matrix that Schwann called the blastema. By contrast, the Virchovian cell was always the product of cell division, and his theory had particular relevance for crucial biological events like the fertilization of the egg, or pathophysiological ones like the origin of the pus cells of inflammation.

As we have seen, Virchow was no narrow specialist but a man whose interests encompassed politics, public health, anthropology, and archeology. Nevertheless, his academic career mirrored much of the university system: the first chair in pathological anatomy was established for him in 1849 in Würzburg, and in 1856 he returned to Berlin to become director of the newly created Pathological Institute. He trained many of the next generation of pathologists and co-founded and edited the leading journal in the field, the *Archiv für pathologische Anatomie und Physiologie, und für die klinische Medizin* (now known as *Virchow's Archiv*). One of Virchow's colleagues at Würzburg, Albert von Kölliker (another student of Müller's) was active in the study of normal histology and his own *Handbook of the Tissues of Man* (1st edition, 1852) has been described as the first textbook of histology. It went through numerous German editions and was translated into the major European languages. What Virchow had done for pathology, von Kölliker did for histology: he placed the cell at the center. As further evidence of increasing specialization within medical science, von Kölliker gave up his joint chair in physiology and comparative anatomy in 1864 to concentrate his energy on microscopical work (in a Microscopical Institute), including embryological and more general zoological problems.

During the middle third of the century, the microscope transformed the foundations of biology, and through it, of medicine. The establishment of cell theory and its application to embryology, histology, pathology, and physiology were done neither overnight nor without a great deal of controversy and debate. Nor was the mere appearance of microscopes capable of magnifying without chromatic or spherical aberration enough. For one thing, cutting, preparing, and staining tissues generated their own technical and conceptual debates. For another, as Virchow's epigram makes clear, seeing microscopically was something that had to be learned, and there was much disagreement about what was seen, to say nothing of the significance of the images the microscope revealed.

Traditionally, English optical makers had led the world, but by the middle of the nineteenth century, German microscopists would have used German microscopes made by companies such as Zeiss and Leitz, and with the standardization and mechanization of production, prices came down, especially in the simple microscope aimed at the student market.

If microscopes were ubiquitous in laboratories, they could occasionally be spotted in consulting rooms as well, especially after the rise of germ theory reinforced the medical importance of the microscopical world. Certainly Robert Koch's career demonstrates how, by the 1880s, fame and fortune could be achieved by the successful medical scientist.

Koch (1843–1910) was a generation younger than Virchow or von Kölliker, and can in fact be called a second-generation pupil of Müller, since it was Jacob Henle (then at Göttingen) who played a key role in Koch's early enthusiasm for medical research. Koch published a scientific paper while he was still a medical student and, following graduation, he spent some months in Berlin, attending Virchow's course in pathology.

He was thus well steeped in the ideology and techniques of the new scientific medicine, though his real career as a scientist did not begin until he had spent about ten years in small-town medical practice. It was as a solitary, country general practitioner that Koch worked out, over about four years, the life cycle and mode of infection of the anthrax bacillus, a common disease of farm animals that occasionally can produce disease in human beings. In 1876 he presented his findings and preparations to Ferdinand Cohn, director of the Botanical Institute of the University of Breslau. The publication of his paper in Cohn's journal *Beiträge zur Biologie der Pflanzen* the following year consolidated his reputation, and after a nibble at work in Breslau, he went to Berlin in 1880 as a salaried scientist in the Imperial Department of Health. His identification of the tubercle bacillus followed in 1882, and he isolated the bacillus of cholera in early 1884, in India. Along the way he introduced numerous technical improvements into bacteriology, and, though his career after the mid-1880s was curiously undistinguished, it goes almost without saying that money was found to build an institute for him: indeed he presided over four, increasingly grand ones.

Details of Koch's career raise issues to be considered in later chapters, but its broad features fit into the pattern of the successful German medical scientists, in its commitment to research (his practice was given up after he moved to Berlin), its technical sophistication, its laboratory and institute orientation, and the number of students who came after.

Institutes with their equipment, furnishings, and salaries did not drop out of the sky, and the story of each new chair or institute would involve negotiations between some university advocate and local or provincial government ministers, or industrial or private philanthropists. Although the creation of new institutes often seemed to have necessitated particular, gifted individuals, their continued viability required a steady stream of students, and in the medical sciences, even those destined for research careers generally came via medical faculties. Much of the routine teaching fell on the shoulders of the *Privatdozenten*, a post that required its holder to present the results of significant research, but that gave him no guaranteed salary, only the right to teach. The *Privatdozent* was a kind of walking embodiment of the values that made the German system tick: proving research capacity before being granted the right to teach, but then having to earn a living by being able to attract enough students to rake in a decent income. For many on the academic ladder, becoming a *Privatdozent* was merely the first step toward becoming a professor, and the director of an institute; for others, especially Jews and those from the margins of the German sphere of influence, it could be the height of their realistic aspirations. For foreign students in particular, the system could be a godsend, for it was the *Privatdozenten* who generally taught them, often in the students' own language.

Students – thousands of them – made the trek to the German universities. They came from all over Europe, including Britain, and from North America as well. In the 1830s, the migration had been a trickle: chemists to Liebig in Giessen, or budding microscopists to Müller in Berlin. Half a century later, it was common for scientifically oriented medical students to want to round off their education by spending some time in the German-speaking universities. For many, probably most, the demands of medical practice when they returned home would have swamped any fleeting ambition to become an English Virchow, or an American Koch. But a remarkably high percentage of the leaders of the new scientific medicine in Britain, Italy, the Scandinavian or Low countries, or the United States, had gone to Germany. Paris might also have been included on the study circuit, although the French themselves were often ambivalent about all things German, even its science, especially after the humiliation of military defeat in the Franco-Prussian war of 1870–1.

III. MEDICAL SCIENCE IN FRANCE

In the 1820s and 30s, a group of British *savants*, led by Charles Babbage, attempted to reform the scientific establishment in Britain. They argued that science in their country was on the decline, that election to scientific societies such as the Royal Society was on social rather than scientific grounds, that neither government nor society valued the results of scientific inquiry, and that neither educational nor employment opportunities in science were adequate. Had Babbage been writing two decades later, he would undoubtedly have looked to Germany to provide him with his foil of a country that valued its scientists. In 1830, though, when he published his *Reflections on the Decline of Science in England*, France still seemed to provide the most obvious model of enlightened science policy. During the Napoleonic period, educational and institutional reforms had resulted in additional academic posts (especially in the new schools of science, engineering, and mining) and figures like Laplace in the physical sciences, and Cuvier in the biological ones had towered over the international scientific scene.

Even as Babbage was writing, however, there were signs that the French star was on the wane. Laplace died in 1827, Cuvier in 1832, and in 1827 Alexander von Humboldt (1769–1859), the German naturalist and traveler, symbolically moved from Paris to Berlin.

The reputation of French hospital medicine had not relied on laboratory-based inquiries, although foreign medical students sometimes went for instruction in chemistry or microscopy as well as experience in the wards and morgues of the Paris hospitals. The career of François Magendie (1783–1855) illustrates aspects of the relationship between science and medicine in the period. He was a product of the medical school, absorbing a distrust of theorizing and system-building and insisting always that well-established facts were all that interested him. Increasingly, these facts were physiological ones gained by animal experimentation. There were other French experimental physiologists in his generation – Flourens and Longet, for instance – but both at home and abroad, Magendie symbolized physiology's struggle to achieve status as an independent discipline, separate from anatomy. He founded in 1821 the *Journal de Physiologie Expérimentale*, to the second volume of which he added the words *et Pathologie*.

Nevertheless, he hardly enjoyed the institutional support that German academics were beginning to achieve. Much of his early teaching was extramural and he was forced to seek a clinical appointment; even that was not officially confirmed until 1826. He used his hospital post to make therapeutic investigations and five years later obtained the chair of medicine at the Collège de France. His optional lectures there expounded the experimental method and discussed the physical phenomena of life as revealed through experimental physiology and pathology. In that sense, he started a tradition that his protégé Claude Bernard (1813–78) continued when he succeeded to the chair after Magendie's death in 1855.

Magendie's career thus encompassed clinical practice and therapeutics as well as experimental work. Although Bernard also came up through the hospital system, working for a year as an intern, he was never happy with the idea of becoming a medical practitioner. In fact, he had turned to medicine out of practical necessity, his youthful dreams of fame as a playwright and literary man coming to naught. Magendie's example showed him an alternative in a life of science. Three years as Magendie's demonstrator allowed him to present his thesis on the chemistry of digestion. However, he failed to pass the examination for a teaching post in the Faculty of Medicine and his marriage – unhappy though it proved – at least gave him a financial respite through his wife's dowry. In 1847 he became Magendie's deputy at the Collège de France and from then on success followed success, including chairs at the Sorbonne and the Museum of Natural History, membership in the academies of science and medicine, a seat in the Senate and the presidency of the French Academy. The last would have been particularly pleasing to Bernard, whose elegant style and clarity of thought elevated this practicing scientist into a man of letters, responsible, with his fellow academicians, for the purity of the French language.

This highly visible career was also extremely French in its trajectory. Unlike his German colleagues, Bernard never headed an institute, and, although he eventually was able to command adequate laboratory facilities, his early years were spent in sparsely equipped and sometimes even privately funded space. Nor was his research ever dependent on much sophisticated laboratory apparatus. Rather, his genius lay in his superb operative techniques, his capacity to keep experimental animals alive through the follow-up and interpretive parts of his investigations, and the elegant simplicity of his experimental designs. His major findings – the role of the liver in synthesizing glycogen and in keeping blood glucose levels within a defined range; the digestive functions of the pancreas; the vasodilator nerves; the site of action of poisons such as carbon monoxide and curare – were characteristically based on simple but compelling experimental evidence.

Bernard had many pupils but never founded a research school in the Germanic sense. Most of his papers and books were published by himself and throughout his career many of those who attended his lectures and demonstrations were foreigners. Unlike Müller, Kölliker, or Ludwig, he never published a textbook; rather, his lectures and ten volumes of published *Leçons* were devoted to science in the making rather than science already made. He was always something of a loner, an individualist who nevertheless recognized the collaborative nature of science: "Art is myself, science is ourselves," he quoted approvingly in his most famous book, *An Introduction to the Study of Experimental Medicine* (1865).[2] More than any other work, this one crystallized the essence and the hopes of science in, and for, clinical medicine.

Bernard drafted this work in the early 1860s, when the first of a series of serious illnesses curtailed his laboratory activities and encouraged him to reflect on and evaluate his own past laboratory life. Always interested in philosophy, he turned the *Introduction* into a general statement of the experimental method as applied to the biomedical sciences: it is in fact one of the most systematic expositions of a philosophy of science ever produced by a practicing scientist. It was also meant to sound a death knell for the exclusively bedside orientation of the hospital medicine in which he had been originally trained.

Hospital medicine had two major limitations, Bernard maintained. As an observational science, it was purely passive, akin to natural history and relying too much on circumstance for the material of its observations. Thus, the repeated correlation of lesions and symptoms had built up good pictures of diseases, for example, the invariable presence of tubercles in phthisis. Such an exercise, valuable as it might be, did not go far enough. These passive observations were limited in a second way: they could not hope to elucidate the causes of the lesions, or the precise conditions under which they were produced. For this, the active observation of the experimentalist was required. At the sickbed, there were too many variables, too many idiosyncrasies to permit rigorous understanding, and the pathological lesion itself was the endstage of disease, formed when all too often effective therapy was unavailable. Only by understanding the dynamics of disease – its pathophysiology – could rational therapeutics be uncovered. This could be achieved only in the laboratory, and only through the use of laboratory animals, in a setting where the general conditions of the animal could be kept constant and the particular feature under scrutiny be minutely examined. Thus, one could not understand disease without understanding the altered functions that had produced the disease. No pathology without physiology, and no scientific therapeutics without both. This triad – physiology, pathology, pharmacology – constituted for him the pillars of experimental medicine, and each was a laboratory science.

Bernard used his own work to illustrate the complex interaction but essential integrity of these three pillars: how, for instance, diabetes could be more comprehensively grasped as a disease after his elucidation of the glycogenetic functions of the liver; or how the pharmacological action of curare (admittedly, a poison rather than a common mainstay of the pharmacopoeia) could be pinpointed to the neuromuscular junction. He was under no illusions that a medical millennium was at hand: the laboratory was just beginning to make its presence felt in medicine.

Bernard was of course well aware of contemporary research in Germany, and in his early days he was a founder-member of an association – the Société de Biologie – whose members looked to Germany for scientific inspiration. This changed in his later years and he discounted the crude reductionism implicit in the research programs of men such as Lüdwig and Brücke. The life sciences were autonomous and would never be mere appendages of physics and chemistry. Nevertheless, the reign of law governed the functions of organisms as surely as the revolution of the earth around the sun. The apparent capriciousness or irregularity of living beings is due to their complexity, not to indeterminacy. Given similar boundary conditions, similar events will occur. Doctors at the bedside have little control over these boundary conditions; the physiologist in the laboratory has much more when operating on or observing his experimental animal. Without the principle of determinism, there can be no science.

Consequently, when the unexpected happens, there must be a reason. Bernard instanced several times in his own career when, by following up unexpected results, important new lines of inquiry were revealed. Further, because determinacy extends to the living world, there can be no uncaused effects and a single instance is always significant. Bernard had little time for statistics in physiology, or for the desire to express everything numerically. Precision was what counted and the use of large series of cases in clinical medicine was a sign of weakness, not of strength: an attempt to counter the lack of control that inevitably accompanies the clinical situation.

Despite the ubiquity of the principle of determinism, animals and human beings are not simply automata, at the mercy of external forces. This is because higher organisms do not live merely in the surrounding environment. Rather, they actively create their own, more intimate environment, the *internal milieu*. Many physiological mechanisms were devoted to keeping within definite limits the salt, sugar, and oxygen concentrations of the blood and tissue fluids, and maintaining a constant body temperature in the face of a variable external one. It was through these mechanisms – called "homeostatic" by the Harvard physiologist W. B. Cannon in the 1920s – that higher organisms achieved a freedom that was nevertheless compatible with the more basic determinism of the universe.

By the time of his death in 1878, Bernard was easily the most famous physiologist in the world. He was given a national funeral, the first scientist to be deemed the equal of a military or political hero. Nevertheless, his fame was modest compared to that of his countryman, Louis Pasteur (1822–95), who was buried with full military honors. For every *Rue Bernard*, there must be at least ten streets called *Rue Pasteur*.

Like Bernard, Pasteur was a patriot who clung even more firmly to the French way of doing things after the humiliations of the Franco-Prussian war. Like him, too, Pasteur retained his roots in the French wine regions, returning each autumn for the harvest. Much of Pasteur's research and publication were done alone, although a devastating stroke in 1868 left him paralyzed down one side and literally forced him to use the hands and feet (but not the brains) of a series of assistants, of whom Emile Roux (1853–1938) was the most distinguished. Unlike Bernard, Pasteur had a happy home life, and Madame Pasteur often acted as his assistant during his early years. Both men prided themselves on the simplicity of their experiments: Pasteur was dubious about the value of many of Koch's technical innovations in bacteriology and Bernard always stressed that complicated experimental equipment increased the potential for error. Great experimenters "made great discoveries by means of simple instruments."

It is indicative of the increasing importance of science for medicine that this most famous of all nineteenth-century medical scientists was not even a doctor, but a chemistry and physics graduate of the Ecole Normale Supérieure, the principal science school in Paris. Even his interest in microorganisms was acquired while studying the optical activity of certain chemical components, especially the tartrates. The capacity of certain compounds to rotate bands of polarized light to either the left or the right had been known for a couple of decades before Pasteur turned his attention to the phenomenon in the late 1840s. This was the first of a series of puzzles that always seemed to lead him straight to microorganisms such as bacteria and yeast. For optical activity, Pasteur determined that such compounds were invariably synthesized by living organisms; if the same compound were made in the laboratory, it would be optically neutral.

Once his attention was focused on this world of the infinitely small, he never looked back. By the time he returned to Paris in 1857 (henceforth his base) after brief stints as professor of chemistry in Strasbourg and Lille, he devoted his research to microbiology: to the age-old question of spontaneous generation; to the nature of fermentation and the role of microorganisms in everyday phenomena like the souring of milk or the rotting of meat; to the manufacture of wine, beer, and vinegar; to the physiology of microorganisms and their place in the diseases of animals such as silkworms, chickens, cattle, pigs, and, finally, human beings; to the nature of infection and immunity; and to the prevention and treatment of infectious diseases.

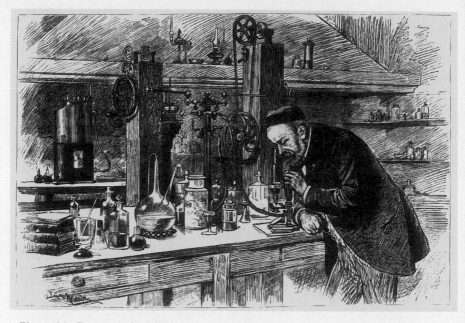

Figure 14. Pasteur in his laboratory, in the familiar pose of looking down his microscope.
The Graphic, *21 Nov. 1885, p. 561.*

In retrospect, at least, there were both a logic and a satisfying unity
to his research career, even if the road from crystals of tartaric acid to
the treatment of rabies could hardly have been forecast in the 1850s.
Nor could the fact that Pasteur ended his life as the Director of that most
Germanic of establishments, a research institute. Nevertheless, despite
its fame or the veneration in which its director was held, the Institut
Pasteur was not endowed on the same lavish scale as Koch's Institute
in Berlin; neither was it the creation of the state or the universities. It
depended on public donations and income from the sale of vaccines to
balance its budget. And Pasteur himself had spent the first twenty years
of his academic career with heavy administrative duties in addition to
his teaching and research responsibilities. No wonder that he looked
enviously at German colleagues and bitterly attributed the French military defeats of 1870 to France's failure to invest sufficiently in science
and technology. He would have been hesitant to separate the two, however: "There are no such things as pure and applied science – there are
only science, and the application of science," he liked to say.[3] Not for
Pasteur some abstract notion of *Wissenschaft*.

His research seemed to bear out that belief, for, despite the theoretical
importance of his ideas, and above all, his germ theory of disease, there
was always immediate practical value to be gained from his work. His

studies on fermentation and brewing benefited the producers of wine, beer, and vinegar; his investigations on the diseases of silkworms saved the French silk industry. Appropriately, for someone who came from science rather than medicine, the infectious diseases that first crystallized his germ theory were those of the silkworms, and this was followed by research on chicken cholera and swine erysipelas (unrelated to human cholera or erysipelas), and anthrax, for all of which he devised vaccines, a word he coined to honor Jenner. His crowning achievement, the rabies vaccine, was for a disease, like anthrax, common to animals and human beings, but its application to victims of dogbites had to be supervised by a medical man.

Later chapters will assess the impact of germ theory on disease concepts and medical practices. What the careers of Magendie, Bernard, and Pasteur point toward is the development, within a French context, of an experimental approach to medicine. This "science empire," as it has been called, was never so well endowed in France as in Germany, and was less entrenched in the medical schools than in the faculties of science. In the hands of someone like Jean-Martin Charcot (1825–93), the clinicopathological orientation remained strong. Charcot was one of the dominant figures in the Paris medical faculty, and, although he would never have considered himself as unscientific, his research axis revolved around the ward and deadhouse. By the late 1880s, experimental microbiology was firmly situated in the *Institut Pasteur* and most of the major French physiologists after Bernard, such as Etienne-Jules Marey (1830–1904) and Paul Bert (1833–86), pursued their careers outside the hospitals and medical schools.

IV. MEDICAL SCIENCE IN BRITAIN

In his *Introduction to the Study of Experimental Medicine,* Bernard referred to seven British figures. All but one were purely historical, like Harvey, Newton, or Bacon. The only contemporary reference was a passing mention to Charles Darwin. Although his comments on the contemporary German scene were not always complimentary, at least men like Müller and Virchow were noticed, as were a dozen or so of his fellow French scientists. British experimental medicine seemed to be beneath his gaze.

This is not to say that the values of science within medicine were not appreciated in Britain, nor that before 1865 the British contribution to the medical sciences had been negligible. Nevertheless, what could be called the vestiges of a career structure in science emerged later in Britain than in Germany or France, and science was more generally pursued on a part-time basis, sandwiched between the demands of clinical practice. Sometimes this was seen as the positive consequence of a productive and creative amateur tradition. At other times it was castigated as the result of three main problems: indifference by the state about the value of research; conservative social and religious values that emphasized natural theology and found vivisection cruel and scientifically worthless; and a series of educational institutions unworthy of a great nation. As T. H. Huxley remarked in the 1850s, doing research in Britain could produce lots of medals and a good many free dinners, but not the wherewithal to pay the cab fare home. The careers of several scientifically ambitious British medical men highlight these themes.

Not surprisingly, William Prout (1785–1850), Sir Charles Bell (1774–1842), and Marshall Hall (1790–1857) each attended the medical school in Edinburgh, though Bell, as a budding surgeon and anatomist, did not take a degree. An early interest in science had directed both Prout and Hall toward medical careers; Bell followed his older brother into surgery. Edinburgh University possessed by far the largest medical school in early nineteenth-century Britain; but London was a magnet for anyone wishing to make his mark in science or medicine. Bell settled there in 1804, Prout in 1812, and Hall in 1826. Each had his scientific aspirations fulfilled by election to Fellowship of the Royal Society. Bell had by far the most successful academic career, as a co-proprietor of the Great Windmill Street School of Anatomy, one of the founders of the Middlesex Hospital School of Medicine, and (briefly), professor of surgery at University College, the original part of what is now the University of London. Despite Prout's considerable Continental reputation, his "academic" career was purely of his own devising: he gave some successful private courses on animal chemistry in his own home, where he maintained his laboratory. Hall, too, did his physiological work at home; intensely ambitious, he applied unsuccessfully for several teaching posts and hospital consultancies, but had to content himself with a brief association with one of the less prestigious private medical schools. He used his researches on neurophysiology, especially the spinal reflexes, to set up himself as a kind of specialist in nervous diseases, particularly of women. Prout's chemical bent led him to gout and the disorders of digestion. Bell was a reasonable operative surgeon in the days before anesthesia and antisepsis.

Each of these men was overtly religious. Prout and Bell each contributed one of the Bridgewater Treatises, that early Victorian flowering of the natural theological tradition. Bell found ample proofs of God's existence and goodness in the design of the hand; Prout sought them in the more varied forms of chemistry, digestion, and (for good measure) the weather. Hall was raised as a Methodist, though his adult religious beliefs were more obscure. Each, too, upheld vitalistic principles in their scientific work. Prout attempted to synthesize urea ten years before its successful laboratory synthesis was hailed by some as the end of vitalism,

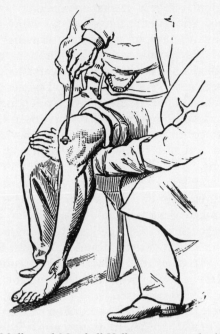

Figure 15. Johannes Müller and Marshall Hall were among the founders of the modern concept of the reflex arc – the integrated, functional unit of a sensory and motor nerve, with connections in the spinal cord. Testing various reflex functions, such as the knee-jerk response, provided clues to neurological diseases if the reflexes were diminished or overactive. Sir William Gowers, A Manual of Diseases of the Nervous System, *3rd ed. (London: J. and A. Churchill, 1899), Vol. 1, p. 21, Figure 2.*

but he always maintained that chemical reactions within a living organism were propelled by irreducible, vital forces. Bell accused Magendie of dark, materialistic aims, particularly during their vitriolic priority dispute about which of them had discovered the functions of the anterior and posterior spinal nerve roots. Although he occasionally operated on a stunned animal, Bell hated vivisection and, indeed, was a bit xenophobic about what he perceived as the disturbing tendencies of Continental science in general. In contrast, Hall was an inveterate animal experimentator (claiming to have spent 25,000 hours in his studies of neurological reflex functions), believed himself to be misunderstood and unappreciated in his own country, and looked instead to France and Germany for scientific approbation, and at the end of his life, to the United States for adulation as a true man of science. Despite the ambiguities of their careers, each achieved a good deal.

Prout brilliantly demonstrated in 1824 that hydrochloric acid is the acid of the digestive juices; he devised a classification of foodstuffs into what became known as carbohydrates, fats, and proteins; and he proposed that the atomic weights of elements might be expressed as integrals of hydrogen, with hydrogen taken as unity. Bell's anatomical studies of the brain and nervous system were aesthetically pleasing and genuinely original; his speculations about neurological functions were shrewd and suggestive, even if he later overstated his claims to the discovery of the spinal nerve root functions. Despite predecessors, Hall and Johannes Müller between them have independent stakes in the elaboration of a modern theory of the nervous reflex. Nevertheless, when compared to contemporaries like Müller and Magendie, their careers were messy and unsettled, at least within the context of their research aspirations.

The next generation, more nearly contemporaries with Bernard and Ludwig, came to their scientific maturity in the 1830s and 40s. By then, King's College London had been founded as an alternative to University College, and together they constituted the teaching portions of the University of London. At University College, William Sharpey (1802–80) was appointed to the chair in Anatomy and Physiology in 1836. Like Bell, Prout, and Hall, he was an Edinburgh product, but he practiced surgery only very briefly before turning to teaching, first extramurally in Edinburgh, then permanently in London. Often described as the father of British physiology, Sharpey was not in the same class as an experimentalist with many of his Continental peers, and his modest original contributions were microscopical in nature. His chief virtues were an up-to-date knowledge of what was going on across the English Channel, and a superb capacity to communicate it to his students. His specially constructed round table, with a groove for mounting a microscope that would be passed from student to student, is still extant. He would frequently demonstrate one of Bernard's recent experimental preparations and helped get what were called practical physiology classes off the ground. Initially practical physiology consisted of little more than microscopy, though eventually students were expected to have rather more hands-on physiology experience, and after 1870, students taking the examinations of either the Royal College of Physicians or Royal College of Surgeons had to have passed a course in practical physiology.

Among Sharpey's students at University College were Joseph Lister (1827–1912) and Michael Foster (1836–1907), whose careers illustrate several features of medical research in late Victorian Britain. Lister became of course the century's leading surgeon, but he combined his primary surgical responsibilities with a substantial commitment to research, microscopical in his early years, then bacteriological in orientation. He published his first paper just after graduation, and his studies of the minute structure and functions of muscles, of lymph flow, and of the dynamics of inflammation secured his scientific reputation and led to his election to Fellowship of the Royal Society in 1860. As is well known, his ideas on fermentation, putrefaction, and postoperative surgical sepsis were partially the result of his familiarity with Pasteur's researches, and for more than a decade after the publication of his initial paper, in 1867, on antiseptic surgery, he was at the forefront of bacteriological research in Britain. Most of this work was done early in the morning, or late at night, in his own home, with his wife as his assistant and amanuensis. On at least one occasion, when he needed a large animal for his research, he worked in a French laboratory, to avoid British antivivisection sentiment.

Lister never actually wished for a full-time career in laboratory research and teaching, and seemed content with his disparate professional activities. In any case, it was around physiology rather than bacteriology that a distinct professional ethos first emerged among the medical sciences in Britain. Many of these scientists had reason to be grateful to Sharpey, although it was perhaps Michael Foster who spearheaded the drive to create in Britain an autonomous, laboratory-based science of physiology.

Like Lister, Foster was a product both of University College and its associated medical school. Like Darwin and Huxley, he spent time on a voyage with the primary aim of making a name for himself as a naturalist. His success was less auspicious than either of the two elder men, and after the voyage Foster spent six years in general practice with his father. Sharpey was able to bring him back to University College in 1867, as instructor in practical physiology. In 1870, partly with Huxley's help, he went to Trinity College Cambridge, as a fellow and praelector in physiology. Not until thirteen years later did Cambridge University officially recognize his importance by making him its first professor of physiology. Characteristically, Foster made it a condition of the chair that its occupant could not engage in part-time medical practice. By then, he had already been a founder-member of the Physiological Society (1876), as well as having established the first British journal in the subject, *The Journal of Physiology* (1878). His *Textbook of Physiology*, first published in 1877, went through several editions and translations and was experimental in its orientation.

Foster was more of a statesman of physiology than a first-rate experimentalist, although he did enough research himself to understand its problems and potentials. He was not even a particularly inspiring lecturer and, in any case, for the last two decades of his life, he could frequently be seen catching the early-morning train from Cambridge to London in order to fulfill his duties at the Royal Society or on various commissions or organizations. Nevertheless, his role in the rise to world prominence of British physiology can hardly be doubted. He presided in Cambridge over what has been described as a "research school," and it was largely its products (C. S. Sherrington, J. N. Langley, Joseph

Barcroft, H. H. Dale, E. D. Adrian) and those of University College (E. A. Sharpey-Schafer, W. M. Bayliss, J. S. Burdon-Sanderson) who established the discipline within the universities and medical schools of Britain. One exception to the indigenous traditions in these two institutions was Ernest Starling (1866–1927), who had trained and taught at Guy's Hospital Medical School before becoming professor of physiology at University College in 1899.

The visibility of British physiology by the final decade of the century should not obscure the fact that, compared to Germany and even France, medical science remained precariously rooted in Britain. After 1876, research on animals had to be done in registered premises by licensed researchers (see Chapter 6); this effectively put an end to the amateur tradition of which men like Marshall Hall had been a part. The alternative structures – endowments, well-equipped laboratories, career structures – were hardly established, despite the efforts of leading scientists like Foster or the existence of a more-or-less organized "Endowment of Science" movement. The German model was widely held up as worthy of emulation, but the State was sluggish to respond and most money to build laboratories or pay those who worked in them came from private philanthropists or students' fees. Science teaching in many of the hospital-based medical schools in London and the provinces continued often to be provided by part-time teachers with clinical appointments and no time or inclination for original research. Nevertheless, by the time of Huxley's death in 1895, the situation was different from what it had been in his youth forty years earlier, even if the medical scientific community in Britain was still small by German standards.

V. MEDICAL SCIENCE IN THE UNITED STATES

It has recently been argued that modern American science was "launched" between 1846 and 1876, those dates spanning the period between the founding of the Smithsonian Institution and the opening of the Johns Hopkins University. As in other national contexts, the medical sciences cannot be divorced from the physical, natural, or biological ones, and throughout the spectrum of the American sciences the influence of Europe, and especially Germany, can be seen. During the earlier century, European travel and education were partial remedies for the cultural inferiority experienced by many American intellectuals and professional people, particularly those living on the Eastern seaboard. The clinical opportunities of Paris had attracted many ambitious young doctors; increasingly, however, it was the laboratories of the German universities that left their mark. Symptomatic of this shift was the contrasting experience in Europe of Henry Ingersoll Bowditch (1808–92) and his nephew Henry Pickering Bowditch (1840–1911).

The uncle was one of many Americans for whom Pierre Louis was the *beau-ideal* of a doctor. He translated several of Louis's works for his American colleagues, published his own *The Young Stethoscopist* (1846), and campaigned for greater public American awareness of preventive medicine and statistics. His two years with Louis (1832–4) colored his whole medical outlook. It was natural that his nephew, from the same leading Boston clan, should also embark for Europe after his graduation from Harvard Medical School in 1868. Paris was his first objective, especially since C. E. Brown-Séquard, the neurophysiologist and neurologist who had stimulated his scientific interests at Harvard, was then teaching in Paris. When Bowditch got there, he discovered that Brown-Séquard had no laboratory, and although he found Claude Bernard inspiring on a personal level, the latter's laboratories were dark, poorly equipped, and ill-provided for students. Consequently, he moved on, first to Bonn and then to Leipzig, where Ludwig's physiological institute had just been opened. Bowditch's father was wealthy and happy for his son to pursue a career in science, even if medical practice would have been more lucrative. This enabled Bowditch to resist the opportunity to return to a physiology post at Harvard in 1870, preferring instead to spend a second year with Ludwig. In the event, the extra year did nothing to diminish Harvard's interest in him, and from 1871 until his retirement thirty-five years later he was intimately involved with the development of science and medicine at Harvard, including a decade as the Dean of its Medical School. He strove to reproduce in his own teaching and research laboratories the ethos he so valued in Ludwig's.

By the 1880s, the number of Americans studying medical topics in German-speaking universities had swelled to a flood: perhaps 15,000 between the mid-nineteenth century and World War I, mostly in Vienna, Berlin, Göttingen, and Heidelberg. Most went for clinical instruction and returned for careers in medical practice, but some, like Bowditch, the biochemist Russell Chittenden (1856–1943) at Yale, or the pathologist William Henry Welch (1850–1934) at Johns Hopkins, went for the laboratories.

No one symbolized the Germanic spirit in American experimental medicine better than Welch, especially since most of his career was associated with the most self-consciously Germanic of American universities, Johns Hopkins. His early life was desultory: he failed to convert his love of classics into an academic career post and his scientific and medical training included an apprenticeship with his father, as well as study at Yale and the College of Physicians and Surgeons in New York City. Europe was his making. During a two-year sojourn (1876–8), he studied physiology with Ludwig and pathology with Cohnheim and Recklinghausen. Returning to New York City, he established a pathology laboratory at Bellevue Hospital Medical School, saw a few private patients, did some miscellaneous writing, and performed a lot of post-mortem examinations. This eclecticism dissatisfied him and he jumped at the offer of the chair in pathology at Johns Hopkins in 1884. It carried a decent salary and enabled him to add bacteriology to his scientific repertoire during a further year's study in Germany with Koch and Pettenkofer.

When Welch took up his post in Baltimore in 1885, the hospital and medical school were still under construction, even though the university itself had been inaugurated in 1876. The Johns Hopkins Hospital opened its doors to patients in 1889, with the medical school following four years later. In all three portions, university, hospital, and medical school, there was an emphasis on advanced teaching and research and, though the money did not last forever, the foundation endowment by Johns Hopkins himself was large enough to allow planning on a generous scale. Welch recruited F. P. Mall (1862–1917), whom he had met in Leipzig, as the first professor of anatomy; J. J. Abel (1857–1938), who had spent six years studying in Germany, got the chair in pharmacology; whereas one of the early products of Johns Hopkins itself, W. H. Howell (1860–1945), took charge of the physiology department. From the beginning, the emphasis was on learning rather than spoon-fed teaching, and on the laboratory, dissecting room, and ward rather than the lecture room. In its stress on learning by doing, the Hopkins ideal had much in common with Paris of half a century before, except that the accessory sciences of the earlier period were now considered basic. A four-year curriculum gave time for these newer subjects; in addition, students were expected to have obtained a bachelor's degree before they began their medical studies.

Compared to the whole, the number of American medical schools prepared to invest in science remained small. But by the end of the century – and this a decade before Abraham Flexner's damning report on the general state of medical education in the United States – there was enough activity in places like Johns Hopkins, Harvard, the University of Pennsylvania, and the University of Michigan, to argue that, if not necessarily by 1876, at least American medical science was being actively launched by 1896. In that year, Welch and Abel founded the *Journal of Experimental Medicine*. The American Physiological Society was established in 1887; its own journal followed in 1898. The pathologists and bacteriologists organized themselves professionally in the 1890s.

The scientifically inclined medical student needed in the 1890s to choose his medical school carefully, and he still would have been in awe of the way science was valued and research provided for in Germany. But the flood tide of study in Germany had already been reached, an indigenous scientific culture within medicine was being established, and the great wave of American scientific philanthropy was just around the corner.

VI. CONCLUSION

By 1900, scientists had established themselves, with varying degrees of success, as a kind of separate estate within medicine. This occurred in different ways and with different timing in the four countries briefly examined. Germany provided the model, but medical science was never completely "Germanized" anywhere else. Mid-century enthusiasm for German science in France was never unambiguous, and political and military events ensured a deepening suspicion later. French scientists tended to be more self-contained, and neither Bernard nor Pasteur really established a research school in the way that Liebig or Ludwig had done.

British medical scientists continued to sing German praises even after the Franco-Prussian War, and far more Britons than Frenchmen went to learn German science and medicine at first-hand. What they and their colleagues established at home was not, however, simply a pale version of German science. The pragmatic orientation of British medicine, the relative lack of state support for medical education and research, and the weakness of the university system in Britain influenced the direction that medical science went.

It was in the United States that the German influence can be most easily seen, even if the diversity of educational standards and licensing practices meant that many doctors and medical schools remained untouched by, or even hostile to, the scientific claims of medicine.

Nevertheless, before the take-off of science in the early twentieth century (to be examined in Chapter 6), a career pattern within the medical sciences had been established. Even when products of the German system were abundant, there was no little Germany in the United States. Full-time posts remained scarce, departments were less autonomous than German institutes, and student fees and private endowments made up important parts of the financial viability of medical institutions.

5

Science, disease, and practice

It is no longer necessary today to write that scientific medicine is also the best foundation for medical practice. It is sufficient to point out how completely even the external character of medical practice has changed in the last thirty years. Scientific methods have been everywhere introduced into practice. The diagnosis and prognosis of the physician are based on the experience of the pathological anatomist and the physiologist. Therapeutic doctrine has become biological and thereby experimental science.

Rudolf Virchow, "Standpoints in Scientific Medicine" (1877), in L. J. Rather, ed., *Disease, Life and Man*, p. 149

T HE scientific estate developed in the nineteenth century alongside a much larger medical profession whose primary concern was the daily round of clinical practice. Early on, many advocates of medical science were also engaged in clinical work, and throughout the century most medical scientists had medical training. They thus worked from within the establishment and their claims for science carried the conviction of those who had grappled with the complexities of diagnosis and treatment. At times, it would have seemed to rank-and-file practitioners that possible benefits lay only in the future, for the translation of chemical, physiological, or bacteriological knowledge from the laboratory to the bedside or consulting room was not straightforward.

A generation ago, medical historians viewed the coming of experimental science within medicine as unproblematic. More recent revisionist accounts have challenged this traditional story, suggesting that science did little for the nineteenth-century patient and that the main beneficiaries were the doctors, who used science as a tool of collective professional advancement and as an aid to achieving a virtual monopoly in health care. There is merit in both points of view, but also a via media, which the following chapters will seek to map. This chapter examines briefly various ways in which science, from chemistry to bacteriology, was incorporated into clinical concepts and clinical practice from the middle decades of the century.

I. CHEMISTRY

At one level, a rudimentary knowledge of chemistry had long been a basic requirement for the practicing doctor, since many of them prepared the drugs they dispensed to their patients. This need not have involved more than simple technical skills, a few pieces of equipment (mortar, pestle, scales, and containers), and access to the ingredients. For much of the century, plants formed the basis of most prescriptions, though mercury was the mainstay of remedies for skin complaints and syphilis, and arsenic was an ingredient of various tonics. As we have learned more about the commercial side of medicine, it has become apparent that proprietary medicines, like Dover's Powder or James's powders, were widely available and commonly taken, usually without consultation with any official medical practitioner. Further, the rise of the dispensing chemist and pharmacist meant that fewer doctors actually compounded their own drugs. The pharmacist himself would generally buy the medicines, or the individual ingredients, from drug wholesalers. Doctors continued to prescribe, of course, and many of them routinely continued to sell bottles of medicine to their patients, but the traditional skills of compounding the medicines themselves became less important.

Instead, doctors could have learned more about the particular effects of specific medicinal agents. François Magendie (see Chapter 4) had first systematically appropriated for medicine the considerable advances in analytical techniques made since the late eighteenth century. His *Formulary* of 1821 attempted to base the pharmacopoeia on chemically pure drugs. It was the result of his own extensive experimental pharmacological work, especially on plant alkaloids such as emetine, quinine, and cinchonine, as well as several decades of analytical investigations by chemists and pharmacists. His approach had many advantages over the old polypharmacy, since the doctor had more control over what his patient was taking and could thus observe therapeutic effects more precisely. The *Formulary* was much admired and frequently revised, but it would be more difficult to demonstrate its influences on the prescribing practices of ordinary doctors.

In fact, even extraordinary doctors like William Prout tended to use chemical knowledge in rather different ways. As noted in Chapter 4, Prout made major contributions to chemistry, nutrition, and digestive physiology, even while earning his living practicing medicine. His major practical work, *On the Nature and Treatment of Stomach and Renal Diseases*, went through five editions under various titles between 1821 and 1848. Few details survive about his private practice, though if the case histories reported in his book are typical, he saw many patients with digestive or urinary disorders. Because "dyspepsia" was a common Victorian complaint, it is hardly surprising that Prout tried to turn his scientific interests to professional account. In a similar way, Marshall Hall used his neurophysiological work as the basis of a practice in "nervous" diseases. Prout's was not simply a patient's guide to dyspepsia, however, but a 500-page monograph written with his colleagues in mind. The last edition provides a convenient focus for examining briefly the ways in which, by the 1840s, chemistry was part of Prout's daily practice.

In the first place, the treatise made ample reference to the European scientific literature in chemistry, microscopy, and clinical medicine: Liebig, Rayer, Berzelius, and Wöhler were all cited, alongside many of his British colleagues. Nevertheless, he chose completely to avoid theoretical issues in chemistry. There was thus no discussion of ways Prout's ideas differed from those Liebig advanced in the latter's *Vegetable and Animal Chemistry*. Nor did Prout use any chemical formulas, even though a good deal of his own treatise dealt with the chemical composition of the urine in disease. However, he provided at the end of the volume directions how other medical men might repeat the chemical and microscopical examinations on which he based his own diagnosis, classification and, to a lesser extent, treatment of digestive and urinary diseases.

It is clear that Prout systematically examined his patients' urine. Few of his case histories neglect to note the color, degree of cloudiness, and, above all, specific gravity of the urine, as well as the presence or absence of sugar, crystals, various salts, and cells. In fact, for him, the urine could provide vital clues to most diseases of both the digestive and urinary systems. His classification of foodstuffs into saccharine, albuminous, and oleaginous (corresponding roughly to our carbohydrates, protein, fats) was duplicated in equivalent pathological urines, as assimilation of food and secretion of urine were intimately connected. Urine analysis was thus fundamental for diagnosing diseases of the stomach and intestines.

Of the diseases of saccharine assimilation and secretion, diabetes was the most important, and the presence of sugar in the urine pathognomonic. He described associated features, such as constant thirst ("an invariable symptom"), voiding of large quantities of urine, and wasting, and was realistic about his therapeutic armamentarium: "no specific remedy is known for this essential symptom of diabetes (sugar in the urine)." He believed that some individuals had inherited a tendency toward the condition, but exposure to cold and damp, or an attack of malaria, might also bring it on. Its pathophysiological defect lay with the stomach and duodenum, where, for largely unknown reasons, the usual appropriation of sugars into fats and albumen failed to take place, leaving the sugar to be secreted by the kidneys. He subscribed to the general view, shortly to be challenged by Claude Bernard, that sugar is not a normal constituent of the blood. Diabetes was, for him, a form of dyspepsia.

Prout's discussion of the nature and diagnosis of diabetes drew on his scientific work: indeed, it was based on it. So was his identification of oxalic acid in the urine of other patients, and his description of what he called the Oxalic Acid Diathesis (i.e., a predisposition to disease associated with oxalic acid). While admitting that on occasion the urine of healthy individuals could contain oxalic acid, a large number of patients could not assimilate this chemical, which, since it could be obtained from the reduction of sugars, was saccharine in its nature. Only a small fraction of such patients developed kidney or bladder stones of oxalates; most simply complained of the cluster of dyspeptic symptoms: flatulence, palpitations, abdominal distension, and bowel irregularities. These symptoms, plus oxalic acid in the urine, clinched the diagnosis. Treatment consisted primarily of dietary management, validated by frequent reference to his research on the nature and digestion of foodstuffs. The diseases of albuminous and oleaginous assimilation and secretion contain similar mixtures of the familiar and the obscure. Prout's diagnostic category of Oxalic Acid Diathesis failed to find much favor among his contemporaries, and would not be found in any modern medical textbook, but it was constructed out of the same combination of clinical practice and scientific analysis of foodstuffs and excretions that characterized his descriptions of diabetes, Bright's disease, and gallstones. He could identify sugar, protein, phosphates, urates, urea, and oxalates in the urine; recognized a variety of cells – mucous and pus, for example – within it; described its physical appearance and measured its specific gravity; and used these findings as a diagnostic aid for a variety of conditions, many of which, like diabetes or oxalic acid diathesis, had no constant pathological changes discoverable at autopsy.

One further instance of the impact of chemistry on the medicine of the 1840s should be mentioned, although it is generally seen from another context: anesthesia. The outlines of the introduction into medicine of what Oliver Wendell Holmes (1809–94) dubbed anesthesia are well known. The control of pain in surgery had long been a desideratum, and various agents and procedures, from alcohol and carbon dioxide to mesmerism, had been employed. None was routinely satisfactory and, in any case, some surgeons felt that pain provided an essential stimulus to recovery.

It is equally well known that the three compounds, nitrous oxide, ether, and chloroform, which in 1846 and 1847 were used with such drama in surgical and dental operations, had all been around for years, and that nitrous oxide, first prepared by Joseph Priestley in 1772, had been recommended by Humphry Davy in 1800 for surgical use, because it was "capable of destroying physical pain." Various ethers, prepared by distilling alcohols with an acid, had been known for centuries and ethyl ether had had a checkered history of medicinal use as an anti-spasmodic as well as the suggestion that it could produce effects similar to those of nitrous oxide. In the 1820s and 30s, the chemical compositions of the whole class of ethers were the subjects of lively debate between the French chemist, Dumas, and Liebig, the latter of whom was one of three chemists independently to prepare chloroform in the early 1830s. When inhaled, nitrous oxide and ether produce lightheadedness and a sense of hilarity and euphoria; hence their casual social use in the early decades of the century.

Two public operations on patients anesthetized with ether, the first at Massachusetts General Hospital on 16 October 1846, the second at University College Hospital in London on 21 December 1846, brought the possibilities of "painless surgery" to both the medical profession and the public. Neither was in any sense a first, and the "discovery" of anesthesia was the subject of acrimonious priority disputes by several individuals with claims. At one level, the whole episode can be reconstructed as a sorry tale of pride, madness, and avarice, of men wise after the event. The facts that Crawford Long (1815–78), who had used ether as an anesthetic in 1842, died a bitter man; that Horace Wells (1815–48), the dentist who had used nitrous oxide in 1844, went insane; or that William Morton (1819–68), the dentist who administered ether on the historic day at the M.G.H., tried desperately to patent the process and died destitute: these facts do not detract from the importance of anesthesia. Recent studies have shown that, despite the rapid spread of knowledge of them, anesthetics were not immediately and universally employed in major surgical operations: their use by military surgeons was restricted, they were thought too expensive for the poor, and their use in obstetrics occasionally questioned on moral grounds. Only one-third of amputations on men at the Pennsylvania Hospital between 1853 and 1862 were performed with anesthesia. As anesthetic deaths began to be reported, anesthetics could no longer be counted as an unmixed blessing. Nevertheless, after 1846, ether and chloroform (first used in 1847) were available, a part of the equation in what has been called "a calculus of suffering."

Equally significant, anesthetics were chemicals produced in the laboratory, of simple composition and already of active interest to chemists. Their ultimate medical use had been incidental to their synthesis, but once that had been demonstrated, closely regulated compounds were scrutinized for anesthetic or other therapeutic properties. John Snow (see Chapter 3), who acquired a formidable reputation in London in the 1850s as an anesthetist, was also an energetic spare-time chemist. He introduced amylene in 1856, and his friend and biographer, Benjamin Ward Richardson (1828–96), produced a series of systematic investigations in the late 1850s and early 1860s on the chemistry and physiological effects of compounds in the amyl, methyl, and ethyl series. He found a couple of useful anesthetics as well as noticing the vasodilatory effects of amyl nitrite, subsequently used in the treatment of angina pectoris.

In 1847, Virchow wrote of chemistry that it "has already accomplished a great deal for us, although thus far very little is useful for practical purposes." He almost certainly was not considering the discovery of anesthetics as a chemical achievement, but chemistry had at least produced those substances and in that sense Virchow had sold the science short, even if his following sentence was more hopeful: "We expect a great deal more from it."[1]

II. MICROSCOPY

If the stethoscope was becoming the symbol of careful clinical practice, it was on the microscope that the scientific authority of medicine rested. Joseph Lister would have been an unusual medical student in the 1850s in owning his own, and fewer still would have kept them after qualifying; but microscopical investigations nevertheless made their impact on much of clinical medicine.

Among mid-century microscopists, Virchow was among the most intellectually agile, and, significantly, his *Cellular Pathology* had as its subtitle "As Based on Physiological and Pathological Histology." Like so much other science of the period, microscopy encouraged doctors to think about the dynamics of disease, about the genesis of lesions rather than their gross, end-stage structures.

Cellular Pathology, though it remains Virchow's best-known book, was not a systematic treatise but the record of a lecture series delivered in early 1858 at the new Pathological Institute in Berlin to an audience composed primarily of practicing doctors. His work was based not simply on the slogan we have already noticed – "all cells from cells" – but three further principles:

1. all diseases are the result of either active or passive disturbances of living cells;
2. cells carry out their functions as a result of physical and chemical processes occurring within them and the microscope can reveal something of this;
3. abnormalities of structure are degenerations, transformations or repetitions of normal structures.

What this meant was that it was theoretically possible to trace every disease back to its primary locus, the cell. Cells were the sites of the pathology because they were also the units of normal functions. Living organisms are not composed exclusively of cells, but even the fluids surrounding many cells (interstitial fluid, or blood serum, for instance)

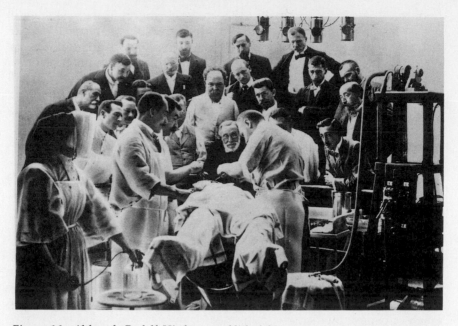

Figure 16. Although Rudolf Virchow established his reputation as a pathologist, he remained keenly interested in clinical issues throughout his professional life. Here the elderly Virchow is observing an operation on the skull during a visit to a Paris clinic. Historischer Bilderdienst, Berlin: August 1900.

lie under the ultimate control of the cells, as part of what Virchow called "cell-territories."

Unsurprisingly, Virchow's lectures did not contain extensive discussions of psychiatric disorders or even functional conditions of the kind that Prout had classed as forms of dyspepsia. Nevertheless, he was clear that any and all diseases had their physical correlates. For instance, diseases too often passed off as general dyscrasias (literally, nonspecific conditions of the blood), such as scurvy, syphilis, or "drunkard's dyscrasia" had their local origins, and it was the task of pathology to elucidate them. Although the primary clinical manifestation of a condition like scurvy might be the blood – oozing from the gums, bleeding under the skin – this did not mean that the blood was necessarily the site of the primary disorder, because the blood was in dynamic relationship with the organs and tissues of the body.

Virchow's comments on the blood carried particular weight, since he had invested much energy in its study. Not only had he worked out pathophysiological explanations for the formation of clots in inflamed veins (thrombophlebitis), and the way such clots can become dislodged to produce a dangerous embolus (a word he coined), but he had also in 1847 described a condition of the white blood cells that he first called leukemia. The latter had involved him in an unproductive priority dispute with John Hughes Bennett (1812–75) in Edinburgh, who a couple of weeks earlier had also published a case history of a patient with an excessive number of white blood cells. Bennett had named the condition leucocythemia, although Virchow's name eventually prevailed. Leukemia was a microscopical diagnosis in the sense that the change in the usual ratio of red to white blood cells usually needed a microscope to recognize. That we still sometimes call them blood "corpuscles" is testimony to the fact that blood was an obvious substance to study with a microscope, thin films of it being easy to make. The older term corpuscles continued to be used even after the cellular nature of the red and white (or colorless) elements in the blood was recognized.

Even though the red corpuscles normally lacked a nucleus – identified as an essential feature of the cell by the botanist Robert Brown (1773–1858) in the early 1830s – Virchow knew that in the embryo or very young infant, many of the red corpuscles possessed nuclei, thus pointing toward their cellular nature. He was not certain where they were formed, but he believed that the spleen and lymph glands were implicated in the production of the white cells. This seemed logical because these organs became much enlarged in leukemia; in fact, Virchow divided leukemia into splenic and lymphatic types, depending on the form of the predominant cell and the relative enlargement of the spleen and the lymph nodes. Virchow was also aware that more modest increases in the number of circulating white corpuscles were encountered in other conditions such as pneumonia. That diseases like pneumonia were also routinely accompanied by an enlargement in lymph nodes (in this case, the bronchial ones) also reinforced his confidence that those nodes were the source of the corpuscles.

Attempts were being made in the 1850s to count the actual number of red and white corpuscles, though this remained a laborious and time-consuming procedure, and Virchow and others relied mostly on their relative numbers, the ordinary ratio being accepted at about 300 red to 1 white. Even a relative count on a blood smear was not routine, and it is not surprising that the reports of patients diagnosed as having leukemia, which gradually accumulated worldwide during the 1850s and 60s, all came from hospitals. It remained an uncommon diagnosis with a grim prognosis.

On the other hand, the white corpuscles themselves were the subject of much observation and discussion. Were they the same as the pus cells of abscesses? What was their relationship to similar kinds of cells to be found in loose connective tissue? What role did they play in inflammation? Did they ever leave the circulation, or did the small arteries, veins, and capillaries form a system ordinarily impervious to cells?

Virchow was by no means the only microscopist with views on these questions, and the answers that he proposed did not always hold sway. Nevertheless, that he devoted so much of his *Cellular Pathology* to discussing them demonstrates their significance for mid-century pathology.

His cellular doctrines required that inflammatory and pus cells had to originate from other cells rather than being formed from some amorphous substance that Schwann and others had called the blastema. Despite the fact that increased numbers of white corpuscles could be seen microscopically in small vessels near a disturbed site (the frog's web was a convenient place to observe this), he believed, contrary to his contemporary William Addison (1802–81) and his student Julius Cohnheim (1839–84), that pus cells were derived from the loose connective tissue rather than the blood. Cohnheim published the classic description of cell movement through the capillary wall (diapedesis) in Virchow's own journal in 1867, but at the time of the *Cellular Pathology*, Virchow still identified the pus cell with the connective tissue.

This had consequences for him beyond simply explaining the steps involved in the inflammatory response or abscess formation. For one thing, Virchow held that the tubercles to be found in the lungs and, often, in other organs, of patients with phthisis, were very much like small abscesses, and the processes involved in their formation thus to be understood. As in abscesses, the inflammatory cells in tubercles eventually began to disintegrate in the center, leaving a middle composed of viscous white material ("caseous metamorphosis," literally, changing into a cheeselike substance), surrounded by a kind of protective ring of cells. Similar events could be seen to occur in the development of cancers, whose origins Virchow also located in cells of the connective tissues. In each case – pus, tubercle, cancer – local connective tissue cells were stimulated by some unknown factor to start dividing, and the metastatic spread of cancer was similar to the spread of tubercles. Why some tumors were malignant, kept growing, and spread, whereas others were benign, and, though they might reach great size, did not metastasize, was difficult to explain. Virchow's answer was mostly descriptive: under different stimuli, cells might reproduce normal structures, as in benign tumors, or they might degenerate or even transform, as in malignant ones.

In practice, decisions about the nature of a particular tumor, and what should be done about it, continued to be based more on clinical than histological grounds. Cohnheim himself introduced in 1870 the technique of quick-freezing tissue, so that the pathologist could examine the tumor quickly and advise the surgeon. Quick-freezing biopsy techniques were rarely used until much later, although Virchow was involved in probably the century's most famous collaboration between surgeon and pathologist, the tragic case of Frederick III, Emperor of Germany. In the 1880s, he developed what in retrospect was laryngeal cancer; his German surgeons wanted to operate, but an English consultant, Morrell Mackenzie (1837–92), after examining him and sending a piece of the lesion to Virchow for examination, decided that the tumor was benign and amenable to medical management. His subsequent deterioration and death, and Virchow's postmortem confirmation of the tumor's malignancy, created an international incident. Incidentally, Frederick's death led to the accession to the throne of his militaristic son, Kaiser Wilhelm II. Whether an operation would have saved his life is unclear, but surgery had been transformed between *Cellular Pathology* and Frederick's death by the emergence of a branch of pathology, bacteriology.

III. BACTERIOLOGY

Virchow believed that his notion of the cell provided a unifying focus for both physiology and pathology, and in particular, demonstrated the common features of inflammation, pus formation, tubercle growth, and cancer. At the same time, another cluster of phenomena, suggestively overlapping with the above pathophysiological quartet, were also the subject of much research and debate. There were striking similarities between fermentation and putrefaction, between the souring of wine and the rotting of meat. Further, the putrefaction of dead organic matter seemed to resemble the suppuration or gangrene to be found in living organisms. Miasmatic theories, which attributed the spread of epidemic diseases to the air-borne poisons of putrefaction, gave additional moment to this gray area of decay, between the living and the dead, the healthy and the diseased.

The dominant mid-century theories of fermentation and putrefaction were chemical, especially those of Liebig. The chemistry of the breakdown of the sugars of the grape into alcohol – or their further transformation into vinegar – was beginning to be understood, as were the compositions of some of the products of putrefaction. Liebig was aware that various fermentations required the addition of yeast, but he held that they acted like catalysts, speeding up what was an ordinary chemical reaction.

Pasteur began to challenge this orthodoxy in the late 1850s with his studies of lactic, alcoholic, and butyric fermentations. His careful investigation of the activities and nutritional requirements of the yeast cells themselves convinced him that fermentation is actually a vital process that required these living microorganisms to occur. Kill the microorganism and fermentation ceases. Extending his researches to putrefaction, he argued that, here, too, the breakdown of larger organic molecules into the fetid products of decomposition also resulted from the activities of living microorganisms: "life takes part in the work of death in all its phases."[2] By the late 1860s, Pasteur had convinced himself (though not the entire scientific community) that both putrefaction and fermentation were always vital processes; he had also shown that two different diseases of silkworms – *pébrine* and *flacherie* – were parasitical, the consequence of infection by specific bacteria. Although he continued occasionally to return to earlier concerns – spontaneous generation, or the fermentation controversy – Pasteur's energies were increasingly focused on what became known as the germ theory of disease.

Pasteur was not the first to study microorganisms in detail, or to suggest that they could be a cause of disease. Prior to his work on silkworms, another of their diseases, muscardine, had been shown by the Italian Agostino Bassi (1773–1856) to be parasitical; the fungal origin of the skin disease favus had been demonstrated, as had the bacterial nature of anthrax. In 1840 Jacob Henle (1809–85) had forecast that many diseases would eventually be shown to be caused by a *contagium vivum* (living contagion). Nevertheless, it is Pasteur and Pasteurization that still have the ring of the familiar.

It is curious that the infectious diseases that Pasteur studied should be dramatic, such as rabies, or economically significant, such as anthrax: but they were not especially significant in terms of human morbidity or mortality. To the public mind, however, Pasteur was the chief architect of the germ theory. Three main reasons may be suggested.

First, Pasteur brought to his medically related researches an extensive range of experimental work and controversy, including, to a generation still getting to grips with Darwin's evolutionary theories, the spontaneous generation question. He had a superb ability to see to the heart of an issue and an unrivaled understanding of the nutritional and environmental requirements of the microorganisms he studied. By the time he began elaborating a systematic germ theory of disease in the 1870s, he was recognized as an authority.

Second, although it would be churlish to suggest that Pasteur was largely a media phenomenon, his career coincided with the rise of the popular press and his reputation was its beneficiary. He appreciated the force of public opinion, and his experiments at Pouilly-le-Fort in 1881, or the extension of his rabies treatment to human beings, were carefully orchestrated affairs. At Pouilly-le-Fort, he invited the press to witness his vaccination of farm animals against anthrax, and to return a few weeks later to contrast the effect of injecting a virulent culture of anthrax into protected and unprotected animals. The timing was perfect, as two of the unprotected animals were actually expiring just as the crowd gathered.

Finally, Pasteur's was no abstract notion of microorganisms as a cause of disease, but one that was almost always attended with therapeutic or specific prophylactic implications. His silkworm studies had led to definite, effective advice, and he developed, in addition to anthrax, vaccines for chicken cholera and swine erysipelas. His techniques varied for attenuating the microorganisms, thereby rendering them noninfectious but still provoking an immune response in the host, but his manipulation of the cultures of the microorganisms went hand in hand with more theoretical speculations on the nature of immunity. These became most evident during his work on rabies, since he was dealing with an active substance that he could not see even with the aid of his microscope. His immunological theories also brought him into conflict with Koch and other bacteriologists, mostly German, who by the late 1880s believed they had wrested the initiative in these matters from Pasteur and his French followers.

Koch certainly occupies, with Pasteur, a place in the pantheon, both for his work with particular diseases such as anthrax, tuberculosis, and cholera, but, equally important, for the technical innovations that he and his students made. Pasteur liked to grow microorganisms in flasks and although this worked very well for him, Koch was right to insist that Pasteur's methods were cumbersome and likely to produce contamination. Koch favored the plate technique, whereby bacteria were grown in a solid medium (first gelatin, then from the early 1880s, agar-agar) in small dishes with rounded edges. (It is no surprise that one of Koch's assistants was named Petri.) This permitted the growth of colonies from single organisms and allowed for quantitative assessments. It was also easier to keep such equipment sterile, especially with the pressurized steam that Koch and his group investigated and recommended. Koch's pioneering of photomicroscopy also helped in the search for standards, which were so important in the last, heady decades of the century, when new pathogenic organisms were being announced every few months. The list of infectious diseases whose causative organisms were then identified includes tuberculosis, cholera, diphtheria, plague, dysentery, gonorrhea, tetanus, and the common organisms of wound infection, staphylococcus, and streptococcus. A number of other disorders, including several forms of insanity, nutritional diseases like beri-beri and scurvy, and various kinds of cancer, were also implicated at some point as consequences of infection. For diseases that have remained in the infectious camp, the first implicated microorganism was not necessarily the one ultimately agreed.

The experimental steps whereby organism A was shown to cause disease B are generally known as "Koch's Postulates." However, there is nothing mysterious about them – they were implicit in the earlier work of Henle, and the clearest explicit formulation of them came not from Koch but his pupil Friedrich Löffler (1852–1915), in connection with his identification of the causative organism of diphtheria in 1883:

If diphtheria is a disease caused by a microorganism, it is essential that three postulates be fulfilled. The fulfillment of these postulates is necessary in order to demonstrate strictly the parasitic nature of a disease:

1. The organism must be shown to be constantly present in characteristic form and arrangement in the diseased tissue.
2. The organism which, from its behavior appears to be responsible for the disease, must be isolated and grown in pure culture.
3. The pure culture must be shown to induce the disease experimentally.[3]

The implication of bacterial toxins in disease processes loosened the requirement for the intact organism to be recovered from the infected tissues and also gave rise to a spate of pathophysiological models based on notions of "auto-intoxication" (diseases caused by the absorption of breakdown products from the intestinal bacteria), ptomaine poisoning, and focal infection (infected teeth, tonsils, or other structures as the source of disease).

The "germ theory of disease" was thus anything but simple and straightforward, but it did produce a new and much more explicit dimension to thinking about the cause of disease. Insofar as the infective organism was perceived to be a sine qua non of a particular disease, this reinforced notions of disease specificity and brought the possibility of somehow equating the disease with the organism. That in turn gave a new cogency to disease classifications based on the botanical analogies of eighteenth-century nosologists. At the same time, the legacy of Claude Bernard's philosophy of discovery, and of much medical research in the century's middle decades, lay in the dynamic conception of disease, with the emphasis on processes and mechanisms, and the continuity between healthy states and diseased ones. It would be a mistake to make too stark a contrast between essentialist and nominalist, pathological and physiological, or static and dynamic, approaches to disease. After all, Virchow, who heralded cellular pathology as the best means of following the dynamic transformations of diseased cells (which could ultimately be traced back to a "normal" state or a healthy mother-cell), ended his life with a much more ontological appreciation of the relationship between the lesion and the disease, while at the same time distancing himself from many of the more exuberant pronouncements of the bacteriologists. Koch, the arch-exponent of germ theory, appreciated the dynamics of infection and immunity and was instrumental in elucidating the notion of the nonsymptomatic carrier-state, particularly in typhoid fever.

The complexity of these issues, and the continuities between pre- and postbacteriological thinking, are shown by tuberculosis. Koch's announcement of his identification of the tubercle bacillus to a meeting of the Berlin Physiological Society on 24 March 1882, and the publication of his lecture three weeks later, created a worldwide stir. Koch's was "one of the great scientific discoveries of the age," announced the *New York Times*. Indeed, Koch's achievement was considerable, since the organism required a good deal of finesse to grow, and special stains to permit its easy microscopical identification. Beginning his research to making his announcement occupied him less than eight months, but the results amply fulfilled the criteria of "his" postulates, including the recovery of the bacillus from guinea pigs that he had experimentally infected.

Koch's demonstrations persuaded many that tuberculosis is an infectious disease. Even so, its hereditary, constitutional nature continued to be widely stressed; the analogy between tubercles and metastatic cancer still seemed apposite; and the statistical association of tuberculosis with poverty and destitution did not go away. As Virchow coolly remarked, "Phthisis has remained what it was." In fact, he was not entirely correct, at least in the medium term. Tuberculosis did become conceived as an infectious disease and thereby generated an extensive public health campaign. What it did not do was lose its emotive characteristics.

The disease's place in the mortality tables – John Bunyan had called phthisis the "captain of all those men of death" – meant that Koch's hint in August 1890 that he had uncovered a substance capable of preventing the growth, in vitro and in vivo, of the tubercle bacillus, was greeted with eager anticipation. Four months later he reported excellent results in patients, though he declined at the time to reveal the substance or how it was prepared. The mystery, and the glowing optimism, not simply from Koch but from several clinicians working with him, heightened the drama and led to a pilgrimage to Berlin of patients and doctors, from all parts of the world. When Koch did make his prized substance public the following year, the scientific community was disappointed, because it turned out to be glycerin extracts of the tubercle bacillus, which several groups had already been working with for years, in an attempt to produce a tuberculosis vaccine. Koch insisted on the unique way in which he prepared tuberculin, as he called it, and remained for several years confident that early cases could be cured by it. Even Koch came to see that tuberculin's therapeutic powers had been greatly exaggerated, although it did prove useful as a diagnostic agent and helped others elucidate some allergic dimensions to tuberculous infection.

Koch's back-to-back discoveries of the causative organisms of tuberculosis and cholera (the latter as part of a scientific mission first to Egypt, then to India) guaranteed him an international status, which was enhanced rather than dented by tuberculin. Less spectacular research in the previous decade, which he had summarized in his first book, *Untersuchungen über die Aetiologie der Wundinfectionskrankheiten* (1878) (translated in 1880 as Investigations into the etiology of traumatic infective diseases), was significant for its application of bacteriological techniques to understand the rationale of the antiseptic surgery that Joseph Lister had publicly introduced eleven years earlier.

IV. ANTISEPTIC SURGERY

As we have seen, surgical anesthesia owed much to chemistry; so, too, did surgical antisepsis, for the substance that Joseph Lister used in his initial antiseptic operations – carbolic acid – was a chemical prepared in the laboratory. It was first isolated and named in the 1830s by a German industrial chemist, Friedlieb Runge (1797–1867), through the distillation and fractionation of coal tar. Like a number of other acids, it was found to have antiseptic properties and carbolic acid (it is also called phenol) acquired an extensive employment in the 1850s in the disinfection and treatment of sewage. Carbolic acid was also tried as a surgical antiseptic in France before Lister began publishing his own account in the 16 March 1867 issue of *The Lancet*.

In fact, antisepsis as a concept and as a desideratum in surgery was not new. Substances that inhibit or retard putrefaction had been called antiseptics since at least the early eighteenth century, and a class of drugs called antiseptics – including tonics and antispasmodics – were regularly used in diseases in which there was a perceived tendency toward putrefaction or mortification. The fact that mortification or gangrene produced fetid smells similar to those of the rotting of meat or dung did not go unnoticed. Surgical wards were a place where such smells could commonly be experienced, especially during outbreaks of erysipelas, pyemia, septicemia, and other postoperative complications.

Sanitarians had noticed this, and it was common knowledge that it was safer to have an operation in your own home than in a hospital. If anyone doubted this, he need only have turned to Florence Nightingale's *Notes on Hospitals* (1859), where the grim hospital statistics were laid out, and surgeons subsequently estimated hospital mortality at three to five times higher than that incurred in private cases. What such figures meant was open to dispute, but the phenomena led the Edinburgh surgeon and introducer of chloroform anesthesia Sir James Simpson (1811–70) to coin the term "hospitalism." This was defined by Sir John Erichsen, surgeon to University College Hospital, as "a general morbid condition of the building, or of its atmosphere, productive of disease."[4] Adherents to the doctrine of hospitalism associated it with large, multistory, old urban buildings and contrasted surgical mortality there with small country hospitals, or new ones built with due attention to cleanliness and fresh air. Nightingale was a great exponent of the pavilion ward, with well-spaced beds and large windows offering cross-ventilation. According to Erichsen, a "pyemia-stricken" hospital ought to be torn down, since its atmosphere, walls, and furniture were irrevocably contaminated. Nightingale thought all hospitals should ideally be taken out of the cities and wondered publicly whether they had not destroyed more lives than they had saved. A succession of temporary sheds would be safer than the permanent edifices people called hospitals.

Such radical solutions were never likely to gain widespread assent, though the opportunity for debating the pros and cons of large urban and small rural hospitals arose when, in the 1860s, the old St. Thomas's Hospital was torn down to make way for a new railway station. Florence Nightingale wanted it moved to the country, whereas John Simon, on its surgical staff as well as occupying his post in government, argued that it needed to remain in London, close to the population it served. Metropolitan surgeons and physicians were unlikely, in any case, to want to commute long distances to see their hospital patients, even if they accepted the arguments of hospitalism, and thus Simon and his allies carried the day. However, pavilion wards were a prominent feature of the new Thomas's, built a couple of miles to the west of the old site, but still squarely in south London. Such ward design not only allowed cross-ventilation, but it also made surveillance of patients by the nursing staff easier. Thomas's was the home of the Nightingale School for training nurses.

The explanatory framework of hospitalism was essentially the older environmental one of the sanitarians, but it is significant that concern over surgical mortality reached such a pitch during the very years when Lister was developing what he called the "antiseptic principle." He had left London for Scotland as a young surgeon in 1853, and returned to the metropolis as Professor of Surgery at King's College Hospital in 1877. In many ways, the Scottish period, in Edinburgh and Glasgow, was the most productive of his life. It was in Glasgow where he developed his antiseptic methods, in Edinburgh where, from 1869, he taught them to large classes. In London, his classes were sometimes pitifully small, but it was there he reaped his personal honors: worldwide fame, the Presidency of the Royal Society, the Order of Merit, elevation to the House of Lords (the first medical man to be so honored). In fact, by the time he returned to London, antiseptic surgery was sometimes known as Listerism, in itself a token of how much he had become a surgical symbol.

Why Lister, especially when we note that French surgeons had already used carbolic acid; that Ignaz Philipp Semmelweis (1818–65) had already developed what can only be called an antiseptic system of midwifery in Vienna; that Marion Sims was busy pioneering the repair of vaginal fistules in the United States and Europe; or that other British surgeons, such as Lawson Tait or Spencer Wells, were beginning to explore, independently of Lister, the surgery of the abdominal cavity, that traditional surgical terra incognita?

Part of the answer, at least, lies in the fact that, more than any of his predecessors, Lister based his antiseptic principle on medical science. His surgical practice rested on an explicit statement of a common origin of putrefaction, fermentation, and wound decomposition following surgery or after a compound fracture (i.e., one in which the bone had broken the skin), and of the source of these processes to the "germs of various low forms of life," as shown by Pasteur's work. Pasteur's experiments on spontaneous generation had demonstrated that air could contain these germs; John Tyndall in Britain was shortly to identify them as being carried on dust particles.

Lister's "system" obviously evolved over the years. Initially, it consisted primarily of soaking his surgical instruments in a solution of carbolic acid, and using carbolic-soaked dressings on the open fracture, both to disinfect and to form a barrier to the atmosphere. This allowed him to reduce the fractures surgically. As an appendix to his paper on treating compound fractures this way, rather than by amputation of the limb, he noted that deep-seated abscesses could also be successfully drained using his antiseptic techniques, though he denied the presence of "septic organisms" in abscesses. Draining them allowed the natural healing process to occur; the carbolic dressings prevented contamination from atmospheric germs. He distinguished between decomposition, an unmitigated evil, and suppuration, which could be part of the healing process. Indeed, he recognized that carbolic acid was a chemical stimulus to suppuration; the difference between carbolic-induced suppuration and the suppuration resulting from decomposing tissue was that the former was self-limited, whereas the latter had a tendency to spread, as in erysipelas and hospital gangrene. In the early 1870s, Lister added the carbolic spray, in an effort to keep the whole surgical atmosphere sterile, and not simply the area immediately around the wound.

Carbolic acid is an unpleasant substance, irritating to the skin, eyes, respiratory tract and, of course, to open wounds. It is not surprising that even Lister, who continued to sing its praises for more than twenty years, also experimented with alternative antiseptics, and with different ingredients to mix with carbolic. The system, as originally described by Lister, was tiresome, and many of Lister's critics thought his attention to detail obsessive, particularly as he continued to make minor modifications in the ritual. Some surgeons gave his methods a trial, found their mortality figures did not improve, and subsequently abandoned them. Others, Thomas Spencer Wells, for example, were converted after using them for a while. In Britain, the most loyal were Lister's pupils themselves, men like Hector Cameron (1843–1928) and William Watson Cheyne (1852–1932), who had been with him in the heroic, Scottish period.

The whole issue of Listerism is complicated in that it coincided with the period of heightened hospital accountability and preoccupation with

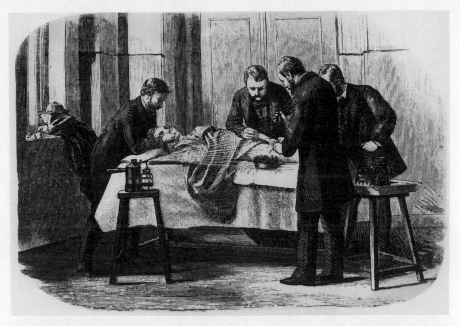

Figure 17. Although this was published in 1882 by Lister's pupil Sir William Watson Cheyne (1852–1932), as an example of an operation "performed with complete aseptic precautions," the surgeons are dressed in their street clothes, without masks and gloves, and the wooden table and tools would have been difficult to sterilize. By 1900, operation rooms looked much more like what we are used to today. Sir William Watson Cheyne, Antiseptic Surgery *(London: Smith, Elder & Co., 1882), p. 71, Fig. 23.*

cleanliness associated with hospitalism. Disinfecting techniques, such as whitewashing walls and bedsteads with nitrous oxide, were commonplace, and the washing that was a byword in the public health movement spilled over into the hospitals. Surgical cleanliness through soap and water, and frequent changing of dressings, was being widely advocated simultaneously to, but independently of, Lister's antisepsis. In the 1860s, "disinfection" was a concept that carried no bacteriological overtones: it meant simply the destruction of the agents – whatever they were – of contagious diseases. Simple cleanliness was part of this. What Lister did was to give "antisepsis" a new theoretical connotation, and if, by the century's end, "antiseptic" and "disinfectant" had become more or less synonymous, this was because germ theory had by then carried the day. But, although Lister made a ritual of antisepsis, he was much less bothered about dirt in the old sanitarian sense. He did not scrub his hands, but merely rinsed them in carbolic solution. He operated in his street clothes. He lived to see surgical gowns, gloves, and masks, but they were first advocated by others. Technically Lister was a gifted surgeon who introduced significant operative changes such as the use of sutures made of catgut that would gradually be absorbed; however, his surgical repertoire remained mostly limited to bones, joints, superficial tumors, and deep abscesses. His results were excellent, but his operations the kind already performed in the pre-antiseptic era. Others pioneered the surgical exploration of the abdominal, thoracic, and cranial cavities.

Lister fiddled with the details of antiseptic surgery, but he never wavered in his insistence that microorganisms were the source of surgical mischief. However, his detailed explanations of the pathophysiological and microbiological causes of suppuration, decomposition, and what came to be called wound infection were complicated and, by the 1880s, outmoded. He followed but did not always accept the researches of people like Koch or the Scottish surgeon Alexander Ogston (1844–1929) on the role of specific microorganisms in the genesis of wound infection. This was partly because Lister clung to his beliefs that abscesses are generally germ-free and that the nervous system is instrumentally involved in the early stages of inflammation; and partly because the two principal bacteria that were implicated in wound infections – named staphylococci and streptococci – appeared to be ubiquitous and often nonpathogenic. Their role was thus difficult to evaluate. Lister's disciple Watson Cheyne had translated Koch's book on wound infection into English in 1880, and Ogston, who also looked to Lister for inspiration, began his work on the etiology of abscesses and other infections about the same time. Curiously, it took Lister some years to accept streptococci and staphylococci as important pathogenic bacteria.

To be sure, some surgeons accepted Lister's antiseptic rituals without the theoretical underpinning. For the most part, however, most surgical skepticism about germ theory was to be found among the anti-Listerians. Academic surgeons in the German-speaking lands adopted Listerian practices on a wider scale than their British colleagues, which was not surprising, perhaps considering how much German science dominated bacteriology by the 1880s. Johann Nussbaum (1829–90), professor of surgery in Munich, sent one of his assistants to work with Lister while the latter was still in Edinburgh; Richard Volkmann (1830–89) from Halle proselytized actively on Lister's behalf. Theodor Billroth (1829–94), whose clinic in Vienna was such a favorite with foreign students, publicly came over during the 1870s; it was Billroth above all who developed operations in the upper abdominal area for cancer of the stomach, perforated duodenal ulcers and strictures of the esophagus. Theodor Kocher (1841–1917) was the chief of an internationally famous clinic in Berne; in addition to his careful attention to antiseptic techniques, he was noted as a slow and deliberate operator whose "physiological surgery" was designed to conserve tissues. He was the first surgeon to win a Nobel Prize, in 1909, for his work on the physiology and surgery of the thyroid gland. In a sense the shift from antiseptic to aseptic surgery was gradual and natural. Lister's disciples could claim that the master had actually been advocating aseptic surgery from the beginning, and "physiological surgery" was a recognition that, bacteria apart, the death of tissue around a surgical wound was to be avoided if at all possible. As one surgeon summarized it, "The great antiseptic is life."

By the century's end, the cult of the surgeon had been well and truly launched. Surgery was associated in the public mind not so much with pain and fetid odors, but with science, drama, and heroics. A new phenomenon, the fashionable surgical disease, had emerged. In Britain, these developments are nowhere better symbolized than with the operation on 24 June 1902, two days before his scheduled coronation, of Victoria's son King Edward VII (1841–1910). Edward had taken ill with fever and abdominal pain several days before. The aging Lister was brought in for a consultation and an emergency operation was advised. The King's Serjeant-Surgeon was Frederick Treves (1853–1923), most remembered today for his association with Joseph Merrick, the "Elephant Man." Treves successfully drained an abscess of the King's appendix, an operation that earned Treves a baronetcy from his grateful monarch and did wonders for the diagnosis and surgical treatment of appendicitis.

V. THE THEORY AND PRACTICE OF SCIENTIFIC MEDICINE

A measure of the extent to which cellular pathology, bacteriology, and the other scientific disciplines were basic to disease formulations by the century's end is provided by comparing Robert Graves's *Clinical Lectures* of 1848 with John Syer Bristowe's *Theory and Practice of Medicine* of 1887.

Graves (1796–1853) was one of the Paris-inspired doctors working in Dublin best remembered for his description of the disorder of the thyroid gland known still as Graves's disease. His *Lectures* are a classic of the bedside approach, mildly disparaging of the student who spent too much time on "the fascinating experiments and doctrines of chemistry, electricity, magnetism, and the polarization of light, to the exclusion of the less fascinating but all-necessary subject of disease and its treatment."[5] The "fevers" occupy much of the first volume and despite vivid descriptions of a number of specific contagious diseases, Graves clearly approached the management of "fever" as a general problem.

Bristowe's world had been transformed through, above all, cellular pathology and bacteriology. Bristowe (1827–95) himself had straddled the worlds of community and hospital medicine, combining a long-term appointment of Medical Officer of Health for Camberwell in South London with a medical consultancy at St. Thomas's Hospital. His textbook went through seven editions between 1870 and 1890. He was one of the group of scientifically informed individuals that Simon had gathered around him; Bristowe and a surgical colleague had produced in the early 1860s a massive sanitary survey of the English hospitals, when Simon was concerned about the implications of hospitalism. The pathology of diphtheria and the specificity of cholera were other subjects that Bristowe had studied on behalf of Simon's office. Despite this emphasis on infectious diseases, and Bristowe's openness to bacteriology, his own particular clinical interests lay more with diseases of the nervous system, on which he also wrote a general monograph in 1888. Indeed, it was in neurology that more traditional clinicopathological methods had continued to pay rich dividends, and Bristowe's textbook is replete with descriptions of diseases such as multiple sclerosis, muscular dystrophy, Menière's disease, and poliomyelitis, which had been newly formulated or provided with sufficient distinctiveness to warrant teaching. Next to Virchow, Jean-Martin Charcot (1825–93) was Bristowe's most frequently cited authority. Compared to Graves, Bristowe devoted proportionately more space to chronic disorders. This was not so much a reflection of their enhanced demographic importance as the simple reaction to a growing list of diagnostic categories deemed worth a mention.

For Bristowe, fever was simply a symptom, to be measured with a thermometer ("to the physician almost as important as the stethoscope"), and, although he appreciated the importance of fever as a prognostic indicator, he had little use for the elaborate fever charts that the German physician Carl Wunderlich (1815–77) had popularized in the 1860s. Wunderlich had developed an elaborate thermometry as a diagnostic aid, arguing that many febrile diseases had identifiable patterns of temperature variation over time. Bristowe was able to place more reliance on bacteriology for his diagnostic help.

He prefaced his discussion of the "Specific Febrile Diseases" with an essay on contagion and the dependence of epidemic diseases on specific contagia. The model for those diseases like diphtheria and cholera, whose causative organisms had been established, fit so beautifully the pattern of diseases like smallpox, mumps, measles, yellow fever, and plague, that he had no hesitation in ascribing the causation of each of these disorders to "a contagion." He expected subsequent research to show these contagions to be microorganisms.

Despite Bristowe's easy acceptance of the germ theory, he was no bacteriological imperialist; each infectious disease had to be carefully judged on its own merits. Koch's researches had removed "all reasonable doubt" that pulmonary tuberculosis was contagious, and, although Bristowe did not describe in detail any possible preventive program, he urged the separation of the sick from the well as a first step. More rigorous isolation of tuberculosis patients was to follow early in the next

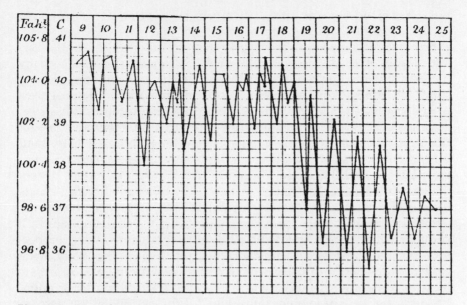

Figure 18. Fever charts have become a routine part of a stay in a modern hospital. They stem from Wunderlich's belief that he could diagnose many specific febrile illnesses by the patterns of the patient's temperature over time. C. A. Wunderlich, On Temperature in Diseases: A Manual of Medical Thermometry *(London: The New Sydenham Society, 1871), Table II, Fig. 3.*

century, though the value of Alpine air was already being touted. In effect, Koch's work justified Bristowe's advocacy of a program of prevention through separation and disinfection, and the importance of prevention was underscored by his therapeutic skepticism: once a diagnosis was made, doctors could do little except treat symptoms as they arose.

Despite the infectious nature of phthisis, Bristowe included it under the diseases of the respiratory organs instead of one of the specific febrile diseases. These latter apart, his arrangement of diseases was entirely system-based: skin and respiratory, cardiovascular, digestive, genitourinary, musculoskeletal, and nervous systems. He included what would shortly be termed as the endocrine glands under the "vascular organs," which also encompassed the heart.

Among diseases of the heart, affections of the valves occupied pride of place, especially because he believed them to be a major cause of cardiac hypertrophy. He provided full stethoscopic guidelines for diagnosing the murmurs of valvular lesions and was aware of what would eventually be called the "physiological murmurs" of increased cardiac output, as after exercise, during pregnancy, or in anemic patients. He regarded cardiac hypertrophy as a compensatory mechanism to some underlying problem; this could include "undue resistance" to the expulsion of blood from the cardiac chambers, but the clinical measurement of blood pressure was not part of his world.

Bristowe recognized the association of pericarditis with pyemia, scarlatina, and other diseases that he identified among those caused by bacteria, but his discussion of both pericarditis and endocarditis was couched entirely in terms of nonspecific inflammation. The prognosis of endocarditis was "very serious," with recovery rarely taking place. This was partly because inflamed valves set up a situation favorable for the formation and expulsion of emboli to the lungs, brain, kidneys, and other vital organs. Myocarditis was, he believed, rarely seen except in consequence of either endo- or pericarditis. However, under "degeneration of the muscular walls," as well as "cardiac aneurysms," "ruptures of the heart," and "cardiac neuralgia" we can recognize both the clinical symptoms and postmortem changes that we now associate with cardiovascular disease and acute myocardial infarctions. "Angina pectoris" was for Bristowe essentially cardiac neuralgia without any direct evidence of a specific cardiac lesion. He advocated the use of amyl nitrate in treating the anginal attack, which, following Thomas Lauder Brunton, he attributed to "spasmodic contraction" of the peripheral arteries.

Although Bristowe described several irregularities of the pulse in his section on heart diseases, he was in many ways less interested in the pulse than Graves had been, or than members of the next generation of physicians such as Sir James MacKenzie (1853–1925) would be. The "new cardiology" that developed, first around MacKenzie and his "polygraph" and later around Sir Thomas Lewis (1881–1945) and the electrocardiograph, was much more functional in its approach to diseases of the heart. MacKenzie's *The Study of the Pulse* (1902) was one of the early salvos in this new approach to heart disease; Bristowe's was a good summary of the older, pathologically oriented tradition.

More generally, Bristowe's whole textbook displayed throughout the extent to which chemistry, microscopy, cellular pathology, and bacteriology had been the key sciences for the clinical medicine of his lifetime. This is not to say that Bristowe had no appreciation of experimental physiology; but the direct impact of the work of Bernard, Ludwig, and their physiological colleagues is harder to discern. Bristowe's physiology of digestion rested mostly on the chemical approach of Prout and his successors; Ludwig's work on the circulation or urinary excretion was never mentioned, and Bernard rated three references, as opposed to thirty-five for Virchow, seven for Pasteur, and five for Koch.

The other striking feature of Bristowe's textbook is its therapeutic realism. Throughout, he emphasized symptomatic management rather than cure, although he recognized that many diseases are self-limited. For only a small handful of diseases could specific medicines or diet "materially alleviate" or cure. As he summarized it: "The great aim of medical art is the cure of disease. Unfortunately, however, a direct cure (at all events a direct cure by means of drugs) in the great majority of cases is totally impossible."[6] In a sense, one of the consequences of his medical science was the recognition of the limitations of his medical art.

6

Medical science goes public

Science is more cosmopolitan than Art.

Lancet, 6 August 1881

I. INTERNATIONALISM AND ITS DISCONTENTS

On 3 August 1881, twenty years before Frederick Treves drained the abscess from King Edward's appendix, the Prince of Wales (as Edward was then known) declared the Seventh International Medical Congress officially open. Like a rite de passage, this ceremony definitively ushered medical science onto the international public stage. The London Congress was not the first such occasion, of course; even before the series of international medical congresses had been inaugurated in Paris in 1867, there had been regular international gatherings in a number of medical and scientific disciplines, including statistics (1851), hygiene and demography (1852), and ophthalmology (1857). Before World War I, most scientific and clinical subjects had their international forums where colleagues could be met, ideas exchanged, and speeches heard proclaiming the capacity of objective scientific knowledge to transcend the divisiveness of multiple languages and the competitiveness of nations. The formation of the Red Cross in 1863 and the signing of the first Geneva Convention in the following year were further testimony to the transnational humanism of medicine and its underlying sciences.

Even within this context, however, the London Congress was special, in both its participation and its visibility. There were more than 3,000 delegates from some seventy countries ("every land in which scientific

Figure 19. Commemorative photographs like this were commonly taken during medical or scientific congresses of the nineteenth century, and were often used as part of the publicity in the reporting of the event. Sometimes they were composed rather than posed, with some individual pictures of delegates cut and pasted onto larger frameworks. There are, however, many actual group photographs of doctors and medical scientists attending meetings. The backdrop of this 1881 International Medical Congress was probably St. James's Hall, in the center of London. It was used for other international gatherings in London. Photographed by H. R. Barraud.

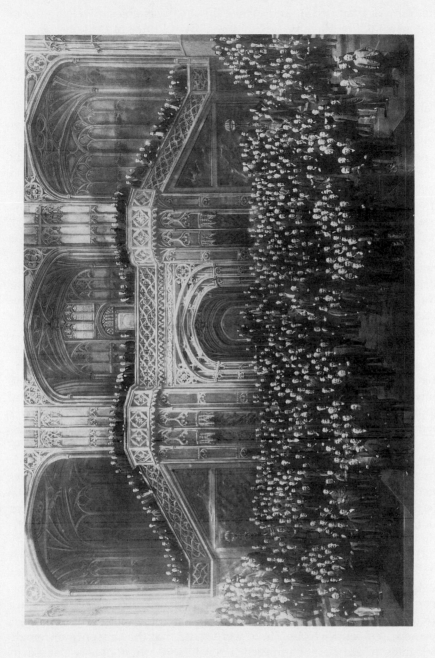

medicine is practised"), and Prince Edward was able to welcome (and dine with) fellow Royalty – Wilhelm, Crown Prince of Prussia – as well as many of the stars of the medical firmament: Virchow, Kölliker, and Koch from Germany; Pasteur and Charcot from France; Lister, Sir James Paget (President of the Congress), and Simon from Great Britain; John Shaw Billings from the United States; and a youthful William Osler from Canada. In addition to several plenary sessions, where men like Virchow and T. H. Huxley spoke, there were fifteen specialist sections representing key areas of medical science and practice. Delegates were entertained in style by prominent citizens, such as the Lord Mayor of London and the wealthy philanthropist Baroness Burdett-Coutts, and by the medical corporations such as the Royal Colleges of Physicians and of Surgeons (although the soirée at the Royal College of Surgeons was something of a failure because the newly installed electric lighting cast an unfamiliar, eerie light on the occasion). There were excursions to Folkestone, Kent, where a new statue of William Harvey was unveiled, and to the Crystal Palace, to which the remains of another international event, the Great Exhibition of 1851, had been removed. Foreign journalists were there, *The Times* (London) devoted some thirty-five columns to reporting it, the medical press even more. Four fat volumes of *Transactions* were published before the year's end.

The message of the Congress was clearly stated by the *Lancet:* "It has demonstrated to the world the progress that medicine has recently made, that it is advancing because it has become more scientific, and that the only great advances yet in store for it must result from the successful application of the same methods."[1] Among other events, David Ferrier had demonstrated his pioneering research on cerebral localization, Richard Volkmann had reviewed the impact of Listerianism on surgical results, Robert Koch had shown his new solid-medium methods for growing bacteria, and Louis Pasteur had reported on his latest achievements in producing vaccines. Charcot was especially impressed with Ferrier's contribution and Pasteur told Koch, "C'est un grand progrès monsieur." Medical science and internationalism could be seen marching hand in hand.

There were, to be sure, a few rough edges. Women, despite a protest "by forty-three duly qualified medical women," were not permitted to register as delegates, and the organizing committee had to issue a statement that the decision to exclude women was not the result of pressure from the Congress's patron (and opponent of medical education for women), Queen Victoria. There were hints that the presence of female delegates might have hampered a resolution, unanimously passed in the closing session, stressing the importance of animals for medical research and deploring any restrictions on their use by competent researchers. The resolution itself was an international show of solidarity behind the British research community still coming to terms with the 1876 Cruelty to Animals Act (see Section VI). Medical research was to benefit further from the Congress, since the surplus generated by the meeting was turned over to a committee, chaired by Lister, which used it to provide expenses for those pursuing research.

At the same time, delegates would have been aware that, beneath the rhetoric of cooperation and collective progress, nationalism and competition could also be part of the medical enterprise. Franco-German rivalries had predated, but also had been intensified by, the Franco-Prussian War of 1870–1. As the State became an increasingly important patron of scientific research and education, and as the research base – especially in German chemical, optical, and pharmaceutical industries – became more obviously tied to economic growth, the political dimensions of science and its technologies came to the fore. King Edward did not live to see World War I, but Kaiser Wilhelm (as the Crown Prince became) did, and formal relationships between Britain and Germany had already deteriorated during the Boer War of 1899–1902. By then, imperialism was in full swing, as most of the major European nations strove to get their share of unclaimed parts of the undeveloped world. Africa was the principal hunting ground, since the British had already managed to claim so much of the rest of the globe.

Consequently, it was in the new specialism of tropical medicine that the competitive spirit was probably most ardent, because it was widely held by the century's close that the successful colonization of tropical latitudes would be furthered by the control of indigenous diseases. Even earlier, however, bacteriology and what was being called immunology had schools and rivalries that had as much to do with personal and national allegiances as they did with science. Pasteur's flattering comments to Koch at the London Congress were undoubtedly genuine, but differences between their approaches, scientific styles, and personalities were beginning to surface, and the two men became irreparably estranged at another international gathering (on hygiene and demography) the following year, 1882, by which time Koch was basking in the glory of his discovery of the tubercle bacillus. Eventually they quarreled about anthrax, about laboratory techniques, about vaccines, about priorities. When the cholera expeditions of 1883 ended with a French death and a German triumph, Pasteurians were appalled on both counts and were indignant when, during a cholera outbreak in France in 1884, the French government had the audacity to ask Koch to investigate it. ("France . . . does not have any need for the services of a German scientist," a leading newspaper proclaimed.) For his part, Koch blocked for a while the use in Germany of Pasteur's rabies vaccine. In general, the French did not send troops of students to the laboratories and polytechnics of Germany, and Pasteur had few German disciples. He made a point of stating publicly that he did not read German, and Koch's spoken French was rudimentary.

At the century's end, Alfred Nobel (1835–96), a Swede who had made his fortune from dynamite and smokeless blasting powder, left his estates to further the cause of internationalism and progress. Three out of five Nobel Prizes were in science (chemistry, physics, medicine or physiology, along with literature and peace). Hitherto, most scientific awards had been national in their orientation, even if foreign scientists were often awarded them (along with honorary membership in local or national groups). Nobel's vision was different, encouraging nominations from abroad (although Scandinavian institutions made the final choice) and seeking deliberately to foster good will among men (the prizes were supposed to be awarded to "those who, during the preceding year, shall have conferred the greatest benefit on mankind"). That the majority of the prizes were for science reflects Nobel's belief that benefit for mankind came principally from that source.

Certainly, Nobel's idea caught on and from the earliest days both the announcement of the recipients and the award ceremony itself have been newsworthy. However, the selection of only the second Nobel Laureate for medicine – Ronald Ross (1857–1932) – raised a storm of protest from both the French and the Italians, who believed that others had been equally or more important in the research for which the Englishman Ross was chosen – the role of the mosquito in the transmission of malaria.

More was at stake than merely reputation in tropical issues, for the bacteriological success of the 1880s encouraged a vision in which colonization and disease control could go together hand in hand. Malaria was one of the most important of these, especially because, unlike some "tropical" diseases such as sleeping sickness and schistosomiasis, which preferentially affected indigenous populations, malaria wreaked havoc among Europeans who found themselves in the malarious districts of the world.

II. TROPICAL MEDICINE

The relationship between climate and patterns of disease had been a medical preoccupation since Hippocratic times, and generations of experience had reinforced the perception that the tropics were many a white man's grave. The cholera pandemics had linked East and West (and the Middle East) in a trail of death and had blunted any comfort Western Europeans could take in the retreat of plague and malaria. The latter, however, was still a problem around the Mediterranean basin and continued to hamper colonial and imperial aspirations in Asia, Africa, and Central and South America. Plague, too, had never disappeared from Asia and the Near East, and an outbreak in China in the 1890s was the beginning of a pandemic that spread devastatingly to India and caused some mortality and much concern in Europe and the United States, where an epidemic in 1900 in San Francisco introduced the dreaded disease to those shores. It returned to San Francisco after the fire of 1906.

Yellow fever was another disease that, though most deadly in tropical and subtropical climates, refused to conform to a simple pattern as a "tropical disease." It had spread along the Eastern seaboard during the early American Republic, and continued throughout the nineteenth century to exert high mortality in the Southern United States, especially in sea and river ports such as Mobile, New Orleans, and Memphis. Occasional outbreaks in French and British ports between the 1840s and 1870s created alarm and puzzlement because its patterns of spread did not conform to any known model. It was always a threat in Western Africa and the Caribbean and Central America, where its prevalence defeated the first attempts to cut a canal through the Isthmus of Panama and where it was a leading cause of death during the Spanish-American War. Leprosy, which had been common throughout Western Europe during the Middle Ages, had curiously retreated to the colder climates of Scandinavia, but also maintained its horrifying presence in Asia, Africa, the Pacific Islands, and the warmer parts of the Americas. Norwegian immigrants even brought it to the American Midwest.

Each of these diseases was "tropical" in the sense that it was more common in warm than cold climates. Other diseases – kala-azar in India and Africa, bilharziasis in the Nile Valley, sleeping sickness in the African savannas – seemed to be confined mostly to hot climates, and mostly to indigenous populations.

Traditionally, explanations had been offered within the broad framework of miasmatic environmentalism, although no easy solutions were apparent to link the distribution and chronicity of a disease like leprosy to the acute manifestations of cholera, seen to originate in India yet spreading, wavelike, to the colder climates of Russia and Northern European cities such as Hamburg. Throughout the nineteenth century, what became known as tropical medicine was literally concerned, despite the anomalies, with "diseases of warm climates." Countries such as Britain, Spain, and Holland, with military, economic, or imperial aspirations in tropical lands, were most concerned with the range of diseases to be found there, especially as they affected the health and lives of their armed forces, civil servants, and businessmen. For example, the East India Company maintained a sizeable medical establishment that became the Indian Medical Service when the British government assumed firmer control of India after the Indian Mutiny of 1857–8. "Western Medicine" had always been considered superior to the indigenous written and oral medical traditions found in Asia, Africa, and the Americas and a few attempts throughout the century were made to establish medical schools and hospitals on Western lines to train and treat non-Europeans; sanitary measures were also applied with various degrees of vigor and success to urban areas of Asia, the Middle East, and Africa. Missionaries had frequently carried medicines and, less frequently, microscopes along with their Bibles – Dr. Livingstone was, if not actually a doctor of medicine, at least trained in medicine. His exploits as an explorer and adventurer made him newsworthy to the *New York Herald* reporter, H. M. Stanley, and his readers, but it was missions and medicine that had taken Livingstone to Africa in the first place.

From the middle of the nineteenth century, two matters helped shape what came to be called tropical medicine. The first was the intensification of imperial rivalries as, somewhat belatedly, other European nations and the United States emulated Britain in creating overseas empires on which their suns, too, might never set. New demands for raw materials and the desire for favored overseas markets, combined with more rapid and cheaper long-distance transport, fostered an intensely competitive spirit in Europe and the United States, which was often pursued in the ideological framework of struggle and social Darwinism. Africa, the Dark Continent, was the largest prize up for grabs, with Germany, France, Holland, and Belgium vying with Britain for a stake in the spoils; the United States feared Spanish influence in the New World and sought actively for its own empire and a controlling share of the seas. Much of the land still available for imperial purposes had tropical climates and tropical diseases.

The second factor was the increased capacity of medicine to aid in Christianizing, civilizing, commercializing, or simply dominating, these vast territories. Doctors of course subscribed to a gospel of medical progress throughout the century; the various successes of the public health movement and, above all, the technological and scientific potentials of bacteriology, impressed even governments of the possibilities of controlling what had previously been called filth diseases but were now germ diseases. If medicine could tame the diseases that were rampant in the tropics, it had undoubted political force as a tool of empire, and the country with the most advanced medical capabilities stood the greatest chance of success in the hostile environments of Africa, Southeast Asia, and the Caribbean. When Joseph Chamberlain (1836–1914) became Secretary of Britain's Colonial Office in 1895, he had no doubt that disease understanding and control was an indispensable part of the imperial mission. One of his earliest moves was to secure the appointment of (Sir) Patrick Manson (1844–1922) as Medical Advisor to the Colonial Office; Chamberlain was also to throw government opinion and resources behind Manson's efforts, a few years later, to establish a School of Tropical Medicine in London.

Manson, a Scot, had gone to the Far East in 1866 as a Customs Medical Officer; during a dozen years in Amoy, off the coast of Southeast China, he published important work on the causative role of *Filaria* – a nematode worm – in elephantiasis, the chronic disfiguring disease that through blockage of lymph flow could lead to massive swelling of the limbs and genitalia. Manson also implicated the bite of the mosquito in the spread of the filarial parasites to human beings, the first time an insect had been shown to be part of a cycle of the natural history of a disease, and his introduction of mosquito nets was useful in preventing elephantiasis.

In 1883, Manson settled in Hong Kong, where he helped establish a medical school and served as the first Dean. Back in England in 1889, he became a successful London consulting physician, specializing in the diseases contracted by Europeans in tropical climates and securing a post as physician to the Seaman's Hospital, a charity that had long provided inpatient care for sick merchant sailors. He turned this association to good advantage, since it offered a clinical facility for the School of Tropical Medicine, which he was instrumental in establishing in 1899. The year previously, he had published a textbook in the subject, *Tropical Diseases. A Manual of the Diseases of Warm Climates*. In the way of these things, the direct descendent of Manson's book is a multiauthored affair, but it is still in print a century later.

Manson was by inclination more a natural historian of disease, and a parasitologist, than a straightforward clinician (despite the fact that he worked as a general practitioner in Amoy), and he stamped his vision of tropical medicine on the specialism, especially in Britain but to a certain extent throughout Europe and America. What was distinct about the discipline was its parasitological dimension. Manson recognized, of course, that diseases like cholera, plague, and even leprosy were bacteriological, but by the end of the century, many of the distinct diseases of warm climates had been implicated with other classes of organisms: schistosomiasis by another class of worms, the trematodes *Bilharzia;* sleeping sickness by a *Trypanosome*, a protozoan; the common form of tropical dysentery by an amoeba; and malaria by another genus of protozoans, the *Plasmodium*. Initially, bacteriology was not even taught in Manson's School of Tropical Medicine, not because it was not an important subject for medical officers destined for service in tropical climates to know, but because it was already available in the various medical schools and departments of public health where potential students would previously have studied.

Nevertheless, the extent to which bacteriology was widely seen as a French or German science gave the British some comfort: tropical medicine was still there to be colonized. Not only were other groups of organisms besides bacteria implicated, the chains of infection were often more complicated than the water, food, milk, or air-borne diseases of temperate climates. Manson never forgot that his most systematic research efforts concerned worms whose complicated disease-causing life cycles also involved mosquitoes.

He was also the patron of the other man who was instrumental in establishing tropical diseases as a medical specialism: Ronald Ross. Manson in 1894 had already announced his conviction that malaria, a disease with much more widespread social, political, and economic implications than elephantiasis, was also spread by mosquitoes. It was the same year that Ross was on furlough in England from the Indian Medical Service, where he had served since 1881. Ross had already been studying malaria, but it was Manson who convinced his younger colleague that the disease was caused by the parasite that the French microbiologist Charles Laveran (1845–1922) had identified in the blood of malaria patients as long ago as 1880, and also that he, Manson, was correct in his hypothesis that the malaria parasite was spread by mosquitoes.

Ross returned to India in 1895, determined to provide the experimental and clinical proof of Manson's ideas. From London, Manson acted as Ross's agent and advisor: writing long and encouraging letters, arranging for the publication of Ross's reports in important medical journals, demonstrating specimens Ross sent home to influential medical men such as Lister, by then President of the Royal Society, and seeking to secure from Ross's superiors resources and, above all, research time from his mundane medical and administrative duties. The problems were hardly straightforward, involving as they did a complicated interaction between the life cycle of the *Plasmodium* and the clinical disease, the existence of more than one form of the organism capable of causing the different forms of malaria (tertian, quartan, etc.), and the slowly dawning realization that not all species of mosquitoes can act as vectors in the chain of disease.

Between 1895 and 1898, Ross succeeded in demonstrating, to Manson and a number of other key scientists' satisfaction, that the mosquito is an invariable agent in the transmission of malaria; in addition, he worked out, in an animal model using birds, the detailed relationship between the *Plasmodium* life cycle and disease. Independently, and virtually simultaneously, Giovanni Grassi (1854–1925), working with his fellow Italian Amico Bignami (1862–1929), related human malaria to the *Anopheles* mosquito and showed that this mosquito becomes first infected itself through feeding off the blood of a human being with the *Plasmodium* parasite in his bloodstream. As Manson had written to Ross in 1895, "Laveran is inclined to take up the mosquito hypothesis, and I have no doubt that by next summer the French and Italians will be working at it. So for goodness' sake hurry up and save the laurels for old England."[2] The priority dispute between Grassi and Ross was hardly solved when, in 1902, the Nobel Committee chose to award the Prize for Medicine or Physiology to Ross alone. Not that the Nobel Prize brought Ross much inner peace: though he had by then settled permanently back in Britain, and though he continued to involve himself in various international malaria eradication programs, Ross remained convinced that medical research in general, and his own talents in particular, were insufficiently appreciated, and inadequately rewarded, by the British government and public. (Incidentally, the Nobel Committee made amends to Laveran by awarding him the 1907 Prize for the original discovery of the malaria parasite; Grassi was never placated.)

The same year (1898) that Ross and Grassi were sparring for laurels in their malaria research, the Spanish-American War pitted an old and a new imperial power against each other. The war lasted less than four months and the Americans got their toehold in the Caribbean, Central America, and the Far East with little damage from Spanish bullets. Typhoid and yellow fever were another matter and the appalling military mortality from disease led to the establishment in 1900 of an Army Yellow Fever Commission. For some years, a local Havana doctor, Carlos Finlay (1833–1915), had been advocating a mosquito-borne theory of yellow fever spread, based on experiments with volunteers, whereby healthy subjects were bitten by mosquitoes that had subsequently fed on yellow fever victims. The volunteers regularly came down with the disease, although it was possible to discount Finlay's evidence, since he had used no controls and had taken only minimal precautions to protect his volunteers from other possible sources of infection between the bite and the development of symptoms. Various bacteria had been proposed as probable causative agents, though no agreement had been reached.

The Yellow Fever Commission, which included among its members Walter Reed (1851–1902), had the cooperation of Finlay and the Chief Sanitary Officer in Havana, the American military doctor William Gorgas (1845–1920). With the work of Ross and Grassi so recent, it is not surprising that the Commission took Finlay's mosquito hypothesis so seriously, operating in the time-honored way of subjecting under controlled conditions, healthy volunteers to mosquitoes that had previously bitten yellow fever patients. This time another species of mosquito, *Aedes aegypti*, was shown to be involved. Despite the accidental infection and death of one of the Commissioners, Jesse Lazear (1866–1900), the laboratory and field studies were sufficiently compelling to encourage Gorgas to begin a mosquito eradication program in Havana. The results there and in the Panama Zone were a dramatic vindication of those who claimed that, without medical science, the conquest of the tropics was impossible.

There were those who still believed that "tropical medicine" was simply the application of the methods and techniques of bacteriology to infectious diseases in the tropics. Against this, Manson always argued that the scientific roots of the discipline lay in biology: in the biology of the flora and fauna of the tropics, in parasitology, helminthology, and entomology, to name but three biological specialisms. Within a few years of the foundation of the London School and its rival in Liverpool, institutions were established in France (three), Germany, Italy, Belgium, and the United States. The imperial dimension often jostled with the idealism of internationalism. Thus, British doctors were annoyed when the British Colonial Office invited Robert Koch to Africa in 1896, and again in 1902, to study outbreaks of economically disastrous diseases in cattle. In fact, Koch spent much of the period from 1896 to 1907 in Africa, with varying success, studying malaria and sleeping sickness as well as several diseases of animals. It was almost as if, for him, the excitement had gone out of simple Old World bacteriology.

Because imperial concerns were public, so was tropical medicine. The discipline's achievements between 1890 and World War I were impressive: so impressive that it was possible at the time to say that medicine itself justified imperialism. If claims that diseases such as malaria, sleeping sickness, and cholera would soon be eradicated were naive; if concern was only slowly and grudgingly shifted from European settlers to whole populations; if the extent to which health and socioeconomic circumstances were inextricably linked was only dimly appreciated; nevertheless, tropical medicine – its concepts, techniques, and technology – showed itself of much more than casual importance. If nothing else, it taught the public still in Europe or America to beware of flies and mosquitoes, ticks and lice, all of which had been shown to be vectors of disease. Among other things, it made window screens and fly swatters a part of modern life.

III. RESEARCH INSTITUTIONS

International scientific jamborees, declining mortality statistics, and dramatic tales of dangerous experiments, a few of which led to martyrs' deaths, were not the only things that announced the public presence of medical science. Bricks and mortar played their part as well. For a generation increasingly comfortable with the idea of warfare between science and religion, or the positivistic ideal that science would dispel superstition and create heaven on earth, the notion of sanctuaries of science would seem quite natural. Between 1890 and World War I, the German research institute took root abroad, though not without adaptation to new habitats.

The German institutes had, as we have seen, grown up with attach-

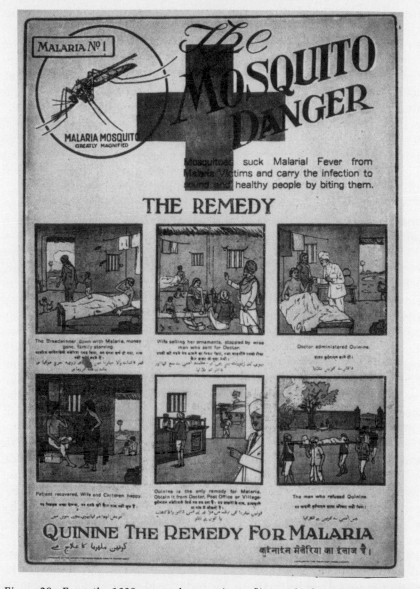

Figure 20. From the 1890s onward, mosquitoes, flies, and other insect transmitters of disease were often pictured in both medical and lay publications. This educational leaflet would have been unusual in the period before World War I, in that its message was directed at the native population. "The Mosquito Danger," anonymous, Malaria and Quinine *(Amsterdam: Bureau for Increasing the Use of Quinine, 1927), p. 48, Plate 29.*

ments to universities and this continued to be a common pattern in the period of further growth and consolidation. Robert Koch was associated with no fewer than four institutes in Berlin, the last three built more or less with Koch in mind. The third, erected at the height of the tuberculosis excitement, was expensive, even lavish; its annual budget equalled the total research budgets of all the other departments of the University of Berlin. Although the money was provided by Parliament, this Institute of Infectious Diseases had a great deal of autonomy, and Koch, as director, was able to resign his formal position with the University to concentrate entirely on research. Elsewhere in Germany, local government was prepared to chip in to attract internationally famous scientists such as Paul Ehrlich (see Section IV) to their communities.

The City Fathers of Paris also recognized that they had a treasure in Louis Pasteur, though the local and national state contribution to the Pasteur Institute consisted primarily of the building site and a fraction of its building costs. Much of the money was raised by public subscription at home and abroad. Major benefactors included the Russian Czar, the Emperor of Brazil, and a Sultan. Because rabies treatment facilities were combined at the Institute with research laboratories, and because British patients could receive rabies treatment there, a campaign was mounted for the British Government to make an official contribution. While this faltered, the Prince of Wales (who had visited the Institute shortly before its official opening on 14 November 1889) made a personal contribution of £100, to which others joined. A British Rabies Commission had examined Pasteur's rabies treatment and although somewhat concerned with the difficulty of evaluating the success of his program (it was impossible to tell how many of the individuals treated with the rabies vaccine would, untreated, have developed the disease), both the dread of the disease and the saintliness of the vaccine's inventor made the Institute an attractive object of philanthropy. The public was not simply supporting the rabies treatment center, of course, but the research laboratories as well, the three sections of which were headed by the devoted Pasteurians, Emile Duclaux, Pierre Roux, and Charles Edouard Chamberland.

Pasteur actually wanted his Institute to be independent of the State and without official attachment to a university medical school, so the fact that it was largely financed by individual gifts and benefactions pleased him. Its structures and functions were duplicated in a series of Pasteur Institutes elsewhere in France and in French dominions overseas. It also provided the principal stimulus for the endowment of an analogous research establishment in Britain, successively named the British Institute for Preventive Medicine (1891), the Jenner Institute of Preventive Medicine (1898), and the Lister Institute of Preventive Medicine (1903). When, in the flush of enthusiasm over the Pasteur Institute

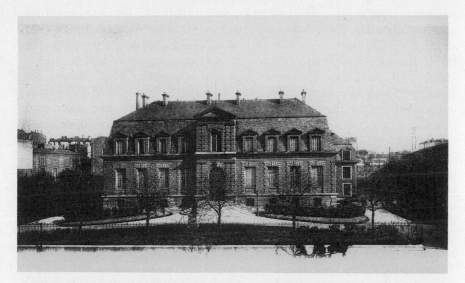

Figure 21. The Institut Pasteur *became Pasteur's monument: the site of his apartment, his laboratories, and, ultimately, his tomb.* Institut Pasteur: Cinquantenaire de la Fondation, 14 Nov. 1888–14 Nov. 1938 *(Paris: 1939).*

in Paris, British doctors, scientists, and well-disposed laymen decided to launch a campaign to endow an institution for medical research in Britain, they considered naming it after the French *savant*. It was decided against, partly because both government and scientific opinion favored the muzzling of dogs, and their quarantine if imported from abroad, as the most effective means of stamping out rabies in island Britain, so any close association with rabies would be inappropriate. In addition, Pasteur, a hero to many, was the object of vilification among antivivisection groups. The inclusion of "Preventive Medicine" in the title was meant to deflect attention from the use of experimental animals that the research activities of the Institute ultimately involved.

Charity giving for hospitals, dispensaries, and other aspects of medical care was well established; not so for medical research, as early targets for endowments were woefully overoptimistic. Under the Jenner banner, less than 6 percent of the target was reached after two years, and almost all of that amount had come from three donations. A single massive benefaction was made in 1898 by Lord Iveagh (1847–1917), the Irish brewer (whose family name was Guinness) and philanthropist. Ironically, his decision was prompted largely because one of his workmen had been bitten by a rabid dog and was successfully treated in Paris.

The Lister Institute was situated in London with no university attachment, although at one stage a close association with the Pathology Department of the University of Cambridge had been on the cards. Since laboratory space was still in short supply in Britain, the Lister Institute accommodated a good many external workers in addition to its own small scientific staff, which in 1900 numbered only a handful. At one level, the Lister was an outstanding success, its very existence as a substantial, purpose-built research facility in a prime location near the Thames in London, financed by private charity, testifying to an increasing awareness by the public of the symbiosis of medical research and practice. The Lister's research record justified the confidence, since some important work in bacteriology, immunology, physiology, biochemistry, and nutrition was produced there. At another level, its failure to raise much money in small donations from ordinary members of the public suggests that medical research, as opposed to its dramatic applications in treating disease, was less valued. Without Lord Iveagh, the Lister might well have disappeared before World War I. The hospitals themselves were also anxious clearly to separate any teaching and research activities from patient care, believing that only the latter was capable of attracting sustained charitable giving.

For the scientifically oriented medical community, this meant it was even more important for the State to provide funds for research. A science lobby began to use the pages of journals such as *Nature* (founded in 1869), the *British Medical Journal*, and *The Lancet* to argue the case for scientific and medical research, often against the backdrop of international competition, and to court sympathetic Members of Parliament. Modest achievements such as a Grant-in-Aid scheme administered by the Royal Society, or the Colonial Office money to assist the School of Tropical Medicine, were capped by the building of a National Physical Laboratory, modeled to a certain extent on the German *Physikalisch-Technische Reichsanstalt*, and opened in 1902 with a staff of twenty-six; and by a genuine British innovation, the creation in 1912 of a Medical Research Committee (now Medical Research Council, MRC), with a budget derived from a fraction of the income collected through the National Health Insurance scheme (see Chapter 7). The clause initiating the MRC seems to have been tacked on as an afterthought to the National Health Insurance Act (it is not even certain whose idea it was), but the money dramatically increased the sums available for medical research in Britain. Originally, the money was to be devoted entirely to tuberculosis research, but the Committee quickly widened the brief and although World War I delayed the building of the laboratories, staff appointments were quickly made, several of whom used the facilities of the Lister Institute during the War.

The structure of institutionalized medical research in the United States was also established in embryo before 1914. As in Britain and France, the American government was early on a reluctant patron of medical research, although the bacteriological laboratory attached to the Marine

Hospital, Staten Island, New York, established in 1866, had a continuous history that, with moves and name changes, became in 1930 the National Institute of Health in Bethesda. Various state governments, notably New York and Massachusetts, started public health laboratories, where, in addition to routine diagnostic and analytical work, some research was carried out.

More than in any other country, however, the medical research ethos in the United States was shaped by private philanthropy and by those who advised the philanthropists, especially Andrew Carnegie (1835–1918), John D. Rockefeller (1839–1937), and his son John, Jr. (1874–1960). Carnegie, Scottish-born, went to Pittsburgh with his family in 1848 and made his fortune in iron and steel. A disciple of Herbert Spencer and his gospel of competitive social evolution, Carnegie was also firmly committed to education, social meliorism, and world peace. He left his name on dozens of public libraries and several research institutes, of which the one in Washington was perhaps the most significant. Medicine itself was never the preoccupation with Carnegie that it became for the various branches of the Rockefeller philanthropic enterprises, but the Carnegie Institution of Washington, founded in 1902, contained facilities and administered grants for research in the life sciences, including embryology, which cut across medicine. In addition, Carnegie sponsored and published the investigations of Abraham Flexner (1866–1959) into the condition of medical education in North America and Europe.

The Carnegie Corporation, established to oversee the various facets of Carnegie's largesse, commanded vast sums, but even these were dwarfed by the size of Rockefeller's pockets. The elder Rockefeller had made his money in oil. A devout Baptist, much of his early philanthropy had been religious in character. The University of Chicago, the object of some of his earliest and most sustained bequests, was a Baptist institution even as it was using Rockefeller money to create a secular research orientation, especially in the sciences and social sciences. It was a Baptist minister, Frederick T. Gates (1853–1929), who guided Rockefeller's early giving and convinced Rockefeller, whose personal physician was then a homeopath, that medical research was a good investment. Gates had read William Osler's *Principles and Practice of Medicine* (1st ed., 1892), with its elegant descriptions of disease and its quietly pessimistic account of their treatments, and decided that money could do something about it.

With the exception that it was endowed by an individual rather than the State, the Rockefeller Institute for Medical Research (1901) was one of the most Germanic of such institutes established outside Germany. Its goals were to be pure research, a prior flirtation with the University of Chicago to be its parent being rejected partly because a university would, potentially, impose pedagogical compromises on staff time. Instead, it became an independent establishment in New York City. Private practice was also strictly forbidden to Rockefeller medical staff, in the greater interests of new scientific discoveries. Abraham Flexner's brother Simon (1863–1946) was appointed director of laboratories, a position that made him de facto director of the Institute itself. Like a good many of the first generation of American medical scientists, Simon Flexner was a student of William Welch, who had followed his master's advice in studying also in Europe. Flexner was a good if not world-class laboratory scientist who had isolated the *Shigella* organism (a common cause of dysentery), and did important work on the serum treatment of meningitis. He succeeded Welch as the editor of the principal American medical journal of international standing, the *Journal of Experimental Medicine*. Even more crucially in the longer run, he encouraged Rockefeller (and Gates) to consider the Rockefeller Institute as an establishment with a wide research brief, and not simply in the infectious diseases, as was more common at the time. Consequently, the Institute found a place for individuals like Jacques Loeb (1859–1924), who approached physiology from the standpoint of general biology, and Peyton Rous (1879–1970), who worked on many aspects of cancer.

Despite the more eclectic approach that evolved at the Rockefeller Institute, most of the independent research establishments founded in the decades after 1880 quite naturally concentrated their activities on the infectious diseases. Even the Rockefeller Institute garnered more publicity through Flexner's work on meningitis and polio than it did from Loeb's researches on biological tropisms or the material basis of behavior. As a by-product of this emphasis, many of the institutes also became engaged in the marketplace, for, even without the rewards of individual private practice, the new discipline of immunology brought with it a train of lucrative prophylactic and therapeutic measures, in the form of vaccines and serum and antitoxin therapy. Medical research could pay dividends, financial as well as conceptual.

IV. IMMUNOLOGY

Most of the early medical research institutes concentrated entirely or in large part on infectious diseases. At the same time, most of them were more than simply research establishments, for by the 1890s, the economic potentials of microbiology had been recognized. The Pasteur Institute was typical in involving itself not simply with research into disease mechanisms but also with the production, sale, and administration of a whole range of "biologicals": vaccines and antisera to prevent or treat infections. Indeed, some research institutes were little more than production units, applying on an enhanced scale the scientific and technological directives of microbiology and the related but increasingly autonomous discipline of immunology. Science and profit were inextricably mixed, even when the income from vaccines and serum products merely went to support the work of the institute itself, as it did at the Pasteur.

The word "immunity" and its Latin roots originally carried the legal connotation of exemption, for example, from military service or taxation. Its medical use, as exemption or freedom from a particular disease, was an obvious extension, though not one commonly adopted until the 1880s. By then, several of the phenomena that immunological theories sought to explain had been encountered in the course of work on the mechanisms of infection and resistance to it. Pasteur, ever sensitive to the delicate nutritional requirements of microorganisms, had originally postulated that both attenuation of a parasite and resistance of a host were related to nutritional circumstances, the microorganism losing its capacity to infect because it could no longer grow and reproduce. Implicit in this was the assumption that the intact microorganism – in the case of bacteria a single cell – was the infective agent and that the more of them there were, the heavier the infection. Anthrax, where the large bacillus could be found relatively easily through the microscopic examination of the blood of infected animals, was an important early model for the germ theory.

Pasteur himself was in the 1870s and early 80s more interested in the techniques of vaccine production than the theoretical reasons why vaccines protected (or immunized). However, in 1884, Elie Metchnikoff (1845–1916) observed a phenomenon, first in the water flea (*Daphnia*), then in the starfish, which he called phagocytosis, and subsequently developed this into a full-blown cellular theory of immunity and resistance. Metchnikoff, a peripatetic and emotional Russian zoologist, observed amoebalike cells in these lower organisms attracted to, and seeming to ingest, foreign substances, such as fungi or pieces of thorn. He had already done much work on evolutionary relationships, and, in a fit of inspiration, it occurred to him that these amoebalike cells in *Daphnia* might be primitive analogues of the pus cells of the inflammatory response of higher organisms. Microscopical observations on animals infected with various microorganisms, among them, inevitably, the anthrax bacillus, revealed white blood cells attacking, ingesting, and appearing to digest, these living germs of disease. Metchnikoff likened the white blood cells to a nation's army, "fighting infection" thereby becoming a literal description of the body's response to disease.

Metchnikoff's ideas had dramatic popular appeal; Pasteur liked them, too, the more so, perhaps, because Koch and most German bacteriologists rejected them, with Koch even suggesting that white blood cells actually provided the vehicle whereby germs spread throughout the organism. Pasteur offered Metchnikoff a post at his Paris Institute; indeed, after Pasteur's death, Metchnikoff became its most visible adornment, a scientific guru whose views on diet, constipation, aging, and the biological future of man were eagerly sought and equally eagerly expounded. He advocated the healthiness of eating yoghurt because he believed that the bacilli used in producing it inhibited bacteria in the human gut, which in their turn were one source of harmful putrefactive by-products. Metchnikoff was the first (but not the last) of the Nobel Laureates in Medicine – he shared the 1908 award – to exploit the status it bestowed in propagating his more general ideas on health and society.

Despite the fact that Metchnikoff worked for three decades at the Pasteur Institute, and died in the apartment built there for the Master himself, Metchnikoff never renounced his Russian citizenship. Nevertheless, cellular theories of immunity became associated predominantly with the French scientific community, rival chemical theories with the German one. Thus did the disciples of Pasteur and Koch perpetuate nationalistic science. The Franco-German divisions were not hard and fast: the Pasteur Institute was to produce important evidence for the chemical aspects of immunity, and a few German scientists became fascinated by phagocytosis. By the turn of the century, too, it was common to see merit in both chemical and cellular aspects of immunity. Nevertheless, Koch's doubts about the immunological significance of phagocytosis counted for a good deal in the German-speaking area, and two of Koch's younger colleagues, Emil von Behring (1854–1917) and Paul Ehrlich (1854–1915), provided significant practical and theoretical muscle to the proposition that immunological battles were waged not so much by the blood cells as in the blood serum.

Two lines of inquiry were especially telling on the chemical side. First, it could be shown that the cell-free serum of immunized animals could kill virulent bacteria when united with them, and that protection could be transferred via serum from animal to animal. This suggested that, whatever the significance of phagocytosis, the white cells were not the beginning and end of immunity. Second, in 1888, two of Pasteur's own pupils, Emile Roux (1853–1933) and Alexandre Yersin (1863–1943), showed that cultures of diphtheria bacilli were toxic to animals even when the cells themselves had been filtered out. This implied that it was not necessarily the bacterial cell itself that caused disease, but some substance, or toxin, which the cell produced. A similar phenomenon was demonstrated about the same time for the tetanus bacillus.

It was from these observations that what became known as serum therapy emerged. Working in Koch's Institute with a Japanese colleague, Shibasaburo Kitasato (1852–1931), von Behring announced in late 1890 that the whole blood or serum (either would do) of an animal, which had been rendered immune to tetanus or diphtheria by injecting the relevant toxin, could effectively treat another animal exposed to an otherwise lethal dose of the bacilli. The preparation of the immune animals (von Behring initially used guinea pigs) was accomplished in the way in which Pasteur had used for other purposes, that is, by challenging the test animal with gradually increasing doses of either bacillus or toxin. Von Behring took his case to an international forum the next year, the Seventh International Hygiene Conference, and trials in human beings, mostly children with diphtheria, were started in late 1891 or early 1892. Occasional instances of miracle cures of children, brought back almost from the dead by the new antitoxin therapy, began to be worth space on front pages of newspapers. The English physiologist, (Sir) Charles Sherrington (1857–1952), reported that after an urgent midnight train ride, he had saved the life of his nephew with the first diphtheria antitoxin administered to a human being in Britain. More than thirty articles appeared in the popular press in the United States between October 1894 and May 1895, by which time the use of the horse to raise antitoxin serum had increased supplies.

Advocates argued that the deathrate from acute diphtheria was more than halved. Despite a fair amount of public excitement, serum therapy was never an unambiguous miracle cure. The cure rates were often difficult to evaluate, because patient selection was often haphazard and epidemic diseases such as diphtheria could be notoriously variable in their virulence. Production standards for antitoxins were, in the early years, impossible to control, so supplies of antitoxin varied in strength and degree of purity from batch to batch. Occasional sudden and unexpected deaths of patients being administered antitoxin were alarming, and the more common appearance of what was called serum sickness, with fever, rash, and joint pains, was shown to be a side effect of serum treatment. The fact that antibodies were derived from animals was distasteful to many.

Nevertheless, both the laboratory and commercial pursuit of serum therapies grew apace in the decades after 1890, with the production of antitoxins for a number of diseases besides tetanus and diphtheria, including pneumonia, plague, cholera, and snake bites. At the same time, the protective possibilities of vaccines seemed to many to offer better possibilities for controlling infectious diseases. Vaccines developed from the killed and treated organisms of typhoid, plague, and cholera were introduced within a few years of each other at the end of the century, the latter two by the Russian-born bacteriologist Waldemar Haffkine (1860–1930). He became a naturalized British subject in 1899, and most of his vaccine work was done in India. Haffkine was convinced that, given sufficient resources, he could rid the Indian subcontinent of both plague and cholera, but his personality did not endear him to many British officials in India, there was much popular resistance to his plans for mass vaccination programs among the Indians (the results of his cholera vaccine were at best equivocal), and, in 1902, nineteen people died of tetanus from a contaminated batch of plague vaccine. He was recalled to Britain and, although supported by Ronald Ross and other prominent members of the British scientific community and ultimately personally exonerated by an official inquiry, the episode generated much controversy.

Equally controversial in his own way was (Sir) Almroth Wright (1861–1947), known to theater-goers as the thinly disguised Sir Colenso Ridgeon in George Bernard Shaw's *The Doctor's Dilemma* (1906), and to his critics as Sir Almost Right. He was high-minded, if pompous and opinionated, and an ardent exponent of the biological inferiority of women. It took him almost a decade to get his typhoid vaccine taken as seriously as he thought it should be, but he was vindicated in World War I, when vaccinated British troops suffered a low incidence of the disease. His work on opsonins, substances in the serum that seemed to prepare bacteria for ingestion by white cells (hence Shaw's ringing phrase "Stimulate the phagocytes!") appeared for a time to reconcile chemical and cellular theories of immunity.

In fact, by the time Wright was trying to popularize such notions as the opsonin index and opsonin therapy, chemical theories of immunity had been systematically formulated by Paul Ehrlich, one of the most gifted scientists of his generation. He developed a love of chemistry during his medical studies, and had his enthusiasm for medical research reinforced by the pathologist Cohnheim, the physiologist Rudolf Heidenheim, and Ehrlich's own cousin, Carl Weigert (1845–1904), a histologist and neuropathologist. Weigert's work in the 1870s, when Ehrlich was a medical student, demonstrated the importance of tissue preparation and staining for microscopical investigations. Ehrlich's doctoral dissertation and subsequent researches applied a series of vital stains to the tissues and, above all, the large blood cells that were now distinguished by their affinities to different kinds of dyes (e.g., basophils were stained by alkaline dyes).

Ehrlich continued throughout the 1880s to explore the physiological and pharmacological properties of various dyes that were being manufactured in commercial quantities by the German chemical industry. He examined cellular aspects of oxygen consumption, developed an important diagnostic test for bilirubin in the urine and demonstrated the affinity of the newly discovered malaria parasite for methylene blue. Throughout his career, he was intrigued by the molecular dimensions of physiological and pharmacological events, applying the stereochemical ideas of organic chemists such as Emil Fischer (1852–1919), several of whose synthetic products (such as the barbiturates) were pharmaceutically potent. Above all, Ehrlich believed that the chemical structures of biologically active compounds were intimately connected with those actions and that they could not affect a cell without being attached or

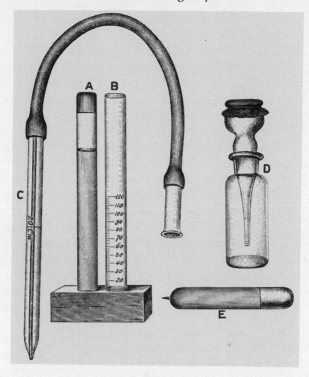

Figure 22. The blood became a much-studied bodily fluid after the improvements in the microscope of the 1830s. Staining techniques made the identification of the different cellular components of the blood easier, and other devices, such as this hemoglobinometer, developed by William Gowers, helped in the diagnosis and therapeutic evaluation of anemia. James Ewing, Clinical Pathology of the Blood *(London: Henry Kimpton, 1904), p. 44, Fig. 13.*

bound to it: *Corpora non agunt nisi fixata* (substances do not react unless they become fixed) was one of his favorite aphorisms.

Certainly that aphorism could be applied to his immunological research. As a Jew, Ehrlich did not find academic advancement easy and some of his earlier posts had not been commensurate with his growing reputation. However, Koch's Institute for Infectious Diseases in Berlin offered him a laboratory (though no salary), and his interest in the field was personal, since Ehrlich had discovered tubercle bacilli in his sputum, spent a year convalescing in Egypt, and received – with apparent effectiveness – a course of Koch's tuberculin therapy. Consequently, Ehrlich was happy to be involved in the administration and evaluation of tuberculin and, following von Behring, in the experimental production of antitoxins. Ehrlich himself demonstrated that various plant toxins could also stimulate antibodies (as they were now being called) in experimental animals. He also undertook the task of providing guidelines whereby the potency of diphtheria and other antitoxins could be measured and expressed in standard units.

By 1895, the scientific and commercial potentials of this line of inquiry were sufficiently promising to encourage specialist institutions, first in an antitoxin control station within Koch's Institute, then as an autonomous center for serum research and testing in a Berlin suburb. Ehrlich headed them both, but was shortly afterward lured to a larger, better equipped institute in Frankfurt, built with a combination of private and public money. There, Ehrlich continued to develop his "side-chain" theory of antigen–antibody interaction, a complicated model of the molecular basis of immunology. Along the way, Ehrlich and von Behring had fallen out over the latter's secret efforts to secure for himself patents for the manufacture of diphtheria antitoxin.

Although the side-chain theory required the fixing of an antigen molecule on a receptor site of a cell before the serum antibody could work, Ehrlich's was essentially a chemical vision of immunity, a part of his molecular vision of reality. That larger vision also included the possibility of pharmacological "magic bullets," the ultimate aim of chemotherapy, a term he both coined and made part of the currency of public medical science.

V. THE PHARMACEUTICAL INDUSTRY

Diphtheria antitoxin was probably the single most important catalyst in the creation of the modern science-based pharmaceutical industry. Tuberculin had preceded it by a few years but its effects remained controversial, and, in any case, slow. Diphtheria antitoxin was not without its shadows, as we have seen, but its effects could be dramatic, especially in desperately ill children. A substratum for the developing pharmaceutical industry was provided by two earlier entrepreneurial traditions, and one academic one.

The first of these was the existence, for at least two centuries, of what were variously called manufacturing chemists or drug importers and wholesalers. The myth that, in earlier, simpler days, doctors prescribed – and their patients used – mostly local herb-based remedies compounded in the doctor's shop or the patient's kitchen, has long been exploded. A vigorous market in medical advice books did provide laymen with instructions for drug remedies for a wide variety of disorders (which ordinary people were assumed to be able to diagnose accurately), and the survival of thousands of manuscript household recipe books testifies to a reliance on self-medication and domestic wisdom. Behind this, however, lay a highly developed network of drug suppliers, selling ingredients in bulk to local practitioners, chemists, and druggists, as well as entrepreneurs advertising their medicines directly to the public.

Examples of the former were the firm of Thomas Corbyn (1711–91), a Quaker drug merchant whose company records have recently surfaced and reveal a remarkable import–export trade in medicines and their ingredients; and the more famous Allen and Hanbury, another eighteenth-century London firm that grew big in the nineteenth by importing and manufacturing drugs and medical equipment and supplies. The latter company did a brisk business in preparations of cod liver oil, throat lozenges, and malt extract, as well as soaps and powdered milk. It did not initially have the technical staff to produce diphtheria antitoxin, which it sold under an agreement with the Lister Institute, where the antitoxin was raised.

At the other end of the market, Thomas Holloway (1800–83) made a fortune out of patent medicines, advertised directly to the public but also available wholesale to druggists and chemists throughout the world, although government regulations of patent medicine sales in France limited his success there. Even patent medicine manufacturers required at least rudimentary laboratory facilities for producing the goods, although advertising claims about purity, efficacy, and therapeutic rationales were aimed at selling medicine rather than telling the truth. Significantly, the language and concepts of bacteriology, immunology, and other innovative medical sciences were assimilated by market-oriented manufacturers, who offered the public such products as Radam's Microbe Killer. Needless to say, an American named Edward Koch (no relation to the bacteriologist) advertised his own remedy called "Dr. Koch's Cure for Tuberculosis." There can be little better evidence of the visibility of medical science in the two decades before World War I than the use of its vocabulary and concepts to sell quack, patent, and secret remedies.

This aspect of pharmaceuticals was big business and it generally circumvented the medical profession, for which economic anxiety and righteous indignation pointed in the same direction. The American Medical Association and the *British Medical Journal* initiated separate inquiries into the murky area, analyzing the ingredients in hundreds of patent medicines, exposing their inefficacy (or even harmfulness), and drawing attention to the staggering profit margins: the contents of patent medicines generally cost but a tiny fraction of the retail price, with most of the manufacturer's costs being absorbed by packaging and advertising.

More obviously relating to science and technology was the other entrepreneurial strand, the chemical industry, which thrived above all on dyes. In Britain, W. H. Perkin (1838–1907) isolated mauve, or aniline purple, from coal tar in 1856, and, although he established a highly profitable chemical factory, it was the Germans who exploited dyes and organic chemistry most effectively. Several of the individual firms that banded together after World War I to form the industrial giant I. G.

Farben dated from the mid-nineteenth century, including such familiar names as Bayer and Hoechst. Solvents, bleaches, fertilizers, explosives, and paints were as important as the synthetic dyes, although the last entered the medical world in histological stains and the therapeutic possibilities of Ehrlich's work on malaria. Friedrich Bayer's (1825–80) firm was originally more concerned with dye manufacture than research, but under Carl Duisberg (1861–1935), it developed research interests into pharmaceuticals, diversified into separate chemical and pharmaceutical branches, and made substantial profits from drugs such as aspirin (1899) and phenacetin (1887), both of which names the firm coined.

In addition to these commercial enterprises, the pharmaceutical industry was also to benefit from the academic discipline that Claude Bernard had called experimental therapeutics, though pharmacology became its more lasting name. Its institutional development followed a familiar path in Germany, where research institutes, notably those at Dorpat and Bonn, produced research schools with close ties to chemists and physiologists and the ultimate aim of explicating the precise physiological effects of compounds with known chemical compositions. In France, Bernard cast a long shadow, and pharmacology remained for the most part a minor adjunct to experimental physiology. In Britain, too, posts in therapeutics and materia medica were held principally by clinicians with broad interests, although T. R. Fraser (1841–1920) in Edinburgh and Thomas Lauder Brunton (1844–1916) in London sought to introduce an experimental dimension to their activities, and Brunton's *Textbook of Pharmacology, Therapeutics and Materia Medica* (1885) emphasized the first of this triad. It was translated into German, French, and Italian. In the United States, John Jacob Abel (1857–1938) established a pharmacology department at Johns Hopkins in 1893, where the German ideals he had absorbed during six years of European study (1884–90) were put into practice.

As an experimental discipline, pharmacology was heavily dependent on both chemistry and physiology for its materials and techniques, for without pure, known substances and definite physiological values, it could not hope for the precision Bernard envisioned for experimental therapeutics. Abel spent his first decade at Johns Hopkins examining the actions of suprarenal gland extracts, the active principle of which was variously called epinephrine and adrenaline. Coming in the wake of the claims of several distinguished scientists that monkey testicles could, when suitably prepared, sexually rejuvenate old men, Abel's isolation from adrenal extracts of a substance that could increase the heart rate and blood pressure seemed modest indeed. Nevertheless, the extent to which the physiological actions of adrenaline seemed to duplicate the functions of the sympathetic nervous system intrigued a number of scientists, and the potential therapeutic uses of "Adrenalin" (the name was patented) were exploited in the marketplace by the American pharmaceutical firm, Parke Davis and Co.

By the end of the century, an increasing number of pharmaceutical manufacturers were eager to turn discoveries made in academic physiological, bacteriological, and pharmacological laboratories to good account. Cooperation between science and commerce was not always easy, however. Patents and commercial secrecy smacked of the bad old days of nostrum selling and often clashed with the ideals of open scientific inquiry. When Abel and some academic colleagues established in 1908 the American Society for Pharmacology and Experimental Therapeutics, they excluded from membership anyone in the permanent employment of any drug firm (a ban not eliminated until 1941). Earlier, the American-born pharmaceutical entrepreneur Henry Wellcome (1853–1936) had run into similar problems in Britain when he sought to obtain registration for animal experimentation for his Wellcome Physiological Research Laboratories, established in 1894. Although Wellcome argued that this establishment and a separate one concerned with chemical research were independent of his commercial drug firm, both laboratories were at the very least financed out of the latter's profits and in practice came to be rather closely linked with the manufacturing firm. Wellcome managed to secure the backing of a number of key members of the British medical establishment and was successful in his second attempt, in 1901, to obtain the necessary Home Office authority for animal experiments to be performed in his physiological laboratories. Other British pharmaceutical firms followed suit, as animals became increasingly used to raise antitoxins, produce vaccines, and test new products.

Connections between science and commerce were less ambiguous in Germany, even if Ehrlich was sometimes disquieted by the crass entrepreneurial activities of colleagues like von Behring. Nevertheless, the research laboratories at Ehrlich's Frankfurt Institute had close connections with industry, especially Farbwerke Cassella and, then, Hoechst, which patented, produced, and marketed the drugs that many saw as the culmination of Ehrlich's career: salvarsan and neosalvarsan. Unlike biologicals such as vaccines and serum products, these were chemicals synthesized in the laboratory and seemed to justify Ehrlich's appellation of *chemotherapy*. Whether salvarsan was quite the "magic bullet" that Ehrlich had defined as the goal of chemotherapy was another matter. His work over three decades on the selective affinities of chemicals for certain kinds of cells (or microorganisms) convinced him that "internal antisepsis" (what he dubbed *therapia sterilisans magna*) was feasible. He had had some success with trypan red in trypanosomal infections.

Ehrlich turned his attention to syphilis after its causative organism had been demonstrated in 1905. He examined a large series of arsenical preparations, of which salvarsan (arsphenamine) was, famously, number 606, as he sought to achieve a balance between toxicity for the parasite and tolerance by the host. Working from 1909 with Sahachiro Hata (1873–1938), a Japanese colleague, first with experimental spiro-chaetal infections in rabbits, and then on human subjects, Ehrlich announced the new chemotherapeutic drug the following year. Much of the remaining five years of his life was spent trying to control the consequences of his medicament: the modification (neosalvarsan, number 914) to improve patient tolerance, the voluminous correspondence and publicity surrounding it, a lawsuit against a reporter who alleged he had experimented on prostitutes against their wills, control of supplies, reports of unsuccessful cases, relapses and allergic reactions to the drug. That neosalvarsan was a treatment for an emotionally charged and morally ambiguous disease such as syphilis, and that Ehrlich was a Jew in a time of growing anti-Semitism, further complicated the reactions.

In a sense, neosalvarsan was both the prototype and the apogee of the chemotherapy of Ehrlich's lifetime and a couple of decades beyond: synthesized in the laboratory, tested on animals, more effective than what had been previously available, and commercially attractive. It was rather more bullet than magic, but it was proof positive that research could pay and it was one of the pharmaceuticals that, when German patents were discounted after the outbreak of World War I, was quickly manufactured by Allied pharmaceutical companies. Other prewar German drugs – chloral hydrate, aspirin, phenacetin, phenobarbital – had greater staying power. Of the nonbiologicals, however, none had generated more excitement and controversy than the 606th arsenical compound that Ehrlich had examined.

VI. EXPERIMENTAL PHYSIOLOGY

While the glamorous sciences of bacteriology, immunology, and Ehrlich's chemotherapy generated most excitement in the decades before World War I, experimental physiology was hardly lost from the public gaze, though sometimes in ways its practitioners would not have wished. Across a broad front, experimental medicine needed animals, and, for some members of the public, an edifice of science built on the apparent sufferings of cats, dogs, rabbits, monkeys, and guinea-pigs was both corrupt and corrupting. Although to many Pasteur and Koch were international heroes, to others they represented all that was cruel and dangerous in a world threatened by materialistic, godless science.

Concern with animal welfare has a long if episodic history and, although vivisection was unfavorably remarked on by various seventeenth- and eighteenth-century literary figures, horse beating, bear baiting, cock-fighting, and similar sports and practices were the principal target of the first organized animal protection group. This was the Society for the Prevention of Cruelty to Animals, established in 1824 by the Irish social reformer Richard Martin (1754–1834) ("Humanity Martin"). It received a royal charter in 1840, decades before the foundation of an organization (still not "royal") to prevent cruelty to children, a fact that provoked the comment that the British love their animals more than their children.

Certainly it was in Britain where the antivivisection campaign was most vocal and powerful. From the middle decades of the century, laboratory animals were an object of increasing concern and two events in the 1870s catalyzed the antivivisection movement. One was the demonstration by a French physiologist of the effects of alcohol injected into two dogs at the 1874 Norwich meeting of the British Medical Association. A prosecution of wanton cruelty was brought against the Frenchman (then safely back in France) and three Norwich doctors who had arranged the demonstration. Though unsuccessful, the trial generated much comment in the medical and general press and placed animal experimentation firmly on the political agenda. A year earlier, a second event had provided antivivisectionists with more ammunition: the publication, in two volumes, of the *Handbook for the Physiological Laboratory*, edited by (Sir) John Scott Burdon Sanderson (1828–1905), then professor of physiology at University College London. At one level, the volumes were tangible evidence that animal physiology was coming of age in Britain, especially at University College and the University of Cambridge, where another of the book's authors, (Sir) Michael Foster (1836–1907), had gone in 1870. Increasingly, practical, hands-on physiology was becoming a routine part of the British medical curriculum and could no longer be brushed aside as a wanton activity indulged in by foreigners. Because the volumes were a handbook for the laboratory rather than simply a textbook, they revealed another level to the enterprise, as specific descriptions of animal experiments ("intended for beginners in physiological work") gave antivivisectionists detailed information about what might be going on in the medical schools and laboratories of Britain.

A strong parliamentary lobby led to the creation of a Royal Commission in 1875 to examine the whole question of experimental medicine, with membership from both scientific and antivivisectionist groups. A good deal of damage to the scientific cause was done by another of the authors of the *Handbook*, E. E. Klein (1844–1925), a German-born bacteriologist who had settled in London and who treated the Commission with contempt ("No regard at all" was his answer when asked what he thought of animals he was experimenting upon). Other representations of the research lobby were more diplomatic before the Commission, although there was private anger that medical research might be legislated out of existence in Britain, and petitions and counterpetitions began to circulate, ranging from calls to abolish all research using live animals to plans to leave the matter completely in the hands of the experimentalists.

By late 1875, the level of public and parliamentary awareness was such that some form of legislation was probably inevitable. Alternative bills were debated in Parliament. The resultant 1876 Cruelty to Animals Act was a compromise that initially satisfied neither the antivivisectionists nor the science lobby. In the end the Act (and subsequent modifications) actually achieved the aim to provide a reasonable framework to "reconcile the claims of science and humanity," and remained on the statute books until 1986, by which time common European legislation was being discussed. It set limits on the use of animals for demonstrations and teaching, required both individual scientists and premises to be licensed with the Home Office before research involving live animals could be performed, discussed anesthesia and painless killing of the animal after the experiment, and set strict criteria for justifying the use of horses, cattle, and other mammals.

No other country produced legislation aimed at regulating animal experimentation until well into the present century, and, as we have seen, the delegates to the 1881 International Medical Congress deplored the fact that their British colleagues had been singled out. In actuality, the Act probably increased professional consciousness of the experimental basis of medicine: the *British Medical Journal*, *Nature*, and other journals vigorously campaigned on behalf of the profession's research minority and the Physiological Society, established in 1876 by Foster and a group of like-minded individuals, had as one of its aims the provision of mutual support against antivivisectionists. Foster's *Journal of Physiology* of 1878 provided an outlet for publishing experimental papers. The Home Office inspectorate, whose job it was to police the Act, consisted of individuals sympathetic to the research cause and antivivisectionists managed to recruit only modest support from within the medical profession. A prosecution against David Ferrier in connection with the monkeys with cortical ablations demonstrated to the Congress failed: although Ferrier was not licensed at the time, it turned out that the operations had been performed by a colleague who was. The medical establishment was horrified that the Act might leave them at the mercy of snooping fanatics; the antivivisectionists were convinced that the trial's unsatisfactory outcome showed that the Act had no teeth to it and wanton and cruel torture of animals in the name of science would continue without control.

Among medical scientists, the physiologists continued to be most wary of anti-vivisectionist activity, because their experiments often involved major surgery on the animal; in fact, only a fraction of animal experiments involved physiologists, and much of the growth in animal use was through the less emotive procedure of injection and evaluation of pharmacological or bacteriological preparations. It was a physiologist who was at the center of the most heated confrontation between scientists and antivivisectionists before World War I. Two Swedish medical students witnessed on 2 February 1903 a demonstration at University College London, organized by (Sir) William Maddox Bayliss (1860–1924) and his colleague Ernest Starling (1866–1927). Published accounts accused Bayliss of flagrant breach of the 1876 Act, of operating on a conscious dog whose pancreas had previously been removed and whose cries pierced the lecture theater. Bayliss promptly sued Stephen Coleridge (1854–1936), Chairman of the National Anti-vivisection Society (and one of the founders of the National Association for the Prevention of Cruelty to Children), for libel. Bayliss won his case and got substantial damages (which he donated to medical research), but the "Brown Dog Affair," as the episode became known, was characterized by heated publicity, mass demonstrations (by both sides), and violent and unruly clashes between police and demonstrators. A statue in Battersea Park, London, near where much of the agitation occurred, still commemorates the event and the brown dog itself.

The antivivisection movement raised a number of salient issues: about the price of experimental knowledge; about its validity in human settings, given its origin in animal models and preparations; about the relationship between experimentation on animals and more subtle forms of experimentation on patients, especially women and paupers; about gender roles in medicine, especially women scientists and vivisectors; about cruelty to animals manifesting itself in cruelty to patients; about medical education as a form of indoctrination; about medicine as a materialistic and, ultimately atheistic, endeavor; about medical motives and medical trustworthiness. Card-carrying members of the dozen or so antivivisection societies never numbered more than a few thousand and it is difficult to believe (if impossible to quantify) that their ardor extended to more than a tiny fraction of the population of Britain. Most of that population would have been unaware of the issues, or if aware, unmoved either way. Nevertheless, the Act and the movement that created it served to consolidate the medical profession, and, in so doing, distance it from the public it served. It was not simply the knowledge doctors possessed, but the methods whereby they collectively achieved it, that created dilemmas that are still cogent.

Neither the 1876 Act nor the depth of antivivisection sentiment prevented physiology in Britain from achieving international status in the decades before World War I. In Cambridge, Foster and his pupils J. N. Langley (1852–1925) and W. H. Gaskell (1847–1914) created a research school that turned out a number of future Nobel Laureates and other scientific success stories, and buttressed Cambridge's reputation as the most progressive medical school in Britain. Foster himself had been interested in the question whether the stimulus of the heartbeat is muscular or neurological; Cambridge-trained physiologists ultimately extended the brief to the anatomy and physiology of the autonomic nervous system, the chemical transmission of nerve impulses, and the integrated control of reflexes and movement. At University College London, Bayliss and Starling presided over another active physiology department, where cardiovascular physiology, the nature of proteins and enzymes, and the actions of what Starling first called "hormones" were high on the agenda.

Bayliss and Starling had initially worked with the important but unspectacular digestive hormone that they named secretin. For the public, however, the thyroid and the testicles were seen to be the glands most potent with promise. The functions of the thyroid had long seemed obscure: perhaps its purpose was merely to give shape to the neck, or to slow the blood flow to the brain. From the 1870s, however, a series of clinical observations and experimental investigations established that the thyroid was essential to life and implicated its malfunction in conditions such as cretinism and goiter. Enlarged glands began to be surgically removed, often with disastrous consequences if insufficient thyroid tissue was left behind. Total removal of the thyroid from an experimental animal led to its death, but this could be prevented by transplanting the extirpated gland elsewhere in the dog or monkey. From this line of inquiry came injection experiments using macerated thyroid tissue. These worked as well as transplantation and by the 1890s, injections and then oral preparations of thyroid gland were being successfully used in human beings whose thyroids had been surgically removed or were judged to be underactive. Since slow growth and sluggish mental functions were two of the features of cretinism, thousands of underachieving children were logically if not always appropriately placed on thyroid extract, and it was recommended for a wide range of symptoms in adults, from constipation and obesity to tiredness and depression.

If thyroid extract was thought to sharpen the bowels, reflexes, and brain, testicular extract might reach other parts. On 1 June 1889, Charles-Edouard Brown-Séquard (1817–94) reported to a distinguished scientific society in Paris that he had rejuvenated himself through subcutaneous injections of extracts of guinea-pig and dog testicles. It was a claim that commanded serious consideration, since Brown-Séquard was a scientist of international renown: Claude Bernard's successor in Paris, holder of a chair at Harvard and a consultancy in London. He had long been intrigued by "glands," especially the adrenals, and had pioneered the experimental injection of gland extracts. In his hands, testicular extracts seemed to promise, if not eternal life, at least extended sexual potency and the amelioration of many diseases of debility and old age. "Organotherapy" was more than a nine-day wonder, with a core that survived some of the early extravagant claims: "In the hands of one experimenter, [a medical reporter wrote] the paralysed immediately walk, the lame throw aside their crutches, the deaf hear and the blind see." The same reporter pointed out that when others administered testicular extract, no benefit seemed to accrue from its injection. The medical profession remained divided about Brown-Séquard's last line of research, and his death not long after he had "rejuvenated" himself punctured the idea of frolicking centurians. Nevertheless, organotherapy shared with serum and vaccine therapy the promise of miracles in a bright new age of science.

VII. THE INVISIBLE REVEALED: X-RAYS

Tuberculin and testicular extract made their headlines; diphtheria antitoxin and neosalvarsan received prominent media coverage; but perhaps no scientific event of the period was so instantaneously newsworthy as Wilhelm Röntgen's (1845–1923) discovery in late 1895 of what he modestly called "a new kind of ray," or "x-rays." Working with the vacuum tubes perfected by the English scientist (and psychical researcher) William Crookes (1832–1919), Röntgen effectively discovered x-rays in early November; on 22 December he x-rayed his wife's hand, which photograph became one of the most potent images of the whole century. On 28 December he communicated his findings to the Würzburg Physical-Medical Society; ten days later newspapers all over the world had been informed of Röntgen's rays, which could pass through wood, paper, clothes, and flesh. Voyeurs were disappointed that the rays went through flesh as well as clothes, although this did not stop the marketing of contraptions supposedly able to reveal the body beneath the garments, and the sale of "x-ray proof underclothing for ladies." The phenomenon was rapidly assimilated into the popular culture of the day. Indeed, because of the timing between Röntgen's communication and the Christmas holidays, combined with Röntgen's retiring personality, the popular rather than the scientific and medical press spread the news.

X-rays thus had immediate popular, scientific, technological, commercial, and medical reverberations. As early as 7 January 1896 a radiograph was taken for clinical purposes, and their use in diagnosing bone fractures and locating foreign bodies and gunshot was obvious and dramatic. Bismuth and barium compounds were quickly shown to be opaque to the rays, soon permitting the diagnostic use of what is now known as "barium swallows" and "barium enemas." Many of the opaque substances used were messy, unpleasant, and potentially dangerous and improved only gradually, mostly through trial and error. Early chest radiographs were even less satisfactory, since exposure times

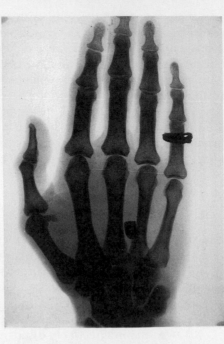

Figure 23. The x-ray of Mrs. Röntgen's hand was one of the familiar medical images of the era, and it became fashionable to have one's hand x-rayed. This radiograph is of Lord Lister's hand, with ring on fifth finger, no date. Provenance: Lord Lister, Sir William Lister. In the Wellcome Institute.

were very long (initially at least twenty minutes) and contrasts not very sharp. Despite widespread interest in tuberculosis and other pulmonary disorders, mass chest x-ray screening programs were not inaugurated until shortly after World War I.

Prolonged exposure to x-rays was quickly observed to have physiological effects, such as browning or even burning the skin, and causing ulcerations, hair loss, and dermatitis. Within a year of Röntgen's discovery, this had been turned to therapeutic account by a Viennese physician who had used x-rays to burn off a hairy mole from a patient. Other doctors began quickly to report success in treating a variety of skin conditions with the new rays, ranging from acne to lupus vulgaris (skin tuberculosis). At precisely the same period, the Danish physician Niels Finsen (1860–1904) burst upon the scene with his work suggesting that ultraviolet light rays were bactericidal and so also offered promise for treating lupus. Many early hospital radiology departments provided both radiation and ultra-violet light therapy, and Finsen's researches stimulated the development of Alpine (i.e., high altitude) tuberculosis sanatoria and incidentally encouraged the popular belief that bronzed skin is healthier than white.

Hard on the heels of these wondrous developments came the discovery in 1896, by Henri Becquerel (1852–1908), of radiation, associated with heavy elements such as uranium. Drama, romance, and human interest were added when the husband-and-wife team of Pierre (1859–1906) and Marie (1867–1934) Curie joined the hunt for other radioactive elements. Before Pierre was tragically killed in a road accident, they had discovered polonium and radium and shared, with Becquerel, a Nobel Prize. Their family life – they had two daughters – made excellent newscopy, as did their dedication to each other and to their joint researches. Following her husband's death, Marie Curie became the first woman to lecture at the Sorbonne.

In and of themselves, x-rays and radiation were phenomena of especial interest to physicists, from which discipline Röntgen, Becquerel, and the Curies came. Their diagnostic and therapeutic implications for medicine simply reinforced the role of science within medicine. By 1900, there were radium institutes, radiology journals and societies, textbooks, and more than a hundred diseases where the new miracle cures had been employed. Even x-ray burns were being treated with more x-rays, but it was for the dreaded if imprecise diagnosis of "cancer" that the new therapies seemed to promise the most. Carcinomas in a variety of sites – breast, head, larynx, abdomen, cervix – sarcomas, lymphomas, leukemias were all reported to respond to x-rays. It is no accident that several major cancer research charities and hospitals date from this period.

As so frequently happens, therapeutic enthusiasm outran caution, and both the limitations and the dangers of radiotherapy were only slowly and painfully realized. The martyrs to x-rays included many patients and not a few of the early workers in the field (including Marie Curie). Early warnings were neglected, monitoring schemes not contemplated, lead shields and common sense absent. The first *medical* Nobel Prize in the field was not awarded until just after World War II, to H. J. Muller for his demonstration that x-rays can cause genetic mutations.

One might hope that the calculus of risks and benefits might be investigated more quickly today than it was a century ago. Nevertheless, the x-ray scenario is a thoroughly modern one: in the rapidity with which news of it spread, and the role of the media in the diffusion; in the mixture of science, technology, and commercialism that attended it; in its internationalism; in the speed with which a specialism formed around it; in the way in which it threw up public scientific figures; in the impact of the physical sciences on medicine; and in the expense the new technology added to medical care.

Coming as they did in the waning years of the nineteenth century, x-rays provided further proof that the old medical order was changing.

7

Doctors and patients

> The public are our employers, and, in the long run, we shall be what our employers make us.
> Robert Brudenell Carter, *Doctors and their Work* (1903), p. 13

A PATIENT seeking medical care on the eve of World War I would have had different expectations from those of his or her grandfather or grandmother in a similar situation around the middle of the nineteenth century. If the complaint were serious, the later patient could anticipate a more extensive diagnostic workup. The stethoscope might have been used in either situation, but the earlier doctor would not have examined the eyes with an ophthalmoscope, the ears with an otoscope, or the throat and larynx with a laryngoscope. The doctor in 1914 would not have had an electrocardiograph in his consulting rooms, though a few doctors in some urban centers might have referred a patient to a hospital where an electrocardiogram could be taken. More common would have been a request for an x-ray, and blood might have been taken for examination but almost certainly not as part of the therapy. Sputum or urine or a swab might have been sent away for bacteriological analysis, and some doctors would have had a microscope and some chemical reagents close to hand.

Although vaginal specula were available in 1850, indeed, were known to the ancients, the later doctor would have been more likely to use it, if the problem were deemed gynecological or obstetrical; and male and female patients alike had a greater chance of having an operation recommended to them. Should surgery have been agreed it would probably have taken place in a hospital, private clinic, or nursing home, regardless of the patient's social class. Even medical conditions might have landed him (or her) in a hospital ward or, if the patient could afford it, room. If the disease were one of several infectious ones, a fever hospital or isolation at home might be in order; if the diagnosis were tuberculosis, the doctor might send the patient to a sanatorium, though these were still scarce in 1914. If the patient were poor, he might well have presented himself to a charitable dispensary or outpatient or emergency service of a charitable hospital, where charges would be minimal or waived. Even for a patient in employment, the visit might well have been paid for in advance or by a third party, through arrangements with the employer, trade union, friendly society or, in Britain and Germany, national insurance schemes.

Some things would have changed but little or not at all. The class and sex of the patient would have influenced how he or she was treated, both at a personal level and often in terms of diagnosis and therapeutic recommendation. The doctor would almost certainly have been male or if female, seeing only women and children as patients. If working outside a hospital or dispensary, he would almost certainly have been in solo practice.

Whether the patient of 1914 would have had more confidence in the doctor than his grandparents would have had in theirs is another matter. From our standpoint, the patient *should* have had, since the medicine of 1914 was diagnostically and therapeutically closer to our own. The profession, too, was more confident, generally better educated, and more tightly regulated. At the same time, there were those even then who mourned the passing of the old-fashioned doctor, who knew his patients and their familial and social circumstances, and dispensed wisdom along with his pills. Crude mortality rates were falling in 1914, although how much was the result of medical interventions, how much medical prevention, and how much social and economic meliorism, is problematic; historical morbidity is even more difficult to get at; and the pastoral functions of medicine are impossible to quantify. Nevertheless, at some level, these matters are related to the educational, professional, institutional, and economic structures of medicine, which this chapter seeks to describe.

I. EDUCATING A PROFESSION

The rise of the science estate within medicine effected changes in some educational priorities, though without obliterating features that had developed during the first half of the century. For one thing, the hospital continued to occupy its central place in the life of most medical students in Europe, and some in the United States. Clinical lectures and demonstrations, ward rounds, and outpatient attendance first exposed them to what for most would be their lifelong professional preoccupation, patients. Science courses might add to the student's total educational experience; they might teach him how better to understand the disease etiology and mechanisms; how better to handle diagnostic technology such as the microscope or Petri dish; how better to evaluate the drugs he prescribed or the papers he read in the increasing number of professional journals at his disposal.

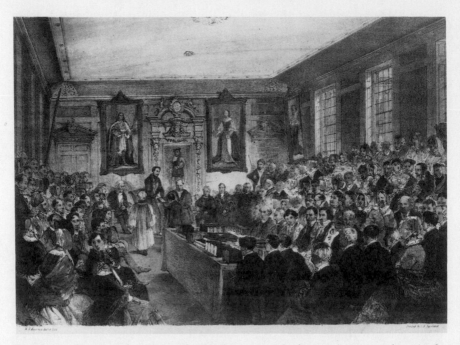

Figure 24. Opening of session and prize-day ceremonies became important dates in the medical school calendar. They usually included inspirational speeches from professional élites and occasionally attracted the great and the good from other walks of life. Here, Queen Victoria's husband, Prince Albert, is distributing the prizes at St. Thomas's Hospital Medical School in the 1840s. Colored lithography by W. H. Kearney. Printed by C. H. Fairland.

If more science was to be taught, the course had to be lengthened or time found within existing requirements. In practice, some medical schools added a year to what had varied between two and four years in earlier decades, though some of the slack was taken up by simply making students attend longer hours. By mid-century, the apprenticeship was rapidly disappearing, which meant that medical students were based wholly at the school. This in turn made it easier for a school to engender loyalty among its pupils and to create a more substantial academic environment. Some schools began to provide accommodations for their students, and student societies, special lectures, and prize-day celebrations helped make the schools feel more "academic."

For the top medical schools, the academic atmosphere was reinforced by association with a parent or affiliated university. The pattern varied from country to country. In France, for instance, the medical schools continued to have a good deal of autonomy, whereas in Germany the university affiliation had already been close by mid-century. In Britain, and especially in London, hospital-based medical schools maintained their independence, but their students were eligible to sit the examinations of the University of London, and thereby qualify (if they passed) for the university degrees of M.B. (Bachelor of Medicine), or Ch.B. (Bachelor of Surgery), C.M. (Master of Surgery), and M.D. From the 1840s, the Universities of Oxford and Cambridge began to take medical education more seriously, though neither city was populous enough to possess a hospital sufficiently large to provide comprehensive clinical training. Consequently, medical students from there had to go to London or elsewhere for their two or three years' clinical work, returning to be examined by and take the medical degrees of, one of the ancient universities. Cambridge in particular became an outstanding place for science, and from half a dozen medical students per year at mid-century, there were about a hundred by 1900. That growth in itself was testimony to the enhanced value placed on the basic scientific training of medical students.

Traditionally, the medical corporations in Britain (the Royal College of Physicians, Royal College of Surgeons, Society of Apothecaries plus the Royal Colleges or Faculties in Edinburgh, Glasgow, and Dublin) had through their examination and licentiate, membership or fellowship schemes provided the commonest route to formal qualification. The Medical Act of 1858 (of which John Simon was a principal behind-the-scenes architect) ratified the pluralistic system, whereby either the corporations or the universities could examine and certify a candidate's fitness to practice medicine. In the eyes of the law, the L.R.C.P. (Licentiate of the Royal College of Physicians) and an M.B. from a university were roughly equivalent, though in reality, the latter was the tougher qualification to achieve.

The 1858 Medical Act did not, as many medical men wanted, outlaw unorthodox practitioners, homeopathists, herbalists, naturopaths, or others with medical cosmologies at variance with the regulars. There was to be no medical monopoly. Rather, the public was allowed to buy the medical services (or cosmologies) they wished. The only proviso was that practitioners not medically qualified by the terms of the 1858 Act could not pass themselves off as a "proper" doctor. Those who had qualified through the approved routes – hospital medical school, medical corporation, university medical faculty – were listed (with their formal qualifications) in an annual *Medical Register*, which members of the public could consult if in doubt. Otherwise, if individuals wished to avail themselves of the services of a healer, of whatever stripe, they were free to do so, so long as that healer had not misrepresented himself. Caveat emptor (let the buyer beware) was the underlying philosophy.

Keeping and policing this Register were the primary functions of the General Medical Council, the policing element encompassing the ethical and professional behavior of registrants: sexual misconduct with patients, blatant advertising (there were subtle, acceptable ways of announcing one's credentials and availability to the public), and misrepresentation. The GMC was also charged with keeping an eye on the facilities and educational standards of the medical schools and examining bodies, although this was an area with a good deal of room for maneuver and debate. Since the Council itself was composed of medical men, Parliament in passing the Act had granted the profession a good deal of autonomy. In addition, only properly qualified medical men could hold a large number of public or quasi-public posts, such as consultancies to hospitals, and employment in the Poor Law Medical Service, prison service, insane asylums, colonial medical service, or public health service.

The educational ideal embodied in the Act was that on the day of being let loose on the public, the medical graduate should be a "safe general practitioner," that is, capable of performing basic medical and minor surgical functions. Obligatory training in obstetrics followed later. Gone were the days when the aspiring consultant physician and the budding surgeon would follow different paths from the beginning. Rather, all students followed essentially the same course and were exposed to each of the major divisions of the profession. This common educational experience improved group solidarity. For some, it also lengthened the period of training, as postqualification positions as dresser, house officer, and resident physician or surgeon were sought by those desiring consultancy careers. Some who subsequently had careers in general practice would have spent time as a postgraduation resident officer, but the very fact that basic qualification was deemed to make a person safe for general practice reflects its lower prestige within professional hierarchies and those aspiring to higher qualifications – M.B., M.R.C.P., F.R.C.S. – had longer hospital training. The British equivalent ("preregistration year") of what in France and the United States was called the "internship" did not become mandatory for all doctors intent on practicing until after World War II.

In the 1850s, most of the science teaching, and virtually all of the clinical, was done by "part-timers": men who also were in private practice. We have already noted that surgeons traditionally taught anatomy and the old-fashioned physiology with which it was frequently combined. Physicians usually dominated the teaching of chemistry and therapeutics; pathology was closely integrated into the clinical portion of the course, as patients who died were given postmortem analyses. It was often the physician who would wield the postmortem scalpel. Teachers generally kept a portion of students' fees, with the remainder of their income derived from private practice or other medical work. As more practical, laboratory experience began to be stressed, science teaching became more demanding of time, knowledge, organization, and resources, and the part-timer was gradually replaced by the new breed of professional scientist, even if those in the science lobby continued to be envious of the more highly structured German situation.

In clinical subjects, the part-time system dominated until long after World War I. Even in the university-based schools, such as Edinburgh, Glasgow, University College London, and some of the provincial English schools, professors of medicine, surgery, obstetrics, and other subjects would regularly retain varying amounts of private practice. In the hospital-based schools, such as St. Bartholomew's, Guy's, and St. Thomas's, the hospital consultants also taught. But consultancy posts were essentially honorary, and both teaching and hospital patient care were sources of prestige but not much direct income. Because income was derived from private patients, conflicts of interest were possible. Some consultants were undoubtedly conscientious in their hospital-related duties; others were less so, but hospitals with medical students also had resident medical officers, on whom the burden of teaching could fall. The remnants of the old apprentice system lived on in hospital teaching, as students followed young, ambitious medical staff on their daily rounds, and consultants on regular, more formal but less frequent trips through the wards. Advanced students took on more responsibility by clerking for a period of months. This could be a prelude to a house appointment and gradual advancement through the ranks to a consultancy. Consultants at a teaching hospital were mostly chosen from among its former students.

Science teaching made the biggest impact on a medical school's finances, as laboratories cost money to build and maintain and full-time salaries were not covered by student fees. These were sufficiently high to ensure that most students entering the profession had reasonable resources behind them, that is, to keep medicine largely in the hands of the middle classes. The growing number of student-oriented textbooks in all subjects attests to more uniformity of curricula and to the importance of examinations. Modern examination structures date principally from the middle of the nineteenth century. Examinations became longer, more likely to be written and practical than oral, more systematic, more searching. Students were tested in their "preliminary" subjects – biology, physics, chemistry – in addition to each of the scientific and clinical subjects. Since students from any of the London medical schools could sit the University of London examinations, and since students from any approved medical school could take those of the Royal Colleges, the exams that really mattered – those that led to registrable qualifications – were generally set and marked by people who had not taught the individual student. This in turn required schools to keep an eye on examining bodies and to respond accordingly, as in 1870 when the Royal College of Surgeons decided to make practical physiology a requirement for students sitting the M.R.C.S. Examiners were paid separately by the examination bodies and this provided welcome income, especially for science teachers without recourse to private practice. Examiners themselves began to be chosen at least partly for competence, not simply by virtue of seniority, as had earlier been the custom.

The private, proprietary schools could not compete in such an atmosphere, although crammers and extramural teachers were still around. In the United States, however, a much wider variation of the kind, cost, and quality of medical school continued into the present century. In the 1840s and 50s, even the dominance of "regular" medicine was in some doubt, as homeopathic, botanical, and eclectic doctors formed professional groups, opened their own schools, and vied for patients. Of these alternative medical cosmologies, homeopathy proved the most lasting. Its German founder, Samuel Hahnemann (1755–1843), had become dissatisfied with the traditional aggressive ministrations of regular doctors. His philosophy of health and disease emphasized "natural" remedies and the capacity of minute doses of drugs to cure the symptoms that, in larger doses, the drugs themselves would produce ("like cures like"). The gentleness of the remedies appealed to many patients and some doctors. A few doctors combined homeopathic treatment for some diseases and ordinary (what Hahnemann called "allopathic" – treatment by opposites) for others, but the more common pattern was exclusively homeopathic remedies by those who subscribed to Hahnemann's teachings. The distinction between "lay" and "professional" was less clear-cut among homeopaths and other alternative healers than in the regular profession, though the existence of schools, societies, and journals among alternative groups mirrored developments within orthodoxy. Even among American states that had them, licensing laws varied widely, though probably not so much as the range of facilities, resources, and even pretensions of the medical schools. Medical degrees were far easier to acquire than a medical education: hundreds of proprietary schools offered doctorates for cut-rate fees in rapid time. Modest premises and two or three part-time lecturers could easily constitute a medical school, and even more strikingly than in Britain, medical teachers could be failed practitioners. In many regions of antebellum America, medicine was closer to an occupation (and a precarious one at that) than a profession; entry was easy and drifting in and out common, as circumstances dictated.

On the other hand, there were always medical schools and medical élites that sought to emulate, in appropriate American ways, the best Europe could offer. The Eastern seaboard was naturally most conscious of Europe, and its educational and professional traditions were successively touched by Edinburgh, Paris, and Berlin (or Vienna). Abraham Flexner's damning *Report* on the majority of American medical schools did not come out until 1910; but long before then, a number of university-affiliated schools, and not only those in the East, had begun systematic building programs, curriculum reorganization, and staff recruiting. As we have already seen, from 1876 the Johns Hopkins University offered a model: decently endowed by its benefactor and consciously Germanic in its emphasis on research and advanced teaching. Building the teaching hospital meant that the medical school itself was not fully operational until 1893, but from its earliest days, the "Hopkins" wanted to compete internationally. It raised admission standards for medical students, requiring a full four-year college or university baccalaureate, and exposed them to a rigorous science-based curriculum and clinical teaching dominated by academic "full-timers," that is, university staff clinicians with little or no private practice.

Few places had the endowment and resources enjoyed by Johns Hopkins, and even there the money did not last forever. Even without the salary costs of full-time teacher-clinicians, a science-based, clinically diverse education was an expensive proposition, and those medical schools besides Hopkins that began to respond to the repeated calls of the American Medical Association and (especially after 1890) the Association of American Medical Colleges, for reform, had to work at finding resources and qualified staff. Even before the Rockefellers entered medical philanthropy in a big way, smaller benefactors had been persuaded to give to the medical schools of Harvard and the University of Pennsylvania, and state legislatures in Michigan and Minnesota permitted public money to be invested in equipping and running progressive medical schools in Ann Arbor and Minneapolis. Newly founded medical schools such as Cornell (1898) sought from the beginning to emulate the spreading academic, scientific orientation of the élite institutions; the incorporation of a private, commercial school in St. Louis into Washington University was a step in the same direction. Symptomatic of the trend were the appointment of the first scientist as a medical school dean at Harvard in 1883, and the imposition of student quotas at a number of places where it was obvious that tuition fees would not cover running costs in the best of circumstances, and quality would suffer from overcrowding.

As more and more states initiated independent licensing examinations, the disparity between students who had attended different kinds of medical schools became obvious. Small, commercial schools without university attachment, minimal or no laboratory and clinical facilities, low tuition fees, and short courses of study came under increasing pressure to change or die, and it was probably in his exposure of the worst rather than in his praising of the best, that Flexner and his *Report* achieved the most. In 1906, four years before the *Report*, the United States possessed almost half (162) of the medical schools of the entire world. Almost half of these failed to survive the aftermath of Flexner, who, despite offending a few potential allies with his harsh analyses, marshaled the support of the AMA, the AAMC, the state examining boards, and the giant philanthropic foundations and secured widespread acceptance of his ideals of scientific medicine, taught in schools with a research ethos. Nothing changed overnight, of course, and the initiative was well underway before 1910, but the publication of Flexner's *Report* probably did more than any other single event to lay open the realities, and articulate the alternatives, of medical education in an age of science.

II. HOSPITALS

No single structure, not even the laboratory, is more closely associated with modern medicine than the hospital. Hospitals come in a variety of sizes and perform a multiplicity of functions, so it is not surprising that the hospital's relation to the medical enterprise is neither simple nor constant. The "hospital medicine" of the first half of the nineteenth century (see Chapter 2) left some indelible marks, but the newer professional, scientific, economic, and diagnostic dimensions of later medicine were also reflected in the design, funding, and operation of these institutions.

In the larger hospitals, and many of the smaller ones as well, one constant was an educational presence. In German teaching hospitals, many of the beds were arranged around what was called the "university clinic," a ward or service of twenty, thirty, or more beds under the direct supervision of a professor or other academic doctor who controlled admissions and directed the teaching and research there. Much of the teaching was through demonstration, and foreign students making the trek to Germany or Austria could be exposed to interesting examples of disease, often in the various specialties, but had fewer opportunities of hands-on participation in examination, diagnosis, and treatment. Many of these wards had laboratories attached where microscopical, bacteriological, and chemical work could be carried out, often directly by the students themselves, thus reinforcing the "scientific" orientation of their study abroad. These academic services would also be associated with outpatient clinics, where patient follow-up occurred and less seriously ill patients were examined and treated. Although many hospitals had earlier possessed limited outpatient facilities, these departments became more active during the second half of the century, providing the kind of care that had previously been the function of dispensaries or general practitioners. As the name suggests, dispensaries were institutions where medicines were dispensed but also where patients not requiring hospitalization could be seen by medical staff.

By the century's end, the academic ideals of the university clinic were beginning to be taken up in a few American teaching hospitals, often in connection with the general development of the "full-time" system. In reality, most clinical teaching there continued to be under the control of part-timers. The teaching hospitals themselves were generally more prestigious than those without medical students, even if the students were not always popular with patients and both the educational and research facilities of hospitals sometimes made fund-raising for its more immediate charitable work difficult.

Four principal features characterized British and American hospitals from mid-century until World War I: their continued growth; an increasing medical dominance within them; greater diversity and complexity of design to accommodate their new range of nursing, diagnostic, and therapeutic functions; and variable success in coping with the economic realities of these ever more expensive institutions.

Throughout the second half of the century, the general trend was simply more hospital beds in more hospitals. Older institutions added more wards and new hospitals were regularly founded. In Britain, the voluntary hospital system continued to expand and provide the backbone of the charitable sector. In London and other large cities, many of the newer hospitals were specialist in their orientation, founded to provide treatment for a particular organ or system (heart, lungs, skin, nervous system, urinary system), region (ear, nose and throat), time of life (children, pregnant women), or disease (cancer, tuberculosis). A general hospital or infirmary became obligatory for all market towns and smaller cities, and it was often a source of civic pride along with the town hall, public library, literary society, and notable ancient building or monument. Regular serial publications detailed the growth of charitable giving, in which health-related institutions took pride of place alongside religious, educational, and provident initiatives. The worldwide survey of Sir Henry Charles Burdett (1847–1920), *Hospitals and Asylums of the World* (1891–3), consisted of four massive volumes and an atlas.

It always proved easier to raise charitable money for children and young adults than old people, for acute disease than chronic, for the "worthy" poor than the residuum, for physical than mental disorders. The slack was taken up by an increasing public investment in medical institutions: Poor Law infirmaries, isolation hospitals, insane asylums. The last in particular grew in number and average size, especially after 1845 when legislation required each county to build and maintain an asylum for pauper lunatics. In 1850, there were twenty-four county and borough asylums in England and Wales, with an average size of just under 300; by 1890 there were sixty-six, averaging more than 800 beds each; at the same time, large numbers of lunatics and others suffering from dementia, paralysis, and chronic neurological disorders were ending their days in the Poor Law infirmaries. As institutions like these filled up and overflowed as fast as they could be built, some of the widespread pride at the growing provision of hospital care was tempered with the fear that insanity and hereditary degenerative disorders were the inexorable result of alcoholism, sexual excess and venereal disease, morphinism, and the increasing pace of modern life.

During the same period, doctors continued to invest more heavily in hospital work, to become ever more closely identified with these institutions, and to enjoy more power within them. Within the charity, or voluntary, hospitals, the basic administrative arrangements remained in place, with those who supported the hospital with voluntary contributions still enjoying a say in the management of the institution and the right to nominate patients for admission. In most voluntary hospitals, the doctors were explicitly barred from positions on the management committees, though by the end of the century this was beginning to change. Patient selection, too, could be manipulated to take account of teaching requirements or the particular interests of consulting physicians or surgeons. As outpatient departments increased in number and activity, so did the size of the medical staff. House surgeon and house physician appointments became more common, and a necessary stage in the career structure of a would-be consultant. This in turn provided for a routine medical presence within the hospital.

In many of the smaller, specialist hospitals, doctors had always enjoyed rather more control of patient selection, if for no other reason that the patient needed to be suffering from a particular condition to be eligible for treatment. The stimulus to establish these institutions in the first place often originated from a doctor with ambitions or interests in a certain direction. Even though aristocratic and upper-class patronage was also part of the charitable specialist hospital, the smaller size and greater homogeneity of patient type tended to give the medical staff more autonomy.

In the public sector – municipal hospitals, Poor Law infirmaries, fever hospitals, psychiatric asylums, military institutions – the patients were generally not there by choice, and the medical staff had even greater control. They still could have an ambiguous relationship with the various employing agencies, such as local or borough councils, or Poor Law guardians. Within the public sector, professional associations of medical men were more in evidence, formed not simply for the usual intellectual reasons of holding meetings, exchanging information, and publishing journals, but to work for improved conditions of service, better pay, security of tenure, and pensions. Doctors particularly objected to the advertising of such posts for tender, since this could lead to unsavory competition between applicants and lower salaries, but equally, they argued, to lower standards of care. Public hospitals never acquired quite the cachet of the private, voluntary ones, although groups such as the

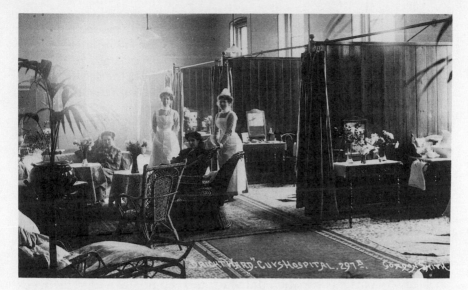

Figure 25. Photographs of hospital wards were frequently used in fund-raising activities of late nineteenth-century hospitals. Medical and nursing staffs were usually much more prominent than the patients themselves. This turn-of-the-century postcard of Bright Ward, Guy's Hospital, London should be compared with the aquatint of the ward in the Middlesex Hospital (see Fig. 7) of a century earlier.

Poor Law Medical Officers' Association and the Medico-Psychological Association began to achieve some of their goals, especially toward the century's close.

If young resident medical and surgical officers achieved increased professional visibility within the hospitals, so, eventually, did the nurse. The rise of modern nursing is no longer seen exclusively in terms of Florence Nightingale and her enigmatic and idiosyncratic career. For one thing, religious orders of nurses were active in hospitals (especially but hardly exclusively in Catholic countries or areas) long before Nightingale was born, much less before she went to nurse soldiers in the Crimean War (1854–6). Consequently, the emphasis on nurses' obedience and service was hardly novel in the mid-nineteenth century. Nor were all or even most pre-Nightingale nurses the drunken, careless, and slovenly hags that Charles Dickens created in Sarah Gamp. Finally, the kinds of nursing reforms that Nightingale advocated, based above all on training and discipline, were already around about the time she went to the Crimea, but independently of her mission. Nevertheless, Florence Nightingale did become the Lady with the Lamp, a public heroine and a potent symbol even before she returned to England in 1856; and the Nightingale Fund Training School for Nurses at St. Thomas's Hospital, established with part of the money that the public subscribed in her honor, bore the stamp of her personality and enjoyed the reflection of her personal prestige. It provided the model that many subsequent nursing schools in Britain, the United States, and the British Empire followed.

Nightingale wanted dedicated, reliable and, above all, respectable young women to enter nursing, and certainly during the second half of the century, nursing became with teaching one of the few occupations a middle-class girl could contemplate. In its hierarchical arrangement and its emphasis on discipline, there was a kind of military ethos in the Nightingale ideal. Although through district nursing, nurse-midwifery, school nursing, and other facets, the profession (as it was increasingly called) became ever more diverse, the initial base was the hospital, where the training schools were located and young trainees were initiated into the duties and skills of their calling.

In the longer term, medical authority was augmented, since even Nightingale herself recognized that ultimately nursing was a collaborative enterprise and much of the nurse's duty was to carry out medical and surgical orders. Besides, the very fact that nursing was becoming so solidly a female occupation did much to keep power within the medical court. However, Nightingale's own ideas of health and disease were broadly environmental and Chadwickian – she had no time for the bacteriological notion of disease specificity – so overseeing a regimen of good diet, cleanliness, and fresh air was central to the nurse's role within the hospital. Further, under the newer dispensation, nurses themselves not only developed a collective identity, but their direct superior was the head nurse, or matron, who was sometimes perceived as a threatening figure by the medical staff. At Guy's Hospital in London, a crisis was reached in 1880, as the matron, Miss Burt, had managed to create a relatively autonomous nursing corps, responsible through her directly to the hospital governors rather than the medical staff. Doctors complained that the regimented rhythm of patient life in hospital – washing, eating, visiting, and so forth – was arranged around the structure of the nurses' day rather than the good of the patient (or the convenience of the medical staff).

The emergence of modern nursing helped make hospitals more medical, not less, even if doctors took a while to adjust to the fact that nurses might come from the same social class as they did and could not be addressed by their Christian names. Nightingale was also an enthusiastic exponent of one of the hallmarks of late nineteenth-century hospitals, the pavilion ward. Such wards possessed two primary assets: the rows of beds in a large rectangular room made surveillance by nursing staff easy, and the tall windows on each side allowed for a generous cross-ventilation, providing fresh air and, so the theory went, preventing the spread of infection. At one level, its rationale still reflected older miasmatic views, when bad smells were sometimes actually equated with disease; and the emphasis on nursing sightlines at the expense of patient privacy is an appropriate reminder that patients mostly came from the lower classes. Nevertheless, the design proved functional and popular and continued to be used even after germ theory had taken away some of its original justification.

More generally, the design of hospitals was the subject of much lively debate, and doctors, nurses, administrators, and architects were all involved. New hospitals were often put to tender, with plans subjected to public inquiry and comment in both the medical press and more general periodicals such as *The Builder*. The state of the art can be seen in volumes such as Sir Douglas Galton's *Healthy Hospitals* (1893). Galton provided detailed discussions on topics such as ward design, ventilation, heating, and lighting, and less than might be expected on the architectural trappings of the newer medical and surgical developments. He considered laboratories necessary only in connection with medical education, and, although a separate operating room "and its adjuncts" would be part of any general hospital by then, Galton had little specific to say about their design. The disinfection room he considered in relation to patients' clothing. He took it for granted that a hospital of any size would have residential accommodations for the nursing staff and probationers, as student nurses were called.

Although Galton was British, no hospital received fuller coverage in his monograph than the recently opened Johns Hopkins Hospital. John Shaw Billings (1838–1913), engaged as the medical consultant, had a large say in its design, and, although its construction had been plagued and delayed by financial problems, it was opened to general acclaim. Billings' military career helped guarantee the dominance of the pavilion ward there, although there was already in the United States more provision for one- and two-bedded wards than was common in Europe. The research and teaching functions of the new institution were reasonably catered for, and the surgical theaters incorporated modern lighting and sterilization equipment. Hopkins' surgeons and gynecologists were to be at the forefront in adopting the modern symbols of the surgeon's craft: the sterilized gown, mask, and rubber gloves.

Needless to say, these characteristics of the late nineteenth-century hospital cost money, and the containment of hospital costs is not simply a contemporary issue. Then, as now, public hospitals felt the pinch of tight budgets, and the private, voluntary ones faced the treadmill of trying to generate ever larger sums from wealthy and not-so-wealthy benefactors. A ward closed not for want of patients but for lack of resources to heat and light, and to pay staff to run it, was a common phenomenon.

Traditional patterns of fund-raising continued. These consisted of such things as personal appeals by prominent aristocratic or wealthy members of the hospital's board of governors, special dinners, soirées or charity balls, sermons with targeted collections in a local church, and the inevitable collection box inside the hospital. Patients who could afford it were often asked to contribute something toward their hospital costs, and the hospitals themselves became increasingly concerned that patients who had the means to pay a private practitioner were abusing the charitable aims of the institution, denying the practitioner his fees and a worthy patient his place in the outpatient department or ward. Clerks were engaged to means-test patients, although this was cumbersome and only modestly successful. It was easy, for example, for patients to give false addresses, which made checking their circumstances very difficult.

To these local initiatives were added several more general medical charities that aimed to raise the profile of the hospitals and to increase participation in charitable giving. In Britain, the Hospital Saturday Fund (so named since Saturday was the common day when the week's wages were paid) encouraged workers to contribute a small sum each week. Similar schemes were adopted in provincial communities. In the sense that such enterprises generated a good deal of money for the hospitals, they were successful, but the worker who contributed a penny a week to the fund naturally assumed that this entitled him and his family to use its facilities, and so increased demand. The Hospital Sunday Fund, started in the 1850s, appealed to middle-class benefactors, through coordinated collections at church services. In London, the Prince of Wales' Hospital Fund of 1897 (it became the King Edward's Hospital Fund for London after Edward ascended the throne) successfully capitalized on the popularity of royalty and spearheaded centralized charitable giving in London for half a century.

These and similar organizations went some way toward keeping voluntary hospitals reasonably solvent, but mounting costs continued to put pressure on them. A second tack was to take middle- and upper-class patients on a full paying basis, thereby partially offsetting the deficits in the charity wards. In the United States, pay beds were common if in the minority throughout the century, as Americans of economic substance accepted the possibility of inpatient care earlier than their British counterparts. Residential medical facilities did exist for the upper classes. Called nursing homes, private medical homes, and convalescent homes, some were run by doctors themselves, though most permitted patients to keep their regular medical attendants. Private madhouses had been common since the eighteenth century, and inebriate houses and institutions for mentally subnormal children and adults advertised their availability to the paying classes. Through most of the century, though, medical and surgical treatment at home was the preferred pattern for those above the status of "deserving poor," and a patient coming to London for an operation by an eminent surgeon might well have it performed in a hotel room. The hospitals kept registers of nurses (which they had trained) available privately.

It is easy enough to assume that the increased usage, from the 1880s, of the voluntary general and specialist hospitals by the wealthier classes was a natural response to the newer diagnostic and therapeutic facilities there; to aseptic surgery and efficient nursing care: in short, for the reasons why sick people still go into hospital. The argument has some purchase, because these very features made the idea possible to sell. But paying patients had to be educated into accepting this as more desirable than treatment at home, in a hotel, or in a small clinic. The hospitals had to prepare for this new type of patient by building private wings or converting older wards, since patient expectations were different from those in receipt of charity. It thus required a capital investment by hospitals, which were for the most part strapped for cash. Private beds were seen as an investment; they were meant to be profitable, not to turn the institution into a commercial enterprise, but to subsidize the hospital's charitable work. Paying patients used common facilities such as x-ray equipment, and they made it easy for the consultant staff to spend more time at the hospital, to keep an eye on their seriously ill patients, and follow them up in the private consulting rooms.

This transformation was well under way by World War I, and it owes much to both the economic realities of the era and the scientific and technological developments within medicine. It represents yet another attribute that links the hospital of 1910 more closely to us than to its ancestor of a century earlier.

III. SPECIALIZATION

The many American or British medical students who spent time in Germany from the 1860s onward would have observed how specialization within the profession might work, at least within the educational context of the teaching hospital. They would already of course have experienced the division of knowledge into separate if overlapping spheres, and seen within both scientific and clinical contexts new pressures on traditional disciplines: the emergence of physiology from the older emphasis on functional anatomy; increasing autonomy for pathology; lectures and/ or clinical work in particular subjects such as medical jurisprudence or the diseases of women and children. There were in addition the traditional division of labor between physicians and surgeons, a growing medical involvement with obstetrics (as male-midwifery was by then commonly called), a group of doctors who concentrated on the insane, and many monographs on disease of a particular kind or a single organ or system. Anyone in the mid-nineteenth century could have simply looked at Western society and seen that increasing occupational diversity was a fact of life.

Nevertheless, specialization within medicine did not seem "natural" or desirable to many doctors. In the first place, it smacked of quackery, or at least of itinerant fringe practice. Bone setters, cataract couchers, and bladder stone cutters were traditional examples of occupational specialization within the healing arts, and those who had earned their living practicing one of these skills had generally worked outside the boundaries of the regular profession, traveling around in search of patients. The anxiety and shame attached to disorders such as syphilis and gonorrhea were also exploited by practitioners offering quick (and expensive) cures. To many regulars, specializing in one operation or disease was tantamount to admitting that you could do nothing else and were thus ill-educated or not properly educated at all.

In addition, specializing entailed putting oneself above one's peers and this went contrary to notions of medical equality. It meant telling the public directly or indirectly that this disease or that operation was best handled by a specialist with greater experience and skill. It could involve poaching patients and thus transgressing the conventions of medical etiquette.

The latter arguments cut both ways, of course: seeing a lot of patients with a particular kind of disorder did enhance experience and patients might prefer being treated by someone who had seen it all before. And the continued founding of specialist hospitals – for diseases of the skin, eye, nervous system, ear, nose and throat, chest, heart – kept the idea in front of the public.

The results of this constant emphasis on more circumscribed bodies of medical knowledge and function are obvious. In the German universities and teaching hospitals, appointments in special branches of medicine and surgery began to be regularly made from about midcentury. These included ophthalmology, dermatology, otolaryngology, pediatrics, obstetrics, gynecology, psychiatry, and neurology. The last two subjects were sometimes combined, though separate posts were the norm by the century's end; by then several universities also had made appointments in orthopedic surgery. Attached to the post would be hospital beds, outpatient clinics, and lecture time; and several of the individuals, for example Albrecht von Graefe (1828–70) in ophthalmology in Berlin, and Ferdinand von Hebra (1816–80) in dermatology in Vienna, taught large numbers of students from home and abroad.

Teaching particular branches of medicine or surgery in special lectures or clinics could be seen as simply providing the all-round training that medical students required, and for most learning to diagnose skin complaints (notoriously difficult despite the fact that the lesion was directly visible), and to use the ophthalmoscope or laryngoscope, were incidental steps to becoming a "safe general practitioner." For those who wanted to spend much or even all their professional life in a special branch of practice, local or national societies began gradually to be formed, and by the end of the century, international congresses had been held in most of the specialisms. More often than not, a specialist periodical in a discipline first appeared in Germany, but the phenomenon was in evidence elsewhere as well. Even in Britain, where élite physicians and surgeons were often vocal in the resistance to specialization, from 1870 to 1900, more new journal titles were aimed at particular groups within the profession than at the profession at large. In the 1850s and 60s, medical or surgical consultants at the general London voluntary hospitals were discouraged or even debarred from simultaneously holding a consultancy at a specialist hospital. By the century's end, the practice had become common, even routine. At the same time, general hospitals began to appoint mostly junior staff members to take responsibility for special departments in skin, eye, throat, and other diseases.

If the phenomenon was clear, the reasons for it were complex. Technological developments could be important, as in otolaryngology or ophthalmology, even if eye hospitals had existed before Helmholtz invented the ophthalmoscope. Competition within a crowded profession also played its part, as ambitious young doctors sought to make a name for themselves by making a limited territory their own. A continuing emphasis on multiple case reporting encouraged doctors to collect and publish whole series of cases, and, as Sir William Lawrence (1783–1867) remarked of the Moorfields Eye Hospital in London, "You may see more diseases of the eye in this institution in three months than in the largest hospital in fifty years."[1] Nor is ours the first generation to believe itself in the middle of an explosion of knowledge, and medical educators a century ago were also concerned at how crowded the medical curriculum seemed to be becoming.

It was easy to decry specialization as artificial and professionally divisive, and to suggest that specialists fell into the trap of seeing not the whole patient but only some favorite organ or disease. Fashions in diagnosis or treatment were blamed on this monomania of the specialist, who was also accused of being too aggressive therapeutically. Gynecologists were singled out as corruptors of female modesty and virtue, through overuse of the vaginal speculum, and of magnifying minor complaints into major ones, creating disease and dependence where it did not exist before. One specialty particularly stood out: psychiatry. The word "psychiatry" was commonly used in its German equivalent (*Psychiatrie*) earlier than in the English-speaking world, where British and American doctors practiced what by mid-century was being called "psychological medicine." They themselves were sometimes referred to as "alienists" (from the French convention), sometimes more starkly as "mad doctors." It was in many ways the earliest medical specialty. It was also the earliest in Britain to associate the private sector with institutional care, through private madhouses, or the "trade in lunacy." Even in the eighteenth century, madhouse keepers ran establishments that catered for the top of the market, as middle- and upper-class families preferred not to cope with the difficulties, embarrassment, and uncertainties of individuals exhibiting "mad" behavior and bizarre thought processes.

Loss of rights and control of wealth and property followed a diagnosis of insanity or mental incompetence, and the possibility of wrongful confinement, following collusion between grasping relatives and unscrupulous madhouse keepers, led to legislation as early as the 1780s to try to provide some checks on the trade in lunacy. Madhouses had to be licensed and a committee appointed by the Royal College of Physicians notified of new admissions. Except for public health, no other area of medicine was to attract so much legislative attention, and even today, psychiatry is occasionally referred to as an "administrative specialty."

The public today sometimes has trouble distinguishing between psychiatry, the medical discipline, and psychology, a nonmedical one, and the roots of this go deep. Madhouse keepers were by no means always medical men, and someone deeply melancholic, or troubled by voices that no one else heard might seek counsel from a clergyman or neighbor. There is a continuous tradition of medical writings stretching back to antiquity that we might label "psychiatric," but also a variety of nonmedical ways of interpreting "crazy" or unusual behavior, and a large body of philosophical literature dealing with the workings of the mind. In addition, the attitudes toward the insane and their treatment, which underpinned so much of the expansion of nineteenth-century "psychiatry," stemmed initially from a response to medical neglect and the inadequacy of medical remedies for mental disturbances.

This was "moral therapy," and, although under the banner of "management" much of what was meant by moral therapy had an older elaboration, early nineteenth-century reformers saw in moral therapy much that was new and hopeful. They associated it with the changes that Philippe Pinel (see Chapter 2) effected in the Paris general hospitals (Bicêtre for men, Salpêtrière for women) during the French Revolution; with the work and writings of Vincenzo Chiarugi (1738–1820) in Italy; and with the foundation, in 1796, of the York Retreat in England. Both Pinel and Chiarugi were doctors, but the therapeutic regimes that they developed downplayed physical remedies and esoteric classification of the varieties of insanity in favor of an approach that stressed a kind of firmness and daily human contact in dealing with their charges. A sympathetic and reliable nursing staff could be just as important as the doctor. In fact, at the York Retreat, the lay resident superintendent and his wife were the central therapeutic figures, and William Tuke (1732–1822), head of the Quaker family that established it, saw it as a nonmedical alternative to Bethlem (Bedlam) and other psychiatric institutions where a medical regimen had dominated. There were to be no whips or chains at the Retreat; rather, a quiet atmosphere to be organized around the ideals of family life and the reward of appropriate behavior. The philosophy of the place was eloquently expounded by Tuke's grandson Samuel Tuke (1784–1857), in his *A Description of the Retreat* (1813), a monograph that put the institution firmly on the world psychiatric map and provided a stark contrast to the public revelations of medical abuse and neglect that emerged in 1815–16 during a Parliamentary Enquiry into the state of madhouses in Britain. Tuke's work was republished in the United States and the institutional ideals copied at the Hartford Retreat and elsewhere.

The extensive publicity given to the Parliamentary hearings (at which, among other reformers, the octogenarian William Tuke was an impressive witness) combined with the alternative to ordinary medical treatment of insanity that the Retreat offered, created the possibility that the insane could have been (to use a barbarous modern term) de-medicalized and their care placed in the hands of well-intentioned lay people. That it did not happen is not surprising in retrospect, for even the Tukes were anxious to use what they conceived as the morally neutral language of a disease model (the insane are ill and deserve to be treated with the same consideration as other sick people), and it proved easy enough for medical men to marry the ideals of moral therapy to the more general aspirations of a medical specialty.

In the middle third of the century, in Germany, France, Britain, and the United States, coherent professional psychiatric groups emerged, with associations, journals, institutions, and reasonably defined roles. That the institutions tended to be called "asylums" rather than hospitals; that the correlation of symptom and lesion, the hallmark of avant-garde clinical medicine, continued to elude the alienists; that the optimistic promises of moral and other therapies did not yield the high rate of cures that seemed so possible in the 1820s and 30s; that the asylums, built with high expectations in tranquil, rural surroundings, became on the contrary, too isolated from general medicine and from society itself; that the medical superintendents, as the head psychiatrists were called, became remote from their patients, preoccupied instead with the daily administration of these gigantic institutions: all these items should be taken into account when evaluating the fortunes of psychiatry and psychiatrists during the century.

They must be balanced, however, against more positive achievements: the reasonably successful campaign to secure public resources for the specialty; a toehold, first in Germany, then in France, Britain, and the

United States, into medicine's academic citadel, as lectures and practical experience in the subject became a part, albeit a minor one, of the medical curriculum; a certain cultural status in the last third of the century, as anxiety, neurasthenia, and other forms of neuroses (as they were increasingly called) seemed to be more prevalent, and new forms of therapy, including hypnosis and suggestion, were being explored. The latter, of course, form part of the background to Sigmund Freud (1856–1939), his early career, and the development of psychoanalysis. The impact of psychoanalysis upon psychiatry is a twentieth-century phenomenon (and was to raise again the questions of psychiatry's relationship to medicine). More generally, though, Freud was able to structure his own career because "office psychiatry" – the treatment of "nervous diseases" outside the asylum – was a late nineteenth-century professional option. In that sense, he was part of the same concatenation of values that permitted George Beard (1839–83), popularizer of the neurasthenia diagnosis, and Silas Weir Mitchell (1829–1914), advocate of the "rest cure" for nervous disorders, to thrive in the United States. Office psychiatry in turn impinged on, and overlapped with, another nascent specialty, neurology, which by the turn of the century was beginning to acquire its own journals, societies, and values.

The process of subdividing medicine broadly conceived into component specialties was hardly complete by World War I; in many ways, it had just begun. Within general medicine, only dermatology and neurology had been split off; within surgery, only ophthalmology, otolaryngology, and, tentatively, orthopedics. Obstetrics and gynecology had consolidated from an amalgam of medical and surgical interests. Cardiology, endocrinology, gastroenterology, neurosurgery, cardiac surgery, and many other specialisms were still unconceived or embryonic. Radiology and anesthesiology were yet poorly differentiated professionally and pediatrics just beginning to acquire an identity. Nevertheless, the idea had been largely accepted by both the public and the profession, and the referral system, on which specialists depended, was beginning to be accepted as part of intraprofessional relations.

IV. PAYING THE DOCTOR

Despite an increasing professional consolidation, and its attendant rhetoric of service, doctors throughout the century were in the business of earning a living in what was actually a very crowded marketplace. Competition could come in many forms: fellow practitioners; hospitals and dispensaries that treated patients who had the means to pay a private doctor; chemists and pharmacists who sold medicines directly to the public; advice books that encouraged every man to be his own doctor; itinerate "specialists," mountebanks, and drug peddlars; shrewd mail-

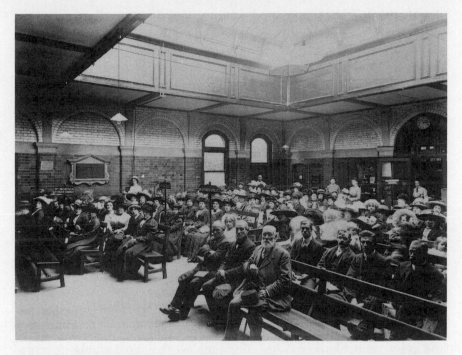

Figure 26. The rapid development of hospital outpatient departments in the late nineteenth century was not universally welcomed by general practitioners, who feared the competition. This scene, from the Great Northern Central Hospital in London, conveys something of how vivid a visit to an outpatient department would have been for a working-class individual.

order merchants; homeopaths and other sectaries who challenged the very basis of medical orthodoxy. Small wonder that many doctors felt themselves beleaguered on all sides, as they sought to earn the income that their professional status should have entitled them. No one tried to sell a career in medicine as an easy option for a young man, but medical commentators, concerned with recruiting a respectable class of person into the ranks, always emphasized that, with good training, integrity, and energy, a decent living and solid social standing could be attained.

Nevertheless, there was always enough competition about to create economic uncertainty among rank-and-file practitioners, and even the urban élite generally had to weather early years of modest earnings. Those who made it to the top had most to lose by any change in the traditional structures of the profession, and in both Britain and the United States fee-for-services continued to be the way in which wealthier patients paid for their medical care. There were guidelines but no rigid rules governing how much a consultation, operation, or home visit should cost, but top physicians or surgeons did very well, particularly if they kept busy and had the occasional grateful patient who paid over the odds. Those who practiced among the less well-to-do, especially the general practitioners, were more precariously placed. So, of course, were their patients, and the modern phrase "medical indigence" has resonances in a nineteenth-century context. The growth of third-party payments for medical care – what we call insurance – had its primary origins in organized labor movements, and ultimately in the increased intervention of the State in the financing and control of medical services.

Various fears haunted working-class people in the century: of the workhouse and the hospital, of unemployment and financial incompetence, of old age and a pauper's burial. It was against these uncertainties that workers' associations began, especially from the mid-century, to collect weekly payments from members, offering benefits in return if injury, unemployment, sickness, or death disrupted the routine of daily life. The size, forms, and functions of these organizations varied considerably, from a loose local association of workers engaged in similar work or employed by the same employer, to larger structures affiliated with the nascent trades union movement. Sometimes, benevolent or paternalistic employers contributed something on their workers' behalf, and the "factory surgeon" became a familiar figure in the industrial landscape, particularly in connection with work-related accidents or injuries, but also with a watching brief on women and children, vulnerable members of the workforce.

Out of this complex mesh of forces and values emerged a new form of medical practice, the contract or club practice. Through what were called friendly societies, workers' clubs, mutual associations, medical institutes, and provident dispensaries, medical men began to be employed on a salaried basis to provide care and medicine for groups of individuals. There were obvious advantages for both parties: for workers, it allowed for weekly budgeting of medical costs (often in a package of income stabilization that also included sickness and unemployment benefits and burial expenses); for the doctors, it gave them a regular, guaranteed salary, plenty of work, and protection against a common problem of those practicing in working-class areas, the nonpayment of medical bills. The capitation system, whereby the doctor was paid a certain annual sum for each patient for whom he was responsible, was the usual method of calculation, and, as George Bernard Shaw suggested, should have encouraged doctors to keep their patients as healthy as possible. Nothing could appear simpler.

In practice, the medical profession qua profession was deeply suspicious of contract practice. Both the BMA and AMA opposed it, and the "battle of the clubs" raged for decades. Doctors argued that it was demeaning for middle-class professionals to be the employees of working-class groups; that the terms and conditions of contract employment were miserly; that the dregs of the profession who deigned to accept such contracts brought the status of the whole down and in any case were often incapable of providing adequate care; and that such arrangements encouraged patients to abuse the system and run to the doctor with every trivial or imaginary complaint.

Despite official resistance, there was generally no shortage of applicants for medical posts within the clubs and associations; younger doctors in particular appreciated the guaranteed income while establishing themselves in a community. Even if the goal of solo private practice remained foremost for most doctors, salaried positions assumed ever larger significance in the closing decades of the century, either through a friendly society, lodge, or club, or through the increasing number of state- or community-funded posts in public health, prison and port authority medical service, psychiatric asylums, and charity clinics.

There was no inevitable passage from contract or salaried service to the forms of national, State-administered medical insurance that were in place in Germany, Britain, and other European countries before World War I. At the end of the nineteenth century, there were striking similarities between Britain and the United States in the varieties of medical practice, medical institutions, and medical competition. The supply of doctors was even larger per head of population in the United States than in European countries, and this in itself heightened competition and potential economic uncertainty among practitioners. In the aftermath of the American Civil War and on into the progressive era of the 1890s and early 1900s, trades unionism gathered strength and a number of social reformers pushed for greater distribution of wealth, enhanced state control of rampant capitalism, and easier access to more and better funded welfare systems. American debates on compulsory national health insurance for workers were most intense in the years surrounding World War I. Pressure groups such as the American Association for Labor Legislation campaigned vigorously, initially with some medical support and the brief cooperation of the traditionally conservative AMA.

Ultimately, however, there was insufficient grass-roots enthusiasm among the doctors, many of whom were by then calling themselves specialists in an effort to augment their prestige and income, and who in any case were unhappy with medical aspects of workmen's compensation acts and other social legislation that did pass Congress. Although contract practice remained associated with a few industries such as the railway, and a few universities began to develop medical services for their staff and students, the movement toward any nationalized scheme of health insurance fell foul of the countercampaign by local, state, and national medical societies, and the fact that World War I made it easy to dismiss national insurance as un-American and undemocratic, because it was pioneered in the very country, Germany, the Allies were then fighting. After the war, the growth in American third-party medical payments was mostly through private health insurance.

The 1883 German system of compulsory national health insurance for large numbers of the workforce was a model for several others instituted in Europe before the century's end (Austria in 1888, and Hungary in 1891), and elsewhere, such as Denmark and Sweden, state funds began to be used to subsidize the existing mutual societies. Several other European countries adopted national insurance plans before World War I. The German scheme, as the first and in a country with growing economic, political, and military muscle, was the most visible. It was often mentioned, in the American backlash against state involvement in medical care, as an example of the horrors of "socialized medicine." Ironically, it was hardly socialistic in intent. Bismarck, its chief political architect, was no friend of the growing tide of collectivist sentiment in the period. In fact, he conceived of State-subsidized, compulsory social insurance as a means of defusing militant working-class agitation and attracting worker loyalty to himself and his grand plans for German industrial, military, political, and imperial advancement.

Bismarck was able to draw on some earlier, more limited experiments with compulsory sickness insurance, and on a well-established German tradition of mutual associations. He ensured that the legislation in the 1880s got maximum publicity abroad, a task made easier by both the increasing international visibility of the German Reich and the steady stream of foreign students in the German universities and medical schools. Countries that subsequently adapted national sickness insurance schemes modified them to suit local demands, traditions, or politics; but the German system contained many features that became common. These included the use whenever possible of the administrative machinery of preexisting mutual associations, to identify participants, collect subscriptions, keep records, assess needs, and dispense payments. The common pattern was a contributory structure (despite Bismarck's desire to make the German scheme entirely State funded), whereby employees, employers, and the State paid varying proportions into the coffers. In general, only industries with large skilled and semiskilled workforces were affected, with no provisions for agricultural and other low-paid laborers. This gave such schemes a predominantly urban orientation and reminds us that they were not the product of philosophies of universal welfare rights. In each country, wage bands of eligibility were created, with those workers falling below an income level forced to seek medical care through charity, the Poor Laws, or other public assistance, and those earning more than the upper limit expected to pay on a fee-for-service basis or obtain private insurance. In some countries workers' dependents were included; in others they were not. In Germany, hospital care was part of the package; in Britain, where earlier mutual associations had been concerned with general practice provision, it was not. In most places, about a quarter of the working population qualified for participation.

The National Health Insurance Act was not passed in Britain until 1911, a generation after comparable legislation in Germany. Nevertheless, with its traditions of individualism and laissez-faire economics, and its traditional ties to the United States, Britain provided the most telling example for American observers. The principal force behind the Act was the Liberal politician David Lloyd George (1863–1945), in 1911 Chancellor of the Exchequer, although soon to be the wartime Prime Minister. It was one of a series of early twentieth-century pieces of British social legislation dealing with pensions, workmen's compensation, unemployment benefits, and the medical inspection of school children.

Lloyd George seems to have been more aware of favorable British comment on the German system than he was of the passion that contract practice had generated in the medical profession, and more eager to pacify the mutual associations than the doctors. A few of the latter were prepared to generalize publicly on the importance of health for the national good, and on how financial considerations should not impinge on access to decent medical care. For the most part, however, doctors were concerned with their collective and individual economic and social positions, and the National Insurance Act seemed to put both in jeopardy: to diminish earnings and to make doctors the servants of their socially inferior patients. In the event, the Act went through Parliament rather quickly, and left the medical profession with the unenviable task of simultaneously trying to organize a collective policy of noncooperation and negotiate the best possible economic terms. The latter succeeded, whereas calls for a strike crumbled in the face of thousands of individual doctors – mostly general practitioners – who recognized that contract practice was already an established fact of life, and the terms under the National Insurance Act were actually better than those obtainable under the old regime. Many of the conditions of practice were comparable to those obtaining under contract or club practice, with the capitation fees a good deal better.

The National Health Insurance Act was, in the best British tradition, something of a compromise. It made special provision for the treatment of tuberculosis and, with the mandatory employer and state contributions, increased the amount of money put into health care. It did nothing to help the perilous financial plight of many of the voluntary hospitals (most of whose governors would have resisted state interference in any case), nor did it provide hospital care, except within a tuberculosis sanatorium. It left intact the medical services under the Poor Law for those who fell outside the remit of the Act, and so failed to satisfy the calls of those who wanted welfare benefits extended to the whole population without the stigma of the workhouse and its humiliating connotations.

Nevertheless, the many European experiments with social legislation were significant, and not simply for the income stabilization that they provided for large segments of the workforce. Within medicine, they strengthened the ties between the profession and the State; made the practice of medicine more public and maybe even more publicly accountable; and extended into the arena of curative medicine some of the concerns that the preventive movement had long since identified. None of the schemes succeeded in marrying preventive and curative medicine; and despite the rhetoric, they were too much sickness than health systems. But for millions of people throughout Europe, they made a visit to the doctor rather more ordinary, if only because it had already been paid for; and they were a reminder that health care had been identified as a social desideratum.

V. WOMEN AND MEDICINE

Until the eighteenth century, organized medicine had relatively little to do with childbirth. It was a social rather than a medical episode, presided over by a midwife, a neighbor, or female relative, and in any case, strictly women's business. If a doctor was involved, it meant that something had gone badly wrong, although the fact that medical men were only exceptionally called in guaranteed that they knew less about the management of labor than the ordinary midwife. In extremis, the male role was often confined to trying to save the mother's life, usually by hacking out the infant, which had become stuck in the birth canal.

The obstetrical forceps began to change this. The design of the forceps was a carefully guarded secret of the Chamberlen family in the seventeenth century, but once made public around 1720, forceps gave doctors a tool to work with. Medical men could then claim to be capable of saving mothers and babies, through assisted deliveries, were they called in early enough. In eighteenth-century London, Paris, and other large cities, a few men began to devote most of their professional energies to obstetrical practice, and it became fashionable among wealthy women to have their babies delivered by man-midwives. William Hunter (see Chapter 1) successfully cultivated obstetrics as well as anatomy teaching. He was appointed accoucheur – the French word seemed to convey gentility on the field – to Queen Charlotte, wife of George III, and actually delivered her fourth child in 1766. (During her previous labors, he had had to wait in the anteroom while a midwife presided over the childbed.) From about the same period, lying-in hospitals, staffed by both midwives and medical men, were established, and designed to

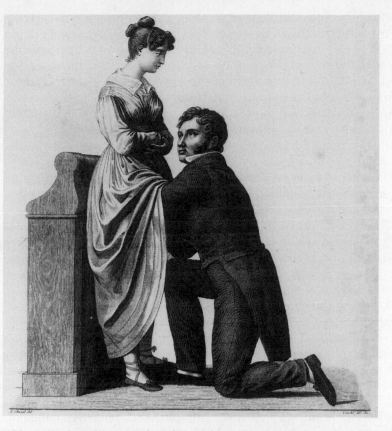

Figure 27. An awkward examination of a woman for signs of pregnancy in the 1820s. From the bemused expression on the woman's face, it is not clear what she wishes the verdict to be. From J. P. Maygrier, Nouvelles démonstrations d'accouchemens *(Paris: Béchet, 1822), Plate xxix.*

provide safe, "advanced" obstetrical care to the deserving poor, either in hospital or (more commonly) through a domiciliary service.

By the end of the eighteenth century, the medicalization of childbirth was under way and many of the issues that continued to exercise doctors, midwives, and mothers in the nineteenth had been broached. These concerned questions of female modesty, the relative competence of midwives and medical men, indications for the use of forceps, and the management of the three stages of labor. Despite the existence of a few lying-in hospitals, childbirth was still overwhelmingly a domestic event, and it was only later in the century that doctors began to argue that childbirth is a pathological (as opposed to a normal, "physiological") process, and therefore by definition required the services of a trained doctor, working in a hospital.

Disputes between midwives and medical men were most acrimonious in the United States, where midwives began to be squeezed out in urban areas by the mid-nineteenth century, and hospital deliveries became more common. In Europe, there were established traditions of licensing and training midwives and the growth of the medical specialty of obstetrics did not threaten to monopolize the childbirth business. By contrast, midwives in the United States never managed during the nineteenth century to achieve formal recognition through a system of licensing, nor did they possess any guilds or larger organizations to speak for them collectively. Although women – paid or unpaid – were still involved in most deliveries, especially in frontier settlements and rural areas, the sustained medical campaign against midwives effectively achieved its goals by the century's end, for several reasons.

First, most midwives came from backgrounds giving them few financial resources, which made training difficult, lowered the social respectability of the craft, and left them vulnerable to medical charges of incompetence and inadequate education. Further, nineteenth-century notions of women's "natural" homemaking role made it difficult in the best of circumstances for genteel women to obtain paid outside employment, particularly in areas of increasing male activity.

Second, many general practitioners actively sought delivery work, even though it could be time-consuming and inconvenient, since successfully delivering the baby would help secure the loyalty and custom of the whole family.

In addition, developments in gynecological surgery had spin-offs in obstetrics. A number of American surgeons achieved fame for their gynecological work. Ephraim McDowell's (1771–1830) backwoods ovariotomies became part of the surgical folklore of the period, and J. Marion Sims (1813–83) acquired a national reputation for his operation to repair vesico-vaginal fistulas, perfected without anesthesia on long-suffering slaves. Sims moved from Alabama to New York City, where he was the driving force behind the establishment, in 1854, of the Women's Hospital. He also conducted two extended trips to Europe, which, by his own testimony, were unqualified triumphs. Certainly he was the most famous American surgeon of his generation. Gynecology and obstetrics were often practiced together as a single specialism, symbolized best by the operation of caesarian section, which by the middle of the century began to be used occasionally as more than a last resort, even if it still ended in the death of both mother and child as often as not.

In the period before antiseptic surgery (see Chapter 5), removing the ovaries became the most important abdominal operation. As surgeons gained more confidence, the range of symptoms they tried to "cure" by removing the ovaries (literally, oophorectomy, rather than ovariotomy) increased. The American Robert Battey (1828–95) advocated the removal of normal ovaries for a variety of conditions, including menstrual difficulties, hysteria, insanity, and epilepsy, and "Battey's operation," popular for about two decades from the 1860s, has achieved much historical notoriety, a symbol of knife-happy surgeons invading the bodies of helpless patients.

Gynecology thus aided the male capture of childbirth, though there was no hiding the fact that throughout the century parturition was safer at home than in a hospital. Prolonged labor would sometimes be successfully terminated by the use of forceps, or the manual manipulation of the infant to ease its entrance into the world, but hospitals continued to offer convenience to the doctors but little to the patients. The major single cause of maternal death was what was called puerperal fever, literally, the fever of childbirth. Although maternal mortality was never actually one of the leading causes of death, even among females, deaths in the flush of youth and at the very time when nineteenth-century women were deemed to have fulfilled their natural destinies were particularly galling. Puerperal fever was particularly so, since it usually set in two or three days after delivery (which could have been uncomplicated) and produced distressing symptoms of headache, vomiting, high fever, and abdominal pain. Mary Wollstonecraft (1759–97) thus died ten days after giving birth to a daughter who, as Mary Shelley, became famous as the wife of the poet and the author of *Frankenstein*. Wollstonecraft had become an ardent champion of the rights of women and her death in childbirth was a poignant reminder of women's lot. The only legitimate daughter of King George IV, Princess Charlotte (1796–1817), also died of complications of delivery, having produced a stillborn son. She was the beautiful heir to the throne and her death shocked the nation and led to the suicide of the royal accoucheur, Sir Richard Croft (1762–1818).

Outbreaks of puerperal fever could be sporadic but cases also tended to occur in clusters, sometimes among the patients of an individual general practitioner but more commonly within the lying-in hospitals or the lying-in wards of general hospitals. Like most epidemic diseases, there was debate about whether it was "contagious" or "miasmatic" in origin. A succession of individuals since Alexander Gordon (1752–99) in Scotland had argued in favor of a specific contagion, spread person to person, but miasmatic contamination associated with crowded hospital wards and putrefaction seemed to many to offer as convincing an explanation.

In 1843, Oliver Wendell Holmes again forcefully put the contagionist case, which, because it implicated doctors in the spread of the disease, found little support within the profession. Shortly after, Ignaz Semmelweis (1818–65) began collecting statistics in the General Hospital in Vienna, which showed that women delivered in the hospital by midwives were much less likely to die from puerperal fever than those delivered by medical staff and students. He argued that decaying organic matter – putrefaction – was the *materia morbi*, conveyed by doctors who went directly from postmortem dissections to the delivery room. He further showed that by enforcing the washing in a chlorinated lime solution of medical hands and instruments before touching a parturient woman, mortality rates in the medical clinic could be reduced to almost the same as that on the midwifery one: from about 10 percent (average, 1841–6) to almost 3.5 percent (average 1847–55). The comparable midwifery figures were about 4 percent and 3 percent.

Semmelweis undoubtedly saved many lives but did not change obstetrical practice outside his immediate sphere of influence. Even that was limited by his being a Hungarian outsider in Vienna, aggressive and polemical in dealing with his superiors, and mentally unstable. His main published work, *The Etiology, Concept and Prophylaxis of Childbed Fever* (1861), was a hard-hitting treatise, but not the brilliant protobacteriological work that later doctors sometimes took it for. It was full of sound practical advice, much of which was in the older sanitarian mold.

Lister came to learn of Semmelweis's endeavors only after he began developing his own ideas of antiseptic practice, which were gradually adopted into obstetrics. By the 1880s, outbreaks of puerperal fever within hospitals were becoming rare, though hospital maternal mortality rates still exceeded those of domestic deliveries, and doctors' rates were worse on average than those obtained by trained midwives. Doctors argued that they got all the difficult cases.

In the United States, obstetrics became increasingly dominated by male practitioners, whereas in Britain, the 1902 Midwives Act assured the continuity of midwifery; and in the Netherlands, Germany, and elsewhere on the Continent, established systems of training and licensing midwives operated throughout the nineteenth century.

Although midwives were disadvantaged when confronted with an increasingly powerful medical profession, they did have one traditional argument in their favor: that natural female modesty was offended by the presence of men in the intimate setting of parturition. It was an argument that also had relevance to women's entry into the medical profession itself. If women were natural healers, full of sympathy, why not teach them medicine, so that a woman could choose to be cared for by one of her own sex?

The argument cut little ice with many members of the medical profession, who maintained that women were too weak physically and intellectually, and too unstable emotionally, to endure the rigors of medical education and the fierce competition of practice. The exploits and struggles of some of the first few intrepid women have long been celebrated: Elizabeth Blackwell (1821–1910), who left England to obtain a medical

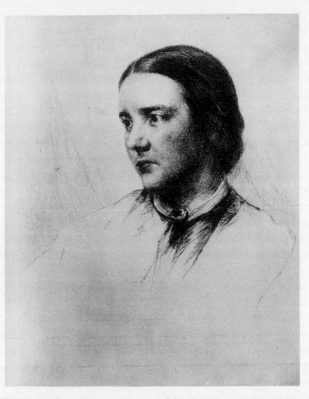

Figure 28. Sophia Jex-Blake (1840–1912), one of the early women medical graduates and a founder (in 1874) of the London School of Medicine for Women, now the Royal Free Hospital and Medical School.

degree in 1848 at a medical college in Geneva, New York; Elizabeth Garrett Anderson (1836–1917) and Sophia Jex-Blake (1840–1912), who battered at the doors of Edinburgh University; Nadezhda Suslova (1842–1918), who graduated from the University of Zürich in 1867, the first modern woman to obtain a medical degree from an established university; or Mary Putnam Jacobi (1842–1906), who followed in Paris four years later. More recent research is beginning to find out more about other women – literally thousands – who followed these pioneers into the medical profession before World War I. Liberal Zürich continued to operate as a magnet, for men and women were educated together there. More commonly, though, it proved easier to establish separate medical schools for women than to find existing institutions and teachers prepared to teach such delicate subjects as anatomy and gynecology to mixed classes. The ease with which American medical schools could be established, and a relatively casual licensing system (in states where it existed at all) made it easier for American women to obtain medical degrees. There were separate medical colleges for women in London, New York, Philadelphia, and Chicago, and only a few top schools, like the University of Michigan, in 1870, opened their doors to women medical students.

Segregated education reinforced the doctrine of separate spheres and meant than many women learned their clinical medicine on women and children only, which directed their subsequent careers in that direction. Medical missionary work was another calling for a large number of early women medical graduates. Some, like Mary Putnam Jacobi, combined medicine and motherhood, as if in defiance of the oft-repeated belief that intellectual activity among women led to atrophied ovaries, masculinization, and sterility. Among early women medical graduates, Jacobi was one of the most distinguished intellectually; her books and articles dealt with neurology, pathology, physiology, and pediatrics. She championed the notion that women should compete on equal terms with men, having absorbed the same scientific spirit, in contrast to Elizabeth Blackwell and others who argued that women should soften the profession, and occupy niches particularly suitable for them, like family practice, obstetrics (but not gynecology), pediatrics, and health education.

In the end, Jacobi's counsel was the more historically prescient. Many of the women's colleges had difficulty surviving the purges of the Flexner era, which meant that some of the battles for women's medical education had to be refought in the twentieth century, in the context of integrated professional training, but in the face of quotas and discrimination.

VI. BEING A PATIENT

For most of the twentieth century, the historical patient has been virtually anonymous. There were two categories of exceptions: patients who contributed to medical discovery by having a peculiar condition or by being the first to receive a new diagnosis or therapy; and the great and good of history, whose ills historically inclined doctors viewed through what they call the "retrospectroscope." A few examples of the first have already been mentioned: James Phipps and Joseph Meister of smallpox and rabies fame, and William Beaumont's patient Alexis St. Martin. Among the latter group are Charles Darwin, probably more diagnosed in death than he ever was in life; St. Paul and his seizures; Napoleon and his piles; and Franklin Roosevelt and his polio, hypertension, and malignant melanoma.

The process of trying to recapture what it was like to be a more ordinary patient has now begun, although we must not fall into the trap of assuming that all working-class people lay desperately ill in hospital, the result of some industrial accident or filth disease; and all middle-class individuals lay in the sunlight on their chaise-longues, discussing with their doctors their ailments, most of which were psychological and to be "cured" by a cruise, a visit to a spa, or a winter in Italy or the south of France. Genteel ladies could and did suffer agonizing deaths from cholera; and hospital case records make it very plain that a good many working-class patients were admitted with mild, self-limited disorders, or simply because they needed a few days' food and rest. Being a patient was (and is) an experience with identifiably universal features and as many nuances as there are instances of sick individuals seeking medical advice and treatment. It made (and makes) a difference if the sick person was male or female; young or old; confronted with minor, serious, shameful, or life-threatening illness (or believed him- or herself to be so); was rich or poor; trusted his doctor or not; was in hospital, outpatient department, doctor's surgery, or at home; was educated or not; was seeing the neighborhood practitioner or a high-powered specialist; was in the hands of a "good" doctor or not. This list could be extended almost indefinitely, for each illness is uniquely experienced.

The patient and his or her illness are unique; the "cure" more routine. The doctors' versions of the doctor–patient encounter are preserved in case records that during the course of the century began to acquire a more formal structure, as teachers sought to instill in their students orderly, methodical habits of observation and physical examination, and hospitals began to use large bound volumes in which the patients' hospital story was described in variable detail on printed forms that encouraged doctors to record specific aspects of the present story, past illness, review of systems, examination, and any diagnostic results. Because of the legal implications of a psychiatric diagnosis and admission to an asylum, the bureaucratic rituals of psychiatry were formalized earlier – by the mid-nineteenth century in many countries – although it is frequently difficult to discover much individuality in psychiatric casebooks, where a patient institutionalized for years or decades might receive less than a page of notes. Often, case registers were literally that: registers of cases rather than histories of individuals. The very fact that medical institutions remained overwhelmingly for those segments of society who were poor and inarticulate means that we usually have only the doctor's side of the story.

The well-trained medical student would have appreciated the value of keeping records, in later life, of his private patients. A good many undoubtedly did, and some private casebooks do survive, even if we can never know how widespread the practice was. Moreover, account books of medical men survive in much greater numbers than casebooks, and some of the latter were as much devoted to the number of visits, fees, and the costs of medicines as to the examination and diagnosis or other medical aspects of the patient's illness. Nor are private medical

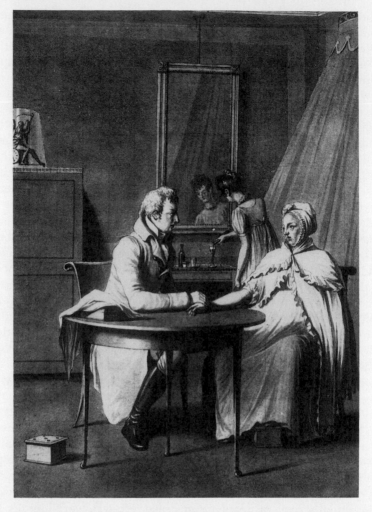

Figure 29. An early nineteenth-century scene of a home visit from the doctor. The patient is fully dressed and there is no evidence that the doctor will base his diagnosis on more than the history, the pulse, and an inspection of the face and tongue. Exhibited: Amsterdam, 6th International Congress of the History of Medicine. Drawing no. 83 (anonymous and as collected by Dr. J. van der Hoefde at Eefdel).

records as systematic in their format as hospital ones, which is not surprising given the specific nature of most doctor–patient encounters outside the hospital, as well as the delicacy of class and gender. Queen Victoria's long-time and trusted personal physician, Sir James Reid (1849–1923), never saw his royal patient's chest and abdomen until her autopsy; indeed, he first saw her in bed only when she was dead. Nevertheless, the private casebooks of Peter Mere Latham (1789–1875) in the 1830s document that he used his stethoscope on his paying patients, just as he did in the wards of St. Bartholomew's Hospital, where he was a consultant. His patients included an archbishop and several peers.

As a kind of abstract concept, "the patient" seems to have acquired a more specific identity among doctors during the century, which is symptomatic, perhaps, of their increasing professional status and the new technologies distancing them from those they treated. More often than not, the abstract patient was referred to as female. Although advice books aimed at the public have a long history, and continued to be regularly produced throughout the century, a slightly different genre of book began to appear. This was the doctor reflecting on, and explaining the nuances of the profession to a lay audience. *Doctor and Patient, The Doctor and His Work, Medicine and the Public* are self-explanatory titles of three such volumes. Another genre of books, with titles such as *Diary of an Invalid* or *Life in the Sick-Room*, explored the other side of the coin. More privately, diaries, journals, and correspondence articulated how individuals a century ago coped with anxiety and uncertainty, experienced illness and pain, and faced dying.

The deathbed scene had long been popular with pious biographers, especially if the subject were devout or at least had died like a Christian. There were no life-support systems, no intravenous feeding, even in hospitals, and, despite the increasing number and importance of the latter, most people still entered and left the world outside of them. A significant part of clinical wisdom was the ability to judge when the patient's condition was hopeless, and to prepare both the patient and the family for the eventuality. Before the doctor decided the time had come, many of them preferred to keep the patient in the dark about the gravity of the condition, believing that hope was literally one of the best medicines available. Depending on his own judgment, and the wishes of the family, the doctor might be discreetly absent for the final moments, leaving the stage to the family, nurse, and clergyman. Many doctors, even religious ones, did not like clergymen hovering around too early or too much, as it might introduce morbid thoughts to the patient, and reduce the chances of recovery. Among Roman Catholics, the timing of the Last Rites was important. Throughout the century, the doctor's task among the dying was probably made easier by the general understanding of the limits of medical power, by the strength of religious belief, and by the rituals surrounding death and mourning.

If doctors at the time often lapsed into the habit of referring to the patient as "she," modern historians have reinforced the trend, for much of the literature on medicine "from below" has concentrated on experiences of childbirth; attitudes toward menstruation and other aspects of female reproductive physiology; gynecological surgery, including clitoridectomy and ovariotomy for a variety of vague, nonspecific complaints; hysteria and other diagnoses made more commonly in females than males; and the series of scientific, cultural, and moral explanations of woman's place in nature: of why she was ruled by the heart (and womb) rather than the head; why she was physiologically suited for the home, marriage, and childbearing rather than occupations in the rough and tumble of the competitive world; why her nervous system was incapable of absorbing too many vigorous impressions or her brain too much rational knowledge; why she was unsuited for the learned professions; why her proper role was as the helpmeet of man, the neutralizing complement to the darker sides of his own aggressive personality. If the path of life led single file, someone had to walk behind.

Versions of this sermon were preached in thousands of ways by thousands of doctors and heard by countless women. Nor were doctors the only ones licensed to preach, nor women their only auditors. Something like this counted for natural knowledge among most – male or female – who thought on these things last century. For the majority of women, marriage was the only really acceptable career. There were positive exceptions, like Elizabeth Blackwell, Florence Nightingale, and Jane Addams; unmarried domestic servants and governesses were necessary, though even they might not remain spinsters forever; and occupations such as nursing, missionary work, and teaching could be admired, and maiden aunts and unmarried daughters fulfill important roles in the domestic economy. A woman's lot might not be easy, but, then, neither was the man's, required as he was to negotiate a world that was perceived as increasingly harsh, cut-throat, and competitive.

Nevertheless, maleness was rarely pathologized; femaleness could be, and was, even in the act of dubbing the universal patient "she."

Many of these issues can be seen in the life and death of one nineteenth-century patient, Alice James (1848–92). In modern times, she has had her life and her death skillfully chronicled, and her diary lovingly edited. In her own short lifetime, she had only a single letter published, and that pseudonymously signed "INVALID." Much of her adult life seems little more than a preparation for death, and of few people does Alexander Pope's poignant poetic line ring truer: "This long disease, my life." Even Alexander Pope, four-foot-six, hunchbacked, and tuberculous, managed a dozen years more than Alice James.

She was hardly typical of the patient in her era, even the female one. Most women, having celebrated their twenty-first birthday, would live past forty-four. Most women married, and the majority of these bore children. Most women kept no diary, or were ever seen by any doctor who contributed to our historical image of the nineteenth-century woman. Most doctor–patient encounters were private and unrecorded.

Nevertheless, Alice James's life is instructive. It links the Old World and the New. It relates a female sufferer to her male doctors. Above all, it provides material insight into a nineteenth-century mind.

That sufficient documents survive to reconstruct a reasonably full biography of Alice James is in itself unusual. But she came from no ordinary family. Her father, Henry James, Sr. (1811–82), was a minor philosopher, writer, and mystic in New England, reasonably prominent in his time but remembered more historically as the father of his children, who included the novelist Henry James, Jr. (1843–1916), and the psychologist and philosopher William James (1842–1910). Alice was the fifth and youngest child, and only daughter. Her two other brothers play only bit parts in history, though major supporting roles in the family drama. They shared family life with their ultimately more famous siblings, fought in the Civil War (unlike William and Henry), married (unlike Henry and Alice), and sired families. All the James children were highly strung and responded in different ways to their parents' desire that each make names for themselves. Such an injunction would have been difficult for the male children, and although it would have not been issued with such force for Alice, she was acutely conscious of family expectations.

But what was a woman reaching adulthood in the 1860s to do, especially if there was no particular financial pressure on her? Get married or devote herself to "good works." Or both. Or retreat into illness. "Choosing" is a harsh word to describe this situation, especially since the Victorians had a precise sense of the way in which a disease diagnosis somehow exculpates the sufferer from "choice." Nevertheless, many of the diagnoses that were given to her carried moral overtones: neurasthenia, hysteria, suppressed gout, cardiac complications, spinal neuroses, nervous hyperaesthesia, and spiritual crisis. As her brother Henry wrote to her in 1883 "Try not to be ill – that is all; for in that there is a failure."

However, by 1883, Alice had already made illness a way of life. Always a sensitive child, she was perceived to be in sufficient difficulty to be sent, at age eighteen, from Cambridge, Massachusetts, to New York City, to spend six months under the care of Dr. Charles Taylor (1827–99), a fashionable orthopedic surgeon and specialist in spinal disorders. A maiden aunt accompanied her, and, as befitted their middle-class status, they lived in rooms provided by Dr. Taylor. Beyond the fact that she was suffering from a "nervous crisis," the family correspondence is unrevealing about her precise symptoms, or about the specifics of her treatment, although Dr. Taylor was known to relate a whole variety of complaints to spinal disorders, and to recommend baths, exercises, and spinal braces in their treatment. Two years before Alice went to him, he had published a monograph entitled *Spinal Irritation or the Causes of Backache among American Women* (1864).

Whatever good Dr. Taylor's course of therapy achieved did not help long, for in early 1865, she suffered a major crisis, with fainting spells, bizarre pains, and prostrations. Writing about it two decades later, she described it as "violent turns of hysteria," and worse than madness, for she still retained the consciousness that she should maintain control of herself and her actions. Her brother William, who was suffering his own physical and spiritual crisis during the same years, would later explore such phenomena as the experience of multiple personality or the fragmentation of self, which was common to their generation and class.

William James claimed to have touched bottom in 1870. By then, Alice had sufficiently recovered to take a grand tour through Europe. Both she and those around her recognized that variety made her better, and after the tour she turned to various social and educational endeavors in Boston, and watched as most of her female contemporaries set out on the adventure of marriage. As for her: "I have to write between thirty and forty letters every month, but I have naught else of importance to do."[2] Her health remained fragile until 1878, the year that her favorite brother, William, became engaged, to another Alice. Alice James then became deeply melancholic, even discussing suicide with her father and afterward insisting that in 1878 she had died spiritually.

Nevertheless, she soldiered on physically, a task made somewhat easier by the coming of Katherine Loring, a strong woman of her own age, and her companion and nurse from the late 1870s. Alice jealously guarded her relationship with Katherine, her illnesses becoming worse whenever there was a danger that other commitments might distract her companion. But even Katherine's ministrations could not do everything, and in 1883 Alice tried two months at the Adams Nervine Asylum, a charitable institution for "nervous people who are not insane." Its doctors were well disposed toward the rest-cure methods of Silas Weir Mitchell (1829–1914), the famous Philadelphia physician. This was a regimen based on a rich diet and withdrawal from all physical and mental activity. Alice put on a bit of weight but got no permanent relief. Instead, she tried the following year a fashionable (and expensive) New York nerve specialist, W. B. Neftel. He emphasized a more vigorous program of exercise and electrical stimulation. She liked him for a while ("the doctor is as kind and easy to get on with as he can be"), though she feared she would return a pauper, such were his fees.

If her pocketbook was dented, it still contained enough to permit her and Katherine to head again for Europe in 1884: Alice was never to return to the United States. She found England rather more to her liking ("The English," she wrote, "so worship the god *Holiday*" that no one there seemed to mind that she never did anything). Among her English doctors was (Sir) Alfred Baring Garrod (1819–1907), a distinguished specialist in gout. He was convinced that her disease was "flying gout," a variant of the more familiar disease in which the gouty tendency expresses itself in dyspepsia and fleeting pains in different parts of the body. Alice was more impressed with the attention she got from Garrod: he listened to her patiently and examined her thoroughly, percussing and auscultating. Indeed, he took such a careful history that she determined to write up her medical history (the "oft-repeated tale") in a booklet she could give to subsequent doctors, to "save breath and general exhaustion." Unfortunately, Garrod's prescription did nothing for her, even seemed to make her legs weaker, and she went off him as she had her earlier doctors.

Other doctors came and went – a Dr. Townsend, a Dr. Torry – and other diagnoses. Meanwhile, the strength in her legs completely failed and she spent most of her days and nights in her bed or on a sofa. Nurses from outside also came and went, but Katherine Loring stayed, as Alice increasingly longed for what she called "the grand mortuary moment." From their side, her doctors thought she would probably improve when she reached menopause. She was not so sure, and her diary, begun in 1889, was as much concerned with death as with life, with the past as with the present or future.

Then, in May 1891, Sir Andrew Clark (1826–93) added a new diagnosis to the formidable list she had acquired. Clark, then the President of the Royal College of Physicians, had looked after the dying Charles Darwin and George Eliot, and was the sometime Prime Minister William Gladstone's longtime friend and doctor. He, too, examined Alice and pronounced the lump she had had on one breast cancerous and beyond treatment. Now that she had a "real" disease, she was morbidly ecstatic.

> To him who waits, all things come! My aspirations may have been eccentric, but I cannot complain now, that they have not been brilliantly fulfilled. Ever since I have been ill, I have longed and longed for some palpable disease, no matter how conventionally dreadful a label it might have, but I was always driven back to stagger alone under the monstrous mass of subjective sensations, which that sympathetic being "the medical man" had no higher aspiration than to assure me I was personally responsible for, washing his hands of me with a graceful complacency under my very nose.[3]

The mental pain had always been harder to bear than the physical: the latter was merely a "grim grindstone"; the former "sears the soul." That was her last judgment, dictated to Katherine the day before she died, eleven months after Clark had made his diagnosis. Consistent to the end, she had resisted asking Katherine to administer a fatal dose of morphine. In the closing months, two other doctors had come, and one had gone, but only Katherine, brother Henry, and a nurse were with her at the grand mortuary moment.

VII. DID SCIENCE MATTER FOR ALICE JAMES?

Did medical science matter for Alice James? After all, she lived through the bacteriological revolution and was the younger contemporary of the giants of nineteenth-century medicine and its scientific basis: of Pasteur and Koch, Virchow, Lister, and all the others. Did their achievements and those of their colleagues help prolong her life or improve her social functioning, or psychological well-being?

In a specific sense, it is hard to escape a negative answer to the first of these possibilities. Nothing that doctors did to her as an individual can be pointed to as likely to have prolonged her life. The rest cure that Dr. Page favored at the Adams Nervine Asylum was probably neither here nor there, when compared to the more vigorous programs of exercise, stimulation, and electrical manipulation that Dr. Neftel advocated in New York City. Dr. Garrod knew as much as anyone about uric acid and gout, but there is no evidence that he ever measured the uric acid concentration in her urine, or that his diagnosis of "flying gout" was one that would make him expect to find anything amiss in her urine, or to be able to do anything about it if he did. Surgery was never contemplated for her breast cancer (that assumes of course that Clark's diagnosis was correct), even though the modern surgical treatment of the disease was currently being pioneered by Halsted at Johns Hopkins. Had she lived ten years later, she might have been operated on, although one doctor subsequent to Clark believed her liver was also involved and if he was correct, an operation would probably have increased her suffering without prolonging her days.

Did her doctors help her to function better during the years that were allotted to her? This is more difficult to evaluate, all the more so because the social function of an unmarried woman in her society was ill-defined. She herself saw the female role essentially in terms of marriage and childbearing and once remarked that if she could find a man who was attracted to her, she would work hard not to lose him. Instead, all she got were brothers and male doctors, and was probably touched in earnest in adult life only by the latter. She experienced variable periods of respite after some of her "cures," but travel, friends, and similar things to preoccupy her mind did more than electrical apparatuses or prescriptions to define positive roles or give her some capacity to fulfill them.

Thirty years later and she would probably have been in psychoanalysis, and several of the nerve specialists she saw might well have been inclined toward it had they been working a generation later. As it was, the psychological support she got from her doctors was not quite what she seemed to need. Reflecting in her *Diary* at the end of her life, she insisted that doctors had failed to take her seriously, because all the diagnoses they gave her were functional. But within the limits of the

medicine of her time, her diseases *were* functional, and the various regimes suggested to her were well within the best offerings of contemporary medical practice. Besides, at times she felt that she had failed
her therapies (and doctors) as much as they had failed her. Her attitudes
toward her doctors were complicated, to say the least, and often went
through a recognizable pattern of initial enthusiasm and subsequent
cooling: "Even the great Sir Andrew Clark faded visibly to the eyes,"
she wrote seven months after he had diagnosed her breast condition,
contrasting the support she got from Katherine with the inadequacies
of her doctors. But that is hardly surprising, given the nature of the
daily, even hourly contact between the two women, to say nothing of
the fact that by then, Alice was actually dictating her diary for Katherine
to write down.

And it was Katherine who was dispensing the formal "psychother-
apy" by way of hypnotism. By 1890, hypnotism and suggestion therapy
were being widely recommended for a whole range of disorders, and
William James had urged her to try it, especially as a form of pain control.
Her last doctor, Charles Tuckey (1855–1925), was an early British exponent of the art. He successfully hypnotized Alice and taught Katherine
how to do so. The sessions did little for her pain but helped, she reported, to calm her nerves and permit sleep.

It would be easy to conclude that science mattered little in the care
that Alice James received, particularly if hypnotism and the related psy-
chotherapies of the period are seen as springing from cultural concerns
that had little to do with laboratory medicine. But the translation of
laboratory discoveries to clinical practice is rarely simple and never instantaneous. And definitions of science, which deny Charcot or Charles
Tuckey any claims to it simply because they became intrigued by the
diagnostic and therapeutic possibilities of hypnotism, can be narrow and
anachronistic. In their various ways, each of Alice James's doctors was
influenced by science, at the very least because each lived in an age of
science and its associated technologies. The concluding chapter will assess briefly the extent to which science had come to matter to medicine
by 1900.

8

Conclusion: Did science matter?

The future belongs to science.
> Sir William Osler, "Introduction" to René Vallery-Radot, *The Life of Pasteur* (London, 1901), p. xvi

I. SCIENCE AND THE DOCTORS

By the end of the nineteenth century, science had become a third estate within medicine, beside the two estates of hospital-approved élite consultants, and their more numerous colleagues who practiced mostly outside the hospitals, and among the lower socioeconomic groups. The details varied from country to country, but a basic structure was in place. These two clinical estates were not homogeneous, of course. Elites ranged from those who held formal academic posts in the medical schools, kept up with the latest literature, and preached the gospel of scientific medicine, to those who acquired fame and fortune by what could be called shrewd clinical skills, personal charisma, pleasing manners, and no knowledge of, or interest in (and even hostility to), the medical sciences. Among the rank and file, there were many who dispensed the same bottle of sweet tasting, colored medicine to all and sundry, never used a stethoscope, and had never looked through a microscope, even in their medical school days. A few doctors joined antivivisection societies, and even in 1900, more than a few of them thought the germ theory overrated, irrelevant, or positively misconceived.

Despite such diversity of attitude and experience, and despite the positive resistance to change by some élite members of the medical profession, that profession had been, was being, and would continue to be, changed by science: and a science that itself was neither monolithic nor static. The diagnostic medicine of the hospital (Chapter 2), and the preventive medicine of the community (Chapter 3), were based on ideals of science just as much as the medicine that was also identified with the laboratory.

Nevertheless, this third estate – the scientific one – was a product of the mid- to late nineteenth century. It consisted of the still small but

218

highly visible cadre of individuals who spent most or all of their professional time in medical research, and in teaching the fruits of research. It was from that group that many of the national and international superstars of medicine came: Bernard and Ludwig, Pasteur and Koch, Virchow and Metchnikoff, Wright and Welch, Ehrlich and von Behring. And it was with that group that most of the international figures within clinical medicine and surgery identified: Lister and Billroth, Kocher and Paget, Osler and Charcot.

The consequence of this was that science did matter to doctors collectively, even if it could be neglected by them individually, and even if much of ordinary medical practice was untouched by it. There are three concrete aspects where this can be seen: medical education, professional identity, and the technology of medical practice.

What was taught and examined in the medical schools was fundamental, and the acceptance of a discipline or approach within the medical curriculum was symptomatic of wider issues. Innovation was easiest in Germany, where the values of *Lehrfreiheit* and *Lernfreiheit* meant that recognized teachers could teach what they wanted and students could follow a course essentially of their own choosing. The State exams were there to guarantee that it added up to a recognized education. In Britain, the variety of examination structures provided some flexibility, but the basic curriculum was prescribed centrally, and the minimum course lengthened, first from three to four years, and then from four to five, to take account of the newer demands of science (especially practical work in histology, physiology, and bacteriology) and introductory teaching in specialist clinical subjects such as ophthalmology and diseases of the ear, nose, and throat. The transformation in education was most dramatic in the United States, both before and after the Flexner Report, where the values of science meant the death of dozens of medical schools without the resources or will to conform. The science lobby was particularly effective there, although it did have ground to make up.

The purpose of this new science teaching was not simply to cram the student with yet more facts: it was to instill in him (and occasionally, her) a critical frame of mind, provide him with the skills and knowledge to adapt to future changes in his discipline, and equip him with the basis of practicing the best medicine. Some of those who resisted the intrusion of science liked to draw on an image of successful practice as a kind of apostolic succession, based on incommunicable knowledge that could not be formally taught, only learned. Proponents of the notion that medicine is an art, and not one founded on science, had the second-best tunes, however, since apostles of scientific practice never denied that many of these indefinable skills were involved in gaining patients' confidences and achieving eminence in clinical medicine. Students were exhorted time and again to acquire these skills, but for the most part within a context in which their scientific knowledge-base was sound and capable of growth. Indeed, Sir Squire Sprigge (1860–1937), editor of *The Lancet*, suggested in 1905 that the new scientific basis of medicine meant that the medical man had to accept the withdrawal from his traditional status as one of the three learned professions and "submit to being classed with other practical workers who have an equal claim with him to be considered men of science."

This was a shrewd observation, the implementation of which would have achieved (in Sprigge's eyes) a raising rather than a lowering of the status of his own profession. It would mean that ordinary practitioners could stand proudly in the shadow of Pasteur and Virchow. It also reflected the extent to which the profession of his generation could be considered as a single one. In the days when medicine was one of the learned professions, it was only the élite physicians who enjoyed that status. Sprigge was speaking of the profession as a whole.

In this process, science played a crucial role. The whole international movement within medicine encouraged the public – and the medical profession – to associate science with the advancement of medicine. International jamborees could border on the merely celebratory, but they were nonetheless effective for all that; and many of the smaller, more specialized ones certainly achieved some of their scientific goals. It would be impossible to quantify how much the image of scientists like Pasteur or scientifically inclined clinicians like Lister did for the profession as a whole. Impossible to quantify, but easy to see. They became public figures and thereby mediated the profession to the public.

The rhetoric of science can sometimes appear as little more than that. Many scientific breakthroughs yielded only shattered glass; many promising avenues led nowhere, many miracle cures cured no one. Therapeutic evaluation was often sloppy, the triumph of hope over reality: the rigorously controlled trial, and double-blind investigations, neither of them perfect, were still in the future. Problems of contamination and standardization dogged the manufacture of biologicals such as antitoxins and vaccines, drug toxicity and allergic reactions were worrisome, debilitating, and sometimes fatal. Legal issues – patents for drugs or procedures, or suits for unforeseen consequences of therapy – began to loom large, as Ehrlich found to his cost. Science and commerce did not (and do not) always happily coexist. Operations with logical scientific justification came and went, often producing only needless operative mortalities and little objective benefit.

Whether science promised more for medicine than it could deliver is a moot point. For many thoughtful individuals who had witnessed the transformation of the late nineteenth and early twentieth centuries, the solution to problems like those just mentioned was not a return to an older order, not less science, but more and better science. The assimilation of scientific concepts and use of scientific-sounding names by patent medicine vendors were in themselves eloquent testimony to the fact that, with the public, the possibilities of science in medicine outweighed the problems.

It would be easy to exaggerate the real impact of laboratory discoveries on daily practice. The business of medicine still preoccupied practitioners of all stripes, and the economic issues, State involvement, and intraprofessional rivalries outlined in Chapter 7 would have loomed far larger to many than the latest physiological or bacteriological announcement. Nor was the promise of constant scientific achievement accepted by all. In the run-up to the century's end, and the inevitable reflective assessments of where medicine had got to, the specter of urban decay, physical deterioration, and increasing hereditary degeneration also loomed large. British centenary celebrations were tempered by the failure of the Boer War, by the high percentage of recruits who had to be rejected on medical grounds, and by the feeling that, as Victoria's long reign moved slowly toward its close, the days of imperial splendor might be closing in. White Americans were beginning to fear the "Yellow Peril," and pogroms in Eastern Europe led to vast migrations and to the dread and reality of typhus and tuberculosis. Alcoholism and venereal disease seemed to be on the increase; secularism, feminism, socialism, materialism, and other "isms" were threatening to many. Science had long marched under the banner of progress, but now evolutionary biology and thermodynamics taught that decay was as much a part of the order of things as progress.

These images were as central to the late nineteenth-century scene as test tubes, microscopes, and Petri dishes. Nevertheless, these latter and hundreds of other tools of the medical trade did matter and help define medicine in the period. Since at least the mid-nineteenth century, it is virtually impossible to separate science and technology. Some artifacts of medicine are very old: medicine bottles, surgical instruments of all kinds, lancets, cups, trusses and splints, braces and urinals, delivery stools, and straitjackets. Even microscopes date from the seventeenth century, and elaborate apothecaries' jars from much earlier. During the nineteenth century, however, to these were added many new artifacts, and many adaptations of older ones: the equipment of the physiological laboratory, such as the kymograph; electrical appliances of all kinds; apparatus to administer anesthetics; new surgical instruments; sterilizing equipment; Bunsen burners; examination and surgical tables; orthopedic beds; new diagnostic aids such as the ophthalmoscope, otolaryngoscope, hemocytometer, sphygmograph, and reflex hammer; x-ray machinery; surgical gowns, masks, and rubber gloves; and finally, the ultimate symbol of the marriage of science and clinical medicine, the white coat, worn first in laboratories from about mid-century, and adopted gradually by medical students and junior doctors toward the century's end; and by their clinical teachers afterward.

Of all the branches of medicine, the one that changed most visibly during the second half of the century was surgery. The outward change was literal, as surgeons switched from operating in frock coats to doing their job in "work clothes," that is, the gowns, masks, and other paraphernalia we still associate with the surgeon's craft. They were still not quite in their modern garb by 1900, but they were getting close to it. Hospitals too, were reflecting this transformation, with their specially constructed operating theaters and their associated changing rooms, disinfectant equipment, and recovery rooms. Interestingly, surgeons increasingly liked to be photographed and painted in their work clothes. Their skills in the theater itself were still essentially of a craft nature, but the surgical enterprise as a whole was presented (and perceived) as one rooted in the new science of medicine. Even physicians who reflected on the course of nineteenth-century medicine emphasized that one of the most striking revolutions had been the post-Listerian surgical one. Modern historians often view this transformation in gynecological terms: of aggressive abdominal surgery and normal ovaries sacrificed on the altar of surgical "science." Nearer the time, even physicians recognized that their surgical colleagues could offer something that was dramatic and might be definitive. Physicians were convinced that they managed patients infinitely better than their medical forebears of a century before: "A chance to cut is a chance to cure." Surgeons increasingly thought in those terms. Their thoughtful medical colleagues generally viewed their own task more modestly. Most diseases, most patients, after all, did not present with a complaint that had an easy surgical solution. Doctors were aware of the way in which the surgery of 1900 was vastly different from the surgery of 1850, but also of the way in which physiology, pathology, bacteriology, pharmacology, and the other basic sciences had impinged on the status of the profession as a whole.

II. SCIENCE AND THE PUBLIC

The doctor of 1900 had reason to be grateful for the scientific medicine of the previous century. His profession was more coherent, more stable, and probably more prestigious than it had been in 1850 or 1800. Although the threats from outside were still there – unorthodox practitioners of various persuasions, self-medication, over-the-counter sales, patent medicine vendors – most run-of-the-mill practitioners would have perceived as much threat to their livelihood from within: from consultants and specialists from medical charities treating patients who should have paid private fees, from overcrowding within the profession. Nevertheless, in the European countries, North America, Australia, and wherever European values had established a cultural hegemony, the medicine that was more-or-less aligned with science and the laboratory had won. The profession had not secured the monopoly that some doctors thought was their right and in the public's best interest. It had, however, secured the patronage of the state, and this was enough in the long run.

Had the victory been fairly earned? Was the public better off putting its faith in an allopath instead of a homeopath or naturopath? Had Listerian surgery really saved the 200,000 lives (some doctors thought this a conservative figure) that was claimed for it in 1900? Were there drugs in the pharmacopoeia that could actually cure disease?

Put in stark, heroic terms like the last of these questions, the answer would seem to be "Not many, maybe only quinine for malaria"; and it is perhaps significant that even physicians surveying the century's medical achievements reserved their warmest discussions about "cure" for the surgeons. One summary article in the 1899 *British Medical Journal* disparaged what its author ironically described as "heaven-born geniuses" who claimed to cure almost every disease. He spoke only of treatment, of an expanding number of useful medicinal agents, better employed than in the past, to which he added improved nursing care and the more knowledgeable management of diet.

No one reflecting in 1900 on the past century's developments could have known that, in the coming three decades or so, Northern European and North American countries would achieve an unprecedented reduction in mortality, a phenomenon that further consolidated the power and status of the medical profession. The end-of-the-century analyses tended to be qualitative ones, but there had been some gains in mortality parameters between 1850 and 1900, with falls in both crude and standardized deathrates. Crude deathrates in England and Wales, for instance, were 20.8 per thousand in 1850, and 18.2 in 1900. Comparable figures for Germany were 25.6 and 22.1, for the Netherlands, 22.2 and 17.9, for the United States 21.4 and 17.2. Exceptionally, French mortality rates hovered in the low 20s for most of the period: 21.4 in 1850 and 21.9 in 1900.

These bald figures do not mean much, and to dissect them completely would require another volume. However, there are reasons to suggest that medicine as an institution had contributed to these real if modest improvements in life expectancy.

Four broad points about which there is reasonable historical agreement need to be made about the figures. First, the improvements in late nineteenth-century mortality were mostly related to children and young adults rather than infants, whereas the dramatic gains in the first third of the twentieth century were heavily influenced by a sharp fall in infant mortality. Second, the continued shift of population from rural to urban areas means that even modest crude gains can be significant, since mortality rates earlier in the century were more sharply weighted in favor of rural populations. Thus, other things being equal, the expectation would be of higher rates at the end of the century, as a greater percentage of the population was living in high-risk urban environments. Third, because of declining birthrates, the relative proportion of infants and children to adults went down, and standardized deathrates are slightly better in 1900 than crude ones. Fourth, mortality improvement was due mostly to declining deathrates from infectious diseases.

Three general explanations can be offered to account for the demographic phenomenon. First, the observed improvements might have occurred solely because of socioeconomic factors that had virtually nothing to do with medicine as knowledge or as practice. Chadwick, Virchow, Villermé, and Shattuck had been well aware, in the 1840s, that rich people lived on average longer than poor ones, and therefore a general rise in the standard of living by the century's end could have produced an improved expectancy of life at birth. Better nutrition has been singled out in one version of this scenario, the argument being that better nourished individuals are more resistant to infection, and better able to survive tuberculosis or gastrointestinal disorders. This argument rests heavily on the fact that deathrates for many of the major killer diseases began to fall before the organized public health movement was sufficiently advanced to have had any significant demographic effect, and the smoothness of the death curves for these diseases from the 1830s or 40s till the century's end points toward a single, continuous operative cause.

Such an explanatory framework would have surprised those who were alive in 1900, although many of them would have recognized the power of a thesis that had a strong socioeconomic dimension to it. And they would have agreed with much of the second broad line of retrospective assessment of nineteenth-century medicine: that the prevention rather than the cure of disease had contributed more to the changing mortality tables. There were continuities between the mid-century sanitary movement and the postbacteriological practice of what was often called scientific hygiene. But there were differences as well, not least in the number and variety of groups that were then devoted to prevention, and the administrative structures within which they worked. Sanitary inspectors, water and food analysts, factory surgeons, inspectors of nuisances, health visitors, surveyors and engineers, public vaccinators, medical officers of health: these were some of the occupational groups already established or becoming visible by the century's end. Whatever may be our historical judgment about their effectiveness, those at the time believed that they were busy applying and teaching others to appreciate the principles of scientific prevention. By 1900, medical science had provided a rationale for water filtration and disinfection; for waste and rubbish disposal; for pest control; for cleanliness; for care in food handling and preparation; for control of building regulations for domestic dwellings and workplaces; for notification and isolation of certain diseases; and for myriad other issues that touched daily life. This is not to claim that many of these goals had not been long argued for, often on other principles. It is to claim that the basic vocabulary of justification by 1900 had become a scientific one.

"The progress which has been made [in preventive medicine] consists essentially in practical applications of Pathological Science," wrote Sir John Simon in 1897. He spoke from within the medical camp, of course, but he also recognized that the implementation of the scientific precepts, which he held dear, involved political, social, economic, and educational matters. But he was in no doubt wherein the basis of what he still called sanitary administration lay: "On the new foundations of Science, a new political superstructure has taken form."[1] The new scientific hygiene, or public health, would not have been possible without success in politics, as members of the science lobby convinced local and national politicians that investment in prevention was worthwhile.

A few specific diseases accounted for much of the decline in mortality in the second half of the century: tuberculosis, scarlet fever, diphtheria, typhus, smallpox, typhoid and cholera, and other diarrheal diseases. Their relative importance varied from country to country, and even region to region. In Britain, most of the decline in smallpox mortality had already occurred before 1850, although this was less true in other parts of Europe, and the worst of all outbreaks of typhus occurred in Russia in the twentieth century, in the aftermath of the First World War.

Tuberculosis is usually taken as the touchstone of the performance of nineteenth-century medicine, and of the modest contribution that the third possibility, curative medicine, might have made to mortality statistics. Tuberculosis was the century's single leading killer in temperate climates, and its decline accounted for a good deal of the perceived mortality decline, and probably had indirect spin-offs, as tuberculous individuals were recorded as dying from other acute diseases that might not have otherwise been fatal. Koch's work gradually gave it the status of a contagious disease and encouraged by the 1930s a series of specific public health measures, ranging from ordinances against spitting in public places to sanatoria where the victim was isolated from the rest of society, from the pasteurization of milk and control of tuberculous cows to mass chest x-ray screening programs. But most of this occurred after 1900, and the existence of a few hospitals before then for consumptives probably had little demographic effect.

Nor, despite the increased diagnostic and etiological insight that bacteriology offered, is it easy to discern much in the vast number of different remedies proposed by clinicians that would have been of positive benefit to tuberculous patients. There seem to be few medicaments that did not at some time or other have an enthusiastic advocate or two for patients with pulmonary tuberculosis: herbs, animal products, chemicals of all kinds. These ranged from the familiar to the bizarre and included mercury, gold salts, quinine, creosote, Chaulmoogra oil, and pig's pepsin, among others. One remedy held up for decades, until well into the twentieth century, was in fact, cod-liver oil: "There is little doubt on the part of practical physicians, none on the part of the public, of the great value of [cod-liver oil] in the treatment of phthisical and scrofulous patients,"[2] wrote J. S. Bristowe. Its benefits were so widely remarked by so many hard-nosed observers that we must discount a great deal of contemporary testimony to assign it to the therapeutic dustbin. However, clinicians like Bristowe and Osler gave cod-liver oil an important supportive role, not a curative one.

The change in attitude was significant. "A great part of the treatment of phthisis usually consists in treating symptoms as they arise," concluded Bristowe. He, and like-minded clinicians at the century's end, *managed* tuberculosis and hundreds of diseases like it. This clinical management, based on an enhanced diagnostic capacity, knowledge of the natural history of disease, and a more critical attitude toward therapeutics, was as much a part of the new scientific medicine as laboratory research or vaccine production. One cannot read the textbooks of Bristowe or Osler without concluding that clinical medicine did have something to contribute to patient care if rarely to patient cure. The contribution of curative medicine to overall mortality figures before 1900 was probably very slight, even if the experience of individual patients or individual doctors may have been different.

Current historical scholarship suggests that the mortality decline between 1850 and 1900 was the result of some combination of socioeconomic improvement and social intervention, of prevention rather than therapy. Nevertheless, the foundations of a more powerful therapeutic effectiveness had been laid; scientific medicine had received the sanction of the state and doctors had become inextricably linked to existing social and welfare movements; and the profession was far more unified than it had been a century before.

Conceptually, and probably in spirit, Osler's *Principles and Practice of Medicine* is closer to us than it is to Cullen's *First Lines of the Practice of Physic*. And a whole series of textbooks of medicine, medical specialties, and medical science in print today are the direct descendants of works first written a century ago. This in itself reflects the extent to which the medicine of our own century is practiced within the professional, institutional, and cognitive frameworks that were largely in place before World War I.

Bibliographical essay

INTRODUCTION

In the bibliographical essay that follows, I have discussed briefly a generous selection of the secondary literature that is concerned with the various themes covered in this volume. In addition, a number of general works are also available. C. C. Gillispie, ed., *Dictionary of Scientific Biography*, 16 vols. (New York, 1970–80), with a two-volume supplement, edited by F. L. Holmes (New York, 1990), contains biographical entries on many of the major figures of nineteenth-century medical science. Roderick E. McGrew, *Encyclopedia of Medical History* (New York, 1985), provides useful summary articles on the most important diseases and medical specialties. John Walton, Paul B. Beeson, and Ronald Bodley Scott, eds., *The Oxford Companion to Medicine*, 2 vols. (Oxford and New York, 1986), has much historical material, even though its principal focus is contemporary medicine. W. F. Bynum and Roy Porter, eds., *Companion Encyclopedia of the History of Medicine*, 2 vols. (London and New York, 1993), offers comprehensive thematic coverage of the field by a distinguished international group of scholars. I have made use of these articles and their bibliographies throughout this volume. The introductory chapter, written by the editors, contains a fuller discussion of general reference sources in the field.

CHAPTER 1. MEDICINE IN 1790

Half a century ago, historians of medicine viewed the eighteenth century as a fallow one, riddled with system building and speculation, pompous doctors and heroic, dangerous therapies. Compared to the achievements of men like William Harvey and Thomas Sydenham in the seventeenth century or the scientific progress of the nineteenth, that of the Enlightenment seemed curiously modest.

More recently, historians have found much to explore. The secondary literature on the physical, natural, and human sciences is analyzed in G. S. Rousseau and Roy Porter, eds., *The Ferment of Knowledge: Studies in the Historiography of Eighteenth-Century Science* (Cambridge, 1980); the chapter on "Health, Disease and Medical Care" by W. F. Bynum (pp. 211–53) has a full bibliography. Two more recent collections of essays contain examples of the continuing scholarly preoccupation with the medicine of the period: W. F. Bynum and Roy Porter, eds., *William Hunter and the Eighteenth-Century Medical World* (Cambridge, 1985);

and Andrew Cunningham and Roger French, eds., *The Medical Enlightenment of the Eighteenth Century* (Cambridge, 1990).

The best general survey of the century's medicine remains Lester King, *The Medical World of the 18th Century* (Chicago, 1958); it is much more balanced than Guy Williams, *The Age of Agony* (London, 1975). The fullest exposition of the major theories of Enlightenment doctors can be found in John Thomson, *An Account of the Life, Lectures and Writings of William Cullen*, 2 vols. (Edinburgh, 1859). These rare volumes are much broader in scope than the title indicates and deserve a modern facsimile edition. Thomson was concerned principally with medical theories; the more practical medical activities of the era have been expertly dissected in James Riley, *The Eighteenth-Century Campaign to Avoid Disease* (London, 1987). Guenter B. Risse, "Medicine in the Age of Enlightenment," in Andrew Wear, ed., *Medicine in Society: Historical Essays* (Cambridge, 1992), pp. 149–95, is a superb concise analysis.

The complex structure of medical care in the old order can be approached through a number of recent works. Roy Porter, *Health for Sale: Quackery in England, 1660–1850* (Manchester and New York, 1989), emphasizes the importance of the medical marketplace for England. Porter has elaborated on several aspects of the theme in articles and chapters in books, including "The Language of Quackery in England 1660–1800," in Peter Burke and Roy Porter, eds., *The Social History of Language* (Cambridge, 1986), pp. 73–103; Roy Porter, "Before the Fringe," in Roger Cooter, ed., *Studies in the History of Alternative Medicine* (London, 1988); *idem*, "Lay Medical Knowledge in the Eighteenth Century: The Evidence of the *Gentleman's Magazine*," *Medical History*, 29 (1985), 138–68; and *idem*, "Laymen, Doctors and Medical Knowledge in the Eighteenth Century: The Evidence of the *Gentleman's Magazine*," in Roy Porter, ed., *Patients and Practitioners: Lay Perceptions of Medicine in Pre-Industrial Society* (Cambridge, 1985), pp. 283–314. The scene in France is dealt with by Matthew Ramsey, *Professional and Popular Medicine in France, 1770–1830: The Social World of Medical Practice* (Cambridge, 1988).

The organization of the orthodox medical profession in the eighteenth century has been described by various scholars. For Britain, a concise exposition is Bernice Hamilton, "The Medical Professions in the Eighteenth Century," *Economic History Review*, second series, 4 (1951), 141–69. Two recent monographs examine the transition of the professional structure from the old tripartite model of physicians, surgeons, and apothecaries to the bipartite one of hospital-based consultants and general practitioners: Irvine Loudon, *Medical Care and the General Practitioner 1750–1850* (Oxford, 1986); and Ivan Waddington, *The Medical Profession in the Industrial Revolution* (Dublin, 1984). Both volumes emphasize the different patterns obtaining in London and the provinces. Provincial medical practice itself has been analyzed by Joan Lane, "The Medical Practitioners of Provincial England," *Medical History*, 28 (1984), 353–71; and the importance of the apprenticeship in the training of surgeons and apothecaries is elucidated by Joan Lane, "The Role of Apprenticeship in Eighteenth-Century Medical Education in England," in Bynum and Porter, *William Hunter*, pp. 57–103.

The vigor of the medical faculty at the University of Edinburgh was appreciated at the time, and the best monograph on it is Guenter B. Risse, *Hospital Life in*

Enlightenment Scotland: Care and Teaching at the Royal Infirmary of Edinburgh (Cambridge, 1986). See also Christopher Lawrence, "Ornate Physicians and Learned Artisans: Edinburgh Medical Men, 1726–1776," in Bynum and Porter, *William Hunter*. Student life in Edinburgh is the subject of Lisa Rosner, *Medical Education in the Age of Improvement* (Edinburgh, 1991).

In addition to M. Ramsey, *Professional and Popular Medicine*, the French scene is well covered in Toby Gelfand, *Professionalizing Modern Medicine: Paris Surgeons and Medical Science and Institutions in the Eighteenth Century* (Westport, Conn., 1980). See also T. Gelfand, "A 'Monarchical Profession' in the Old Regime: Surgeons, Ordinary Practitioners, and Medical Professionalization in Eighteenth-Century France," in Gerald L. Geison, ed., *Professions and the French State 1700–1900* (Philadelphia, 1984), pp. 149–88; and Charles Coulston Gillispie, *Science and Polity in France at the End of the Old Regime* (Princeton, N.J., 1980), especially Chapter 3.

For the old German states, see Johanna Geyer-Kordesch, "German Medical Education in the Eighteenth Century: The Prussian Context and its Influence," in Bynum and Porter, *William Hunter*, pp. 177–205. The monograph by Theodor Puschmann, *A History of Medical Education*, trans. E. H. Hare (London, 1891, reprinted New York, 1965), is still of value. Hermann Boerhaave and the medical school at Leiden were the longtime preoccupation of G. A. Lindeboom, whose biography of Boerhaave is sound: *Herman Boerhaave: The Man and His Work* (London, 1968).

For the medical professions and their education in colonial and early Republic America, see Martin Kaufman, *American Medical Education: The Formative Years, 1765–1910* (Westport, Conn., 1976); William F. Norwood, *Medical Education in the United States before the Civil War* (Philadelphia, 1944); and several of the essays in Whitfield J. Bell, Jr., *The Colonial Physician and Other Essays* (New York, 1975).

Most Enlightenment doctors subscribed to some form of vitalism, a subject easily approached through Thomas S. Hall, *Ideas of Life and Matter*, 2 vols. (Chicago, 1969). William Hunter and Alexander Monro *secundus* were the foremost teachers of anatomy in eighteenth-century Britain. For the former, see Roy Porter, "William Hunter: A Surgeon and a Gentleman," in Bynum and Porter, *William Hunter*; for the latter, R. E. Wright-St. Clair, *Doctors Monro: A Medical Saga* (London, 1964). One point of dispute between these two concerned the lymphatic system: see Nellie B. Eales, "The History of the Lymphatic System with Special Reference to the Hunter-Monro Controversy," *Journal of the History of Medicine*, 29 (1974), 280–94. Gelfand, *Professionalizing Modern Medicine*, provides good accounts of both formal and extramural anatomy and surgical teaching in Paris.

The role of the nervous system in mid-century thinking about health and disease is analyzed by Christopher Lawrence, "The Nervous System in the Scottish Enlightenment," in Barry Barnes and Steven Shapin, eds., *Natural Order* (Beverly Hills, Calif., 1979), pp. 19–40; and Roy Porter, "Introduction" to facsimile reprint of George Cheyne, *The English Malady (1723)* (London, 1991). The whole theme has now been expertly examined by G. J. Barker-Benfield, *The Culture of Sensibility: Sex and Society in Eighteenth-Century Britain* (Chicago and London, 1992). For an exposition of Haller's views on irritability and sensibility, see John D. Spillane, *The Doctrine of the Nerves* (Oxford, 1981); and Karl Figlio, "Theories of Perception and the Physiology of Mind in the Late Eighteenth Century," *History of Science*, 13 (1975), 177–212. For John Hunter, see François Duchesneau, "Vitalism in Late Eighteenth-Century Physiology: The Cases of Barthes, Blumenbach and John Hunter," in Bynum and Porter, *William Hunter*, pp. 259–95; and Stephen Cross, "John Hunter, the Animal Oeconomy and Late Eighteenth-Century Physiological Discourse," *Studies in the History of Biology*, 5 (1981), 1–110.

L. J. Rather, *Mind and Body in Eighteenth-Century Medicine: A Study Based on Jerome Gaub's "De regimine mentis"* (London, 1965), is an excellent study and translation of an important pathologist; and the chapters on the eighteenth century in E. R. Long, *A History of Pathology* (New York, 1965), provide a clear summary of the subject. For nosology, see Lester S. King, *Medical World; idem, Medical Thinking: A Historical Preface* (Princeton, N.J., 1982), Chapter 5; and Julian Martin, "Sauvages's Nosology: Medical Enlightenment in Montpellier," in Cunningham and French, *Medical Enlightenment*, pp. 111–57.

Eighteenth-century therapeutics in general is given short shrift, with the exception of the work of James Lind and William Withering. However, for a sympathetic assessment of the period, see Christopher Booth, "Clinical Science in an Age of Reason," in his *Doctors in Science and Society* (London, 1987), pp. 1–25. Both prevention and the important status of Hippocratism in the period are well treated in Riley, *Eighteenth-Century Campaign*.

The antiestablishment implications on much of the advice literature of the period are explored in a number of articles, including C. J. Lawrence, "William Buchan: Medicine Laid Open," *Medical History*, 19 (1975), 20–35; Charles Rosenberg, "Medical Text and Social Context: Explaining William Buchan's 'Domestic Medicine,' " *Bulletin of the History of Medicine*, 57 (1983), 22–42; G. S. Rousseau, "John Wesley's 'Primitive Physick' (1747)," *Harvard Library Bulletin*, 16 (1968), 242–56; and Mary E. Fissell, *Patients, Power, and the Poor in Eighteenth-Century Bristol* (Cambridge, 1991).

The eradication of smallpox is one of the satisfying achievements of modern medicine and cooperative social policy. A general survey, but including a reasonable account of its eighteenth-century impact, is Donald R. Hopkins, *Princes and Peasants: Smallpox in History* (Chicago, 1983). The standard monograph on inoculation is Genevieve Miller, *The Adoption of Inoculation for Smallpox in England and France* (Philadelphia, 1957). For the Suttons, see David van Zwanenberg, "The Suttons and the Business of Inoculation," *Medical History*, 22 (1978), 71–82. The claim that smallpox inoculation might have been so successful that it was demographically significant is made by Peter Razzell, *The Conquest of Smallpox* (Firle, Sussex, 1977).

The fevers literature is briefly discussed in Riley, *Eighteenth-Century Campaign* and King, *Medical World*. See also W. F. Bynum and V. Nutton, eds., *Theories of Fever, Antiquity to the Enlightenment, Medical History*, Supplement No. 1 (1981), especially Dale Smith, "Medical Science, Medical Practice, and the Emerging Concept of Typhus in Mid-Eighteenth-Century Britain" and W. F. Bynum, "Cullen and the Study of Fevers in Britain, 1760–1820." King, *Medical Thinking*, Chapter 2, has a useful discussion of the vocabulary and diagnostic criteria surrounding consumption/tuberculosis.

CHAPTER 2. MEDICINE IN THE HOSPITAL

Hospitals have long been a popular topic for historical work, and few hospitals of much antiquity have not had their history written. Much of this literature is celebratory rather than analytical and the results are rarely of more than local interest. An excellent sample of recent scholarly work has been brought together in Lindsay Granshaw and Roy Porter, eds., *The Hospital In History* (London, 1989). A standard survey of the subject is John D. Thompson and Grace Goldin, *The Hospital: A Social and Architectural History* (New Haven, Conn., and London, 1975). Several aspects of hospital life in Old Regime France are expertly considered in Colin Jones, *The Charitable Imperative: Hospitals and Nursing in Ancien Régime and Revolutionary France* (London, 1989).

The phrase "hospital medicine" has connotations of the education and practice that developed in Revolutionary France. The classic account of E. H. Ackerknecht, *Medicine at the Paris Hospital, 1794–1848* (Baltimore, 1967), is full of information; and French hospital medicine was, inter alia, a focus for Michel Foucault, *The Birth of the Clinic: An Archaeology of Medical Perception*, trans. A. M. Sheridan Smith (London, 1976). This was one of several volumes in which Foucault analyzed the relationships between knowledge and power in the modern world. The needs of the military and the impact of army medicine on French educational institutions are stressed by David M. Vess, *Medical Revolution in France, 1789–1796* (Gainesville, Fla., 1975). Owsei Temkin's "The Role of Surgery in the Rise of Modern Medical Thought," in his *The Double Face of Janus* (Baltimore, 1977) is the seminal essay on the integration of surgical and medical ideas in the French hospitals and elsewhere.

The works just mentioned interpret the reestablishment of the French medical schools in 1794 as revolutionary. On the contrary, Othmar Keel, "The Politics of Health and the Institutionalization of Clinical Practices in Europe in the Second Half of the Eighteenth Century," in Bynum and Porter, *William Hunter*, pp. 207–56, argues that the methods and ideas underlying clinical teaching before 1794 had much in common with those adopted by the French.

No one would deny that many of the leaders of the early Paris school had been active long before the Revolution. Martin S. Staum, *Cabanis: Enlightenment and Medical Philosophy in the French Revolution* (Princeton, N.J., 1980), provides a full account of the man who could be called the philosopher of the new school. Another of the school's father figures, Philippe Pinel, has long been the focus of Dora Weiner's scholarship and she is preparing a full-scale biography. Her introduction and translation of Pinel's 1793 essay, *The Clinical Training of Doctors* (Henry E. Sigerist Supplements to the *Bulletin of the History of Medicine*, New Series, No. 3, 1980), is particularly valuable. See also Louis Greenbaum, " 'Measure of Civilization': The Hospital Thought of Jacques Tenon on the Eve of the French Revolution," *Bulletin of the History of Medicine*, 39 (1975), 43–56. For the 1803 law that introduced the new system of licensing, see Robert Heller, "*Officiers de Santé*: The Second-Class Doctors of Nineteenth-Century France," *Medical History*, 22 (1970), 25–43.

The background to earlier ideas of the anatomical basis of disease can be approached through Malcolm Nicolson, "Giovanni Battista Morgagni and Eighteenth-Century Physical Examination," in Christopher Lawrence, ed., *Medical*

Theory, Surgical Practice (London, 1992). Bichat is a major figure in the general literature on French medicine, including the monographs by Ackerknecht and Foucault. A full-length study in English is Elizabeth Haigh, _Xavier Bichat and the Medical Thought of the Eighteenth Century_ (_Medical History_, Supplement No. 4, 1984); see also the historiographically informed essay by John Pickstone, "Bureaucracy, Liberalism and the Body in Post-Revolutionary France: Bichat's Physiology and the Paris School of Medicine," _History of Science_, 19 (1981), 115–42. A fine monograph on French and British pathology of the period is Russell C. Maulitz, _Morbid Appearances: The Anatomy of Pathology in the Early Nineteenth Century_ (Cambridge, 1987). It is strong on both conceptual and institutional issues.

The modern history of physical diagnosis is the theme of Stanley J. Reiser, _Medicine and the Reign of Technology_ (Cambridge, 1981). Also still useful is Kenneth D. Keele, _The Evolution of Clinical Methods in Medicine_ (Springfield, Ill., 1963), with good discussions of the auscultation of the heart sounds. Much of the more recent literature is concerned with the social history of physical diagnosis, and its implications for professional power and doctor–patient relationships. Most of this literature starts from the formulations of N. D. Jewson, "Medical Knowledge and the Patronage System in Eighteenth-Century England," _Sociology_, 8 (1974), 369–85; and _idem_, "The Disappearance of the Sick Man From Medical Cosmology, 1770–1870," _Sociology_, 10 (1976), 225–44. See also Roy Porter, "The Rise of Physical Examination," in W. F. Bynum and Roy Porter, eds., _Medicine and the Five Senses_ (Cambridge, 1993), pp. 179–97.

The spread of the techniques of percussion and auscultation has been examined separately by several scholars, including Saul Jarcho, "Auenbrugger, Laennec, and John Keats: Some Notes on the Early History of Percussion and Auscultation," _Medical History_, 5 (1961), 167–72; and Malcolm Nicolson, "The Introduction of Percussion and Stethoscopy to Early Nineteenth-Century Edinburgh," in Bynum and Porter, _Medicine and the Five Senses_, pp. 134–53. Two important essays on Laennec explore the value he placed on auscultation: Jacalyn Duffin, "The Medical Philosophy of R. T. H. Laennec (1771–1826)," _History and Philosophy of the Life Sciences_, 8 (1986), 195–219; and _idem_, "The Cardiology of R. T. H. Laennec," _Medical History_, 33 (1989), 42–71.

Pierre Louis's "numerical method" is put into context in Ulrich Tröhler, "Quantification in British Medicine and Surgery 1750–1830, With Special Reference to its Introduction Into Therapeutics" (Ph.D. thesis, University of London, 1978); in Alvan Feinstein, _Clinical Judgment_ (Baltimore, 1967); and in T. D. Murphy, "Medical Knowledge and Statistical Methods in Early Nineteenth-Century France," _Medical History_, 25 (1981), 301–19. Louis's radical empiricism is examined through the eyes of one of his American disciples, Elisha Bartlett, in Erwin H. Ackerknecht, "Elisha Bartlett and the Philosophy of the Paris Clinical School," _Bulletin of the History of Medicine_, 24 (1950), 43–60.

The general therapeutic attitudes of the French are elaborated in Erwin H. Ackerknecht, _Therapeutics: From the Primitives to the 20th Century_ (New York, 1973), Chapter X; and the pharmacological work of Magendie examined in John E. Lesch, _Science and Medicine in France: The Emergence of Experimental Physiology 1790–1855_ (Cambridge, Mass., 1984).

Georges Canguilhem, _On the Normal and the Pathological_, trans. C. R. Fawcett

(Dordrecht, Holland, 1978), analyzes, inter alia, the tensions between functional and structural approaches to health and disease. Broussais figures largely in Canguilhem's monograph. Broussais has also been the subject of a recent monograph: J. F. Braunstein, *Broussais et le Matérialisme* (Paris, 1986).

A number of the key works of the French school were quickly translated into English, and several of these have been reprinted. See, in particular, J. N. Corvisart, *An Essay on the Organic Diseases and Lesions of the Heart and Great Vessels* (orig. trans. 1812; New York, 1962); and R. T. H. Laennec, *A Treatise on the Diseases of the Chest* (orig. trans. 1821; New York, 1962). The French school is also well represented in Ralph H. Major, *Classic Descriptions of Disease*, 3rd ed. (Springfield, Ill., 1948).

John Harley Warner has long been concerned with the impact of French medicine on British and American students who went there in such numbers. See, for example, J. H. Warner, "The Idea of Science in English Medicine: The 'Decline of Science' and the Rhetoric of Reform, 1815–45," in Roger French and Andrew Wear, eds., *British Medicine in an Age of Reform* (London and New York, 1991), pp. 136–64; *idem*, "The Selective Transport of Medical Knowledge: Antebellum American Physicians and Parisian Medical Therapeutics," *Bulletin of the History of Medicine, 59* (1985), 213–31; and *idem*, "Remembering Paris: Memory and the American Disciples of French Medicine in the Nineteenth Century," *Bulletin of the History of Medicine, 65* (1991), 301–25. Other recent explorations of the topic include Russell Maulitz, *Morbid Appearances;* and Stephen Jacyna, "Robert Carswell and William Thomson at the Hôtel-Dieu of Lyons: Scottish Views of French Medicine," in French and Wear, *British Medicine*, pp. 110–55. A particularly good biography of one of Laennec's English students is Amalie and Edward Kass, *Perfecting the World: The Life and Times of Dr. Thomas Hodgkin* (Boston, 1988). Steven Peitzman, "Bright's Disease and Generation: Towards Exact Medicine at Guy's Hospital," *Bulletin of the History of Medicine, 55* (1981), 307–21, looks at the integration of pathology and clinical practice in another of the "Great Men of Guy's."

In addition to the monographs of Loudon and Waddington cited above, several works examine the evolution of hospital-based education and practice in Britain, and the rise of London as the major teaching center. The Ph.D. thesis of Susan Lawrence ("Science and Medicine at the London Hospitals: The Development of Medical Lecturing in London, 1775–1820" [Ph.D. Thesis, University of Toronto, 1985]) is shortly to appear as a revised monograph; and her articles are exemplary. See especially Lawrence, "Entrepreneurs and Private Enterprise: The Development of Medical Lecturing in London, 1775–1820," *Bulletin of the History of Medicine, 62* (1988), 171–92; and *idem*, "Medical Education and the Apothecaries' Act" in French and Wear, *British Medicine*, pp. 45–73. For the slightly later period, Jeanne Peterson, *The Medical Profession in Mid-Victorian London* (Berkeley, 1978), is the standard work; and Charles Newman, *The Evolution of Medical Education in the Nineteenth Century* (London, 1957), is still useful.

For the United States, the essays in the collection edited by Ronald L. Numbers, *The Education of American Physicians* (Berkeley, 1980), are of a consistently high standard; and the first half of the nineteenth century is covered in two fine histories of medical education: William G. Rothstein, *American Medical Schools and the Practice of Medicine* (New York and Oxford, 1987); and Kenneth M. Ludmerer, *Learning to Heal: The Development of American Medical Education* (New York, 1985). William Rothstein's earlier monograph, *American Physicians in the Nineteenth Century: From Sects to Science* (Baltimore, 1972), is particularly good on the threat to the mid-century profession posed by the various medical sects.

Erna Lesky, *The Vienna Medical School of the 19th Century*, trans. by L. Williams and I. S. Levij (Baltimore, 1976), is the definitive history of its subject. Robert Miciotto, "Carl Rokitansky: A Reassessment of the Hematohumoral Theory of Disease," *Bulletin of the History of Medicine*, 52 (1978), 183–99, looks at the early Rokitansky.

CHAPTER 3. MEDICINE IN THE COMMUNITY

The medical advice literature on both treatment and hygiene can be easily approached through Roy Porter, ed., *The Popularization of Medicine* (London, 1992); especially the articles by Matthew Ramsey, "The Popularisation of Medicine in France, 1650–1900," and Norman Gevitz, " 'But all these Authors are Foreigners': American Literary Nationalism and Domestic Medical Guides"; and B. Haley, *The Healthy Body and Victorian Culture* (Cambridge, Mass., 1978). An older overview of both hygiene and public health is still useful: René Sand, *The Advance to Social Medicine* (London, 1952). George Rosen, *A History of Public Health* (New York, 1958); and *idem*, *From Medical Police to Social Medicine* (New York, 1974), are also indispensable, as is C.-E. A. Winslow, *The Conquest of Epidemic Disease: A Chapter in the History of Ideas* (1943; reprinted Madison, Wis., 1980).

A distillation of Frank's monumental work, in translation, is Erma Lasky, ed., Johann Peter Frank's *A System of Complete Medical Police*, trans. E. Vilim (Baltimore, 1976). Its underlying environmentalism can be approached through Clarence J. Glacken, *Traces on the Rhodian Shore* (Berkeley, 1967); and the context of many of Frank's Enlightenment ideals is brilliantly examined in Peter Gay, *The Enlightenment: An Interpretation*, 2 vols. (New York, 1966–9). See also George Rosen, "Cameralism and the Concept of Medical Police," and *idem*, "The Fall of the Concept of Medical Police, 1780–1890," both in his *From Medical Police to Social Medicine*; and for Scotland, Brenda White, "Medical Police. Politics and Police: The Fate of John Roberton," *Medical History*, 27 (1983), 407–22. James Riley, *Eighteenth-Century Campaign*, has much about infectious diseases and their control. Vicq d'Azyr's French schemes are analyzed by Caroline Hannaway, "The Société Royale de Médecine and Epidemics in the Ancien Régime," *Bulletin of the History of Medicine*, 46 (1972), 257–73; and J.-P. Peter, "Disease and the Sick at the End of the Eighteenth Century," in R. Forster and Orest Ranum, ed., *Biology of Man in History* (Baltimore, 1975). See also Daniel Roche, *The People of Paris*, trans. A. Montaigne (Berkeley, 1987). French poverty in the Old Regime is comprehensively examined in Olwen H. Hufton, *The Poor of Eighteenth-Century France, 1750–1789* (Oxford, 1974).

The old English Poor Laws are concisely explicated by Paul Slack, *Poverty and Policy in Tudor and Stuart England* (London, 1988); and J. D. Marshall, *The Old Poor Law 1795–1834*, 2nd ed. (London, 1985). The general demographic issues are easily approached through Michael W. Flinn, *The European Demographic System, 1500–1820* (Brighton, Sussex, 1981).

The role of religion in early nineteenth-century social reform in Britain is dealt with in Ford K. Brown, *Fathers of the Victorians: The Age of Wilberforce* (Cambridge, 1961) and John Roach, *Social Reform in England, 1780–1880* (London, 1978). The early fever hospital movement is described by W. F. Bynum, "Hospital, Disease, and Community: The London Fever Hospital, 1801–1850," in Charles E. Rosenberg, ed., *Healing and History* (New York, 1979), pp. 97–115.

A general survey of public health in nineteenth-century Britain is Anthony S. Wohl, *Endangered Lives: Public Health in Victorian Britain* (London, 1983). Edwin Chadwick's role in the movement has been elucidated in three monographs: R. A. Lewis, *Edwin Chadwick and the Public Health Movement 1832–1854* (London, 1952); S. E. Finer, *The Life and Times of Sir Edwin Chadwick* (London, 1952); and Anthony Brundage, *England's "Prussian Minister": Edwin Chadwick and the Politics of Government Growth* (University Park, Pa., 1988). The modern reprint of Edwin Chadwick, *Report on the Sanitary Condition of the Labouring Population of Great Britain (1842)* (Edinburgh, 1965), has an excellent introduction by M. W. Flinn. *The Poor Law Report of 1834* has also been edited and well introduced by S. G. and E. O. A. Checkland (Harmondsworth, 1974). Gertrude Himmelfarb, *The Idea of Poverty: England in the Early Industrial Age* (New York, 1984), analyzes the debates on poverty and pauperism in Britain in an age of Malthus and Chadwick. D. Fraser, ed., *The New Poor Law in the Nineteenth Century* (London, 1984), is a good collection of essays on the consequences of the New Poor Law. Ruth Hodgkinson, *Origins of the National Health Service: Medical Services of the New Poor Law, 1834–1871* (London 1967), examines the medical services, and M. A. Crowther, *The Workhouse System* (London, 1981), the hated central feature.

There is an extensive historical literature on cholera. R. J. Morris, *Cholera 1832: The Social Response to an Epidemic* (London, 1976), focuses on the first epidemic, as does Michael Durey, *The Return of the Plague* (Dublin, 1979). Margaret Pelling, *Fever, Cholera and English Medicine, 1825–1865* (Oxford, 1978), concentrates on the theoretical debates about the cause of cholera and reminds us that "fever," however defined, was a far greater cause of mortality during the "cholera years." Both Durey and Ruth Richardson (*Death, Dissection and The Destitute* [Harmondsworth, 1989]) stress the importance of the fact that the first cholera epidemic (1832) occurred in the same year that the Anatomy Act made the corpses of paupers more readily available for dissection. Richardson's arguments are summarized in her article, " 'Trading Assassins' and the Licensing of Anatomy," in French and Wear, *British Medicine*, pp. 74–91. The statistical movement, which encouraged individuals to count cholera deaths and a myriad of other social "facts," has been described by M. J. Cullen, *The Statistical Movement in Early Victorian Britain* (Brighton, 1975). William Farr's place in the movement is the subject of John M. Eyler, *Victorian Social Medicine: The Ideas and Methods of William Farr* (Baltimore, 1979).

John Snow, *On the Mode of Communication of Cholera*, has been reprinted in modern times (W. H. Frost, ed., *Snow on Cholera*, New York, 1936), and his work, as well as that of Budd, are considered in detail in Pelling's monograph. The more general problem of water analysis has been expertly described in Christopher Hamlin, *A Science of Impurity: Water Analysis in Nineteenth-Century Britain* (Bristol, 1990). For an English-language exposition of Pacini's ideas, and their failures to make much impact on the international scientific community, see Norman Howard-Jones, *The Scientific Background of the International Sanitary*

Conferences 1851–1938 (Geneva, 1975). One of the best studies of any modern medical man is Royston Lambert, *Sir John Simon and English Sanitary Administration* (London, 1963). Simon's own writings can still be read with profit: *English Sanitary Institutions* (London, 1897); and *Public Health Reports*, 2 vols., ed. E. Seaton (London, 1887).

For Edward Jenner and the origins of vaccination, see Richard Fisher, *Edward Jenner* (London, 1987), and Derek Baxby, *Jenner's Smallpox Vaccine* (London, 1981). Lambert, *Simon*, has a good discussion of Simon's role in the development of compulsory vaccination in Britain, for which, also, see Royston Lambert, "A Victorian National Health Service: State Vaccination," *Historical Journal*, 5 (1962), 1–18; Roy Macleod, "Law, Medicine and Public Opinion; The Resistance to Compulsory Health Legislation 1870–1907," *Public Law* (Summer and Autumn, 1967), 107–28 and 189–211; and Dorothy Porter and Roy Porter, "The Politics of Prevention: Anti-Vaccinationism and Public Health in Nineteenth-Century England," *Medical History*, 32 (1988), 231–52. See also Donald R. Hopkins, *Princes and Peasants*.

The American experience of cholera is the subject of the classic monograph by Charles E. Rosenberg, *The Cholera Years* (Chicago and London, 1962). A good survey of the history of public health in the United States is John Duffy, *The Sanitarians: A History of American Public Health* (Urbana, Ill., 1992). Excellent local studies include John Duffy, *A History of Public Health in New York City, 1625–1866* (New York, 1968); *idem, A History of Public Health in New York City, 1866–1966* (New York, 1974); Barbara Rosenkrantz, *Public Health and the State: Changing Views in Massachusetts, 1842–1936* (Cambridge, Mass., 1972); and Judith Walzer Leavitt, *The Healthiest City: Milwaukee and the Politics of Health Reform* (Princeton, N.J., 1982). For the religious motivation of some of the early reformers, see Charles E. and Carroll S. Rosenberg, "Pietism and the Origins of the American Public Health Movement," *Journal of the History of Medicine and Allied Sciences*, 23 (1968), 16–35. There is much on Shattuck and the early statistical movement in the United States in James Cassedy, *American Medicine and Statistical Thinking, 1800–1860* (Cambridge, Mass., 1984); and in Gerald Grob, *Edward Jarvis and the Medical World of Nineteenth-Century America* (Knoxville, Tenn., 1978). A broad-ranging comparative Anglo-American survey is Elizabeth Fee and Dorothy Porter, "Public Health, Preventive Medicine and Professionalization: England and America in the Nineteenth Century," in Andrew Wear, *Medicine in Society*, pp. 249–75. William Coleman's study of Louis Villermé provides an excellent introduction to public health in nineteenth-century France: *Death is a Social Disease: Public Health and Political Economy in Early Industrial France* (Madison, Wis., 1982). See also A. F. La Berge, "The Paris Health Council, 1802–1848," *Bulletin of the History of Medicine*, 49 (1985), 339–52; and T. D. Murphy, "The French Medical Profession's Perception of its Social Function between 1776 and 1830," *Medical History*, 23 (1979), 259–78. The urban context is powerfully evoked in Louis Chevalier, *Labouring Classes and Dangerous Classes in Paris during the First Half of the Nineteenth Century*, trans. Frank Jellinek (London, 1973); and the French experience of cholera analyzed by F. Delaporte, *Disease and Civilization* (Cambridge, Mass., 1986); and J. P. Goubert, *The Conquest of Water*, trans. A. Wilson (Princeton, N.J., and Oxford, 1989). For the later period, Jack D. Ellis, *The Physician-Legislators of France: Medicine and Politics in the Early Third Republic* (Cambridge, 1990) is excellent. Evelyn Bernette Ackerman, *Health Care in the Parisian Countryside, 1800–1914* (New Brunswick, N.J., and London, 1990) is wide-ranging in its concerns.

Rudolf Virchow's role in the German public health movement was well described by Erwin H. Ackerknecht, *Rudolf Virchow: Doctor, Statesman, Anthropologist* (Madison, Wis., 1953), and Virchow's extensive writings in the field have been collected and translated into English: Rudolf Virchow, *Collected Essays on Public Health and Epidemiology*, ed. L. J. Rather, 2 vols. (Canton, Maine, 1985). Richard Evans's magisterial *Death in Hamburg: Society and Politics in the Cholera Years, 1830–1910* (Oxford, 1987) examines public health politics and much more in Hamburg.

CHAPTER 4. MEDICINE IN THE LABORATORY

Joseph Ben-David, *The Scientist's Role in Society: A Comparative Study* (Chicago and London, 1984), is both sociologically and historically informed, and its early chapters consider the institutionalization of science in the seventeenth and eighteenth centuries. Chapter 7, "German Scientific Hegemony and the Emergence of Organized Science," is especially important for the nineteenth century. The evocative characterizations of the "scientific spirit" in France, Germany, and England, in John Theodore Merz, *A History of European Thought in the Nineteenth Century*, 4 vols. (orig. pub. 1904–12; New York, 1965), is still valuable. An important modern study of the German university system is C. E. McLelland, *State, Society and University in Germany, 1700–1914* (Cambridge, 1980). See also R. Steven Turner, "The Growth of Professorial Research In Prussia, 1818 to 1848 – Causes and Context," *Historical Studies in the Physical Sciences*, 3 (1971), 137–82; Steven Turner, Edward Kerwin, and David Woolwine, "Careers and Creativity in Nineteenth-Century Physiology: Zloczower Redux," *Isis*, 75 (1984), 523–29, and Claudia Huerkamp, "The Making of the Modern Medical Profession, 1800–1914: Prussian Doctors in the Nineteenth Century," in Geoffrey Cocks and Konrad H. Jarausch, eds., *German Professions; 1800–1950* (New York and Oxford, 1990), pp. 66–84.

For Liebig, see Steven Turner, "Justus Liebig versus Prussian Chemistry: Reflections on Early Institutes – Building in Germany," *Historical Studies in the Physical Sciences*, 13 (1982), 129–62; J. B. Morrell, "The Chemist Breeders: The Research Schools of Liebig and Thomas Thomson," *Ambix*, 19 (1972), 1–47; W. H. Brock, "Liebigiana: Old and New Perspectives," *History of Science*, 19 (1981), 210–18; Frederic L. Holmes, "The Complementarity of Teaching and Research in Liebig's Laboratory," in Kathryn M. Olesko, ed., *Science in Germany: The Intersection of Institutional and Intellectual Issues, Osiris*, 2nd ser., 5 (1989), 121–64; and Timothy O. Lipman, "Vitalism and Reductionism in Liebig's Physiological Thought," *Isis*, 58 (1967), 167–85.

For the continuing influences of romantic ideas on the life and medical sciences in Germany, see Timothy Lenoir, *The Strategy of Life* (Dordrecht and Boston, 1982). On scientific materialism, see Frederick Gregory, *Scientific Materialism in Nineteenth-Century Germany* (Dordrecht and Boston, 1977). The 1847 "manifesto" of Helmholtz, du Bois-Reymond, Brücke, and Ludwig is analyzed by Paul Cranefield, "The Organic Physics of 1847 and the Biophysics of Today," *Journal of the*

History of Medicine and Allied Sciences, 12 (1957), 407–23. For the institutionalization of physiology, see the excellent collection of essays edited by William Coleman and Frederic L. Holmes, *The Investigative Enterprise: Experimental Physiology in Nineteenth-Century Medicine* (Berkeley and London, 1988). The main achievements of Müller and other nineteenth-century German physiologists are assessed in Karl E. Rothschuh, *History of Physiology*, trans. Guenter Risse (Huntington, N.Y., 1973). A generous sample of Helmholtz's writings have been collected in Russell Kahl, ed., *Selected Writings of Hermann von Helmholtz* (Middletown, Conn., 1971).

Ackerknecht, *Rudolf Virchow*, provides an excellent account of the background of Virchow's own cell theory. See also L. J. Rather's introduction to Rudolf Virchow, *Cellular Pathology as Based Upon Physiological and Pathological Histology*, trans. Frank Chance (New York, 1971); and L. J. Rather, trans. and ed., *Disease, Life and Man: Selected Essays by Rudolph Virchow* (Stanford, Calif., 1958). Russell Maulitz, "Schwann's Way: Cells and Crystals," *Journal of the History of Medicine and Allied Sciences, 26* (1971), 422–37, and *idem*, "Rudolph Virchow, Julius Cohnheim, and the Program of Pathology," *Bulletin of the History of Medicine, 52* (1978), 162–82, provide additional intellectual and institutional context. The career and ideas of Robert Koch are well described in Thomas D. Brock, *Robert Koch: A Life in Medicine and Bacteriology* (Madison, Wis., 1988).

For France, see Lesch, *Science and Medicine*, and Robert Fox, "Science, The University and The State," in Geison, *Professions and the French State*. There is an extensive literature on Claude Bernard. His early research career is comprehensively assessed in Frederic L. Holmes, *Claude Bernard and Animal Chemistry* (Cambridge, Mass., 1974). William Coleman, "The Cognitive Basis of the Discipline: Claude Bernard on Physiology," *Isis, 76* (1985), 49–70, is an outstanding recent evaluation. Bernard's *An Introduction to the Study of Experimental Medicine*, trans. H. E. Greene (New York, 1957) should be read by anyone with an interest in nineteenth-century medical science.

The broader institutional context in which both Bernard and Louis Pasteur worked can be usefully approached through the essays in Robert Fox and George Weisz, *The Organization of Science and Technology in France, 1808–1914* (Cambridge, 1980); Harry W. Paul, *From Knowledge to Power: The Rise of the Science Empire in France, 1860–1939* (Cambridge, 1985); and George Weisz, *The Emergence of Modern Universities in France, 1863–1914* (Princeton, N.J., 1983).

The literature on Pasteur is even more extensive than that on Bernard. The best place to start is the monographic-length entry on him by Gerald Geison in the *Dictionary of Scientific Biography*, with an extensive bibliography. The popular biography by René Dubos, *Louis Pasteur: Freelance of Science* (New York, 1986), is sound and readable, and a shorter popular account is W. F. Bynum, "Louis Pasteur: The Pursuit of the Infinitely Small," in Roy Porter, ed., *Man Masters Nature* (London, 1987), pp. 149–62. Bruno Lateur, *The Pasteurization of France*, trans. A. Sheridan Smith and J. Law (Cambridge, Mass., 1988), is a stimulating analysis of the consequences of Pasteur's ideas.

A fundamental analysis of the status of science and scientific careers in early Victorian Britain is J. B. Morrell and Arnold Thackray, *Gentlemen of Science: The Origins and Early Years of the British Association for the Advancement of Science* (Oxford, 1981). The standard survey of the century as a whole is Donald Cardwell, *The Organization of Science in England*, 2nd ed. (London, 1980). For medical comment on the early Victorian scientific scene, see Warner, "The Idea of Science in English Medicine," in French and Wear, *British Medicine*. The careers of the exemplars I have chosen, Prout, Bell, and Hall, are described in biographical studies, the best of which is W. H. Brock, *From Protyle to Proton: William Prout and the Nature of Matter, 1785–1985* (Bristol, 1985). See also Gordon Gordon-Taylor and E. W. Walls, *Sir Charles Bell, His Life and Times* (London, 1958); and Charlotte Hall, *Memoirs of Marshall Hall, M.D., F.R.S.* (London, 1861). Hall's work on the reflex concept is well described in Edwin Clarke and L. S. Jacyna, *Nineteenth-Century Origins of Neuroscientific Concepts* (Berkeley and London, 1987). The Bell-Magendie dispute is conveniently approached through Paul Cranefield, ed., *The Way In and The Way Out: François Magendie, Charles Bell and the Roots of the Spinal Nerves, With a Facsimile of Charles Bell's Annotated Copy of His "Idea of a New Anatomy of the Brain"* (Mount Kisco, N.Y., 1974). Gerald Geison, *Michael Foster and the Cambridge School of Physiology* (Princeton, N.J., 1978), Chapter 1, has a good account of the problems facing anyone wishing to pursue a research career in early Victorian Britain. For William Sharpey, see Douglas W. Taylor, "The Life and Teaching of William Sharpey (1802–1880): 'Father of Modern Physiology' in Britain," *Medical History*, 15 (1971), 126–53; 241–59; and L. S. Jacyna, ed., *A Tale of Three Cities: The Correspondence of William Sharpey and Allen Thomson* (*Medical History*, Supplement No. 9, 1989). A recent reliable biography of Lister is Richard B. Fisher, *Joseph Lister* (London, 1972). Peter Alter's excellent monograph, *The Reluctant Patron: Science and the State in Britain 1850–1920*, trans. Angela Davies (Oxford, 1987), looks at the emergence of a scientific career structure in the later part of the century.

Robert V. Bruce, *The Launching of Modern American Science, 1846–1874* (New York, 1987), cogently argues for the mid-century foundation of an autonomous scientific tradition in the United States. See also John C. Greene, *American Science in the Age of Jackson* (Ames, Iowa, 1984). The German impact on American medical education and medical science is considered by Thomas N. Bonner, *American Doctors and German Universities: A Chapter in International Intellectual Relations 1870–1914* (Lincoln, Nebr., 1963). For Bowditch, see W. Bruce Fye, *The Development of American Physiology: Scientific Medicine in the Nineteenth Century* (Baltimore, 1987). For Chittenden, see Robert E. Kohler, *From Medical Chemistry to Biochemistry: The Making of a Biomedical Discipline* (New York and Cambridge, 1982). For Welch, see Donald Flemming, *William H. Welch and the Rise of American Medicine* (1954; reprinted Baltimore, 1987); and Simon Flexner and James T. Flexner, *William Henry Welch and the Heroic Age of American Medicine* (New York, 1941). The foundation and first decades of the medical school at Johns Hopkins are covered in Alan M. Chesney, *The Johns Hopkins Hospital and the Johns Hopkins University School of Medicine: A Chronicle. Volume I. Early Years, 1867–1893* (Baltimore, 1943). The monographs by Ludmerer, *Learning to Heal* and Rothstein, *American Medical Schools*, also provide good accounts of the impact of science in the pre-Flexner years.

CHAPTER 5. SCIENCE, DISEASE, AND PRACTICE

John Harley Warner, "Science in Medicine," *Osiris*, 2nd ser., 1 (1985), 37–58, is a thoughtful analysis of the theme, with a splendid bibliography. See also S. E. D. Shortt, "Physicians, Science and Status: Issues in the Professionalization of

Anglo-American Medicine in the Nineteenth Century," *Medical History*, 27 (1983), 51–68. Several of the essays in Morris J. Vogel and Charles E. Rosenberg, eds., *The Therapeutic Revolution: Essays in the Social History of American Medicine* (Philadelphia, 1979), also address the issues surrounding science and medical practice.

W. H. Brock, *From Protyle to Proton*, has a little bit on Prout's medical practice; see also Elizabeth Haigh, "William Brande and the Chemical Education of Medical Students," in French and Wear, *British Medicine*. Peterson, *The Medical Profession*, provides the general professional context. W. D. Foster, *A Short History of Clinical Pathology* (Edinburgh, 1961), is still useful, and Reiser, *Medicine and the Reign of Technology*, discusses the development of urine analysis.

F. F. Cartwright, *The English Pioneers of Anaesthesia* (Bristol, 1952), is a standard account of the period before 1846. Good summaries of the early public operations using ether and chloroform can be found in *idem*, *The Development of Modern Surgery From 1830* (London, 1967); and Owen H. and Sarah D. Wangensteen, *The Rise of Surgery: From Empiric Craft to Scientific Discipline* (Folkestone, Kent, 1978). Martin S. Pernick, *A Calculus of Suffering: Pain, Professionalism and Anesthesia in Nineteenth-Century America* (New York, 1985), is a fine social history.

In addition to the literature on Virchow, cited in Chapter 4, see, on microscopy, Arthur Hughes, *A History of Cytology* (London, 1959), for an account of ideas about cell structure and function. For the priority dispute between Virchow and Bennett on Leukemia, see F. W. Gunz, "The Dread Leukemias and the Lymphomas," in M. M. Wintrobe, ed., *Blood, Pure and Eloquent* (New York, 1980), pp. 511–46, and more generally, L. J. Rather, *Addison and the White Corpuscles: An Aspect of Nineteenth-Century Biology* (London, 1972). For mid-century ideas about the nature of cancer, see *idem*, *The Genesis of Cancer: A Study in the History of Ideas* (Baltimore, 1978). The last illness of Emperor Frederick III has been described several times, including P. W. J. Bartrip, *Mirror of Medicine: A History of the BMJ* (Oxford, 1990), pp. 83–87. See also Sir Morrell Mackenzie, *The Fatal Illness of Frederick the Noble* (London, 1888).

The "conquest of infectious diseases," as an earlier generation of doctors and historians optimistically phrased it, has attracted a vast literature, including, of course, that on Pasteur and Koch already cited in the previous chapter. Wesley W. Spink, *Infectious Diseases: Prevention and Treatment in the Nineteenth and Twentieth Centuries* (Folkestone, Kent, 1978); and William Bulloch, *A History of Bacteriology* (Oxford, 1960), are two traditional surveys of the field. Several articles by Codell Carter reexamine aspects of the germ theory in relation to notions of disease causation: "The Germ Theory, Beriberi, and the Deficiency Theory of Disease," *Medical History*, 21 (1977) and *idem*, "Ignaz Semmelweis, Carl Mayrhofer, and the Rise of the Germ Theory," *Medical History*, 29 (1985), 33–53. See also Owsei Temkin's fundamental essay, "An Historical Analysis of the Concept of Infection," in *Double Face of Janus*, pp. 456–71.

Recent work on tuberculosis includes F. B. Smith, *The Retreat of Tuberculosis, 1850–1900* (London, 1988); Linda Bryder, *Below the Magic Mountain: A Social History of Tuberculosis in Twentieth-Century Britain* (Oxford, 1988); Michael E. Teller, *The Tuberculosis Movement: A Public Health Campaign in the Progressive Era* (New York, 1987); and Barbara Bates, *Bargaining For Life: A Social History of Tuberculosis 1876–1938* (Philadelphia, 1992). For Lister's life, see Richard Fisher,

Joseph Lister. A recent analysis of the complexities of Lister's thinking is Christopher Lawrence and Richard Dixey, "Practising On Principle: Joseph Lister and the Germ Theories of Disease," in Christopher Lawrence, ed., *Medical Theory, Surgical Practice* (London, 1992), pp. 153–215. The spread of antiseptic practice is considered in Lindsay Granshaw, " 'Upon This Principle I Have Based A Practice': The Development and Reception of Antisepsis in Britain, 1807–1890," in John Pickstone, ed., *Medical Innovations in Historical Perspective* (London, 1992), pp. 17–46. David Hamilton, "The Nineteenth-Century Surgical Revolution – Antisepsis or Better Nutrition?" *Bulletin of the History of Medicine,* 56 (1982), 30–40, reexamines records contemporary with Lister and challenges the traditional interpretations of the fall of surgical mortality. See also N. J. Fox, "Scientific Theory, Choice and Social Structure: The Case of Joseph Lister's Antisepsis, Humoral Theory and Asepsis," *History of Science,* 26 (1988), 367–97.

Charles Rosenberg, "Florence Nightingale on Contagion: The Hospital as Moral Universe," in Rosenberg, *Healing and History,* pp. 116–36, is an excellent introduction to the "hospitalism" debates. See also Lambert, *John Simon,* pp. 478–85. A useful contemporary summary is Timothy Holmes, "Hospitalism," in Richard Quain, ed., *A Dictionary of Medicine,* new ed., 2 vols. (London, 1895), I, 874–77.

The expansion of surgery after antisepsis is described in Wangensteen and Wangensteen, *The Rise of Surgery;* Gert Brieger, "From Conservative to Radical Surgery in Late Nineteenth-Century America," in Lawrence, *Medical Theory, Surgical Practice,* pp. 216–31; and Ulrich Tröhler, "Surgery (Modern)," in Bynum and Porter, *Companion Encyclopedia of the History of Medicine,* pp. 980–1023. For Treves, see Stephen Trombley, *Sir Frederick Treves: The Extraordinary Edwardian* (London, 1989).

My analysis of Graves and Bristowe is based on my own reading of their works. There is no good modern study of the "Dublin School" of the 1830s and 40s. Graves's work on the thyroid gland is described in Humphry Davy Rolleston, *The Endocrine Organs in Health and Disease* (London, 1936); and V. C. Medvei, *A History of Endocrinology* (Lancaster, 1982). Charcot as a scientific physician can be seen in Christopher G. Goetz, *Charcot The Clinician: The Tuesday Lessons* (New York, 1987). Bristowe the clinician remains unexamined. His work as a Medical Officer of Health is assessed in Anne Wilkinson, "The Beginnings of Disease Control in London; The Work of the Medical Officers of Health in Three Parishes, 1850–1900" (D. Phil. thesis, Oxford, 1981), and, in less detail, in Anne (Wilkinson) Hardy, *The Epidemic Streets: Infectious Disease and the Rise of Preventive Medicine* (Oxford, 1993). For the "new cardiology," see Christopher Lawrence, "Modern and Ancients: The 'New Cardiology' in Britain 1880–1930," in W. F. Bynum, C. Lawrence, and V. Nutton, eds., *The Emergence of Modern Cardiology* (*Medical History,* Supplement 5, 1985), 1–33.

CHAPTER 6. MEDICAL SCIENCE GOES PUBLIC

Aspects of international health initiatives are described in N. M. Goodman, *International Health Organizations,* 2nd ed. (Edinburgh, 1971); and Howard-Jones, *The Scientific Background.* Paul, *From Knowledge to Power,* Holmes, *Claude Bernard,* and Brock, *Robert Koch,* discuss the rivalry between French and German scientists from the middle decades of the century. My own description of the 1881 London Conference is drawn principally from contemporary accounts. See also Bartrip, *Mirror of Medicine*, Chapter 6. Paul Greenhalgh, *Ephemeral Vistas: The "Exposition Universelles," Great Exhibitions and World's Fairs, 1851–1939* (Manchester, 1988), is a stimulating discussion of the vagaries of internationalism in the period.

Two recent collections of essays bring together samples of scholarship in tropical and imperial medicine, a topic of much contemporary interest: Roy Macleod and Milton Lewis, eds., *Disease, Medicine and Empire* (London, 1988); and David Arnold, ed., *Imperial Medicine and Indigenous Societies* (Manchester, 1988). Both contain useful historiographical introductions. Alfred W. Crosby, *Ecological Imperialism: The Biological Expansion of Europe, 900–1900* (New York and Cambridge, 1986), examines the spread of European plants, animals, and diseases, along with people. Philip D. Curtin, *The Image of Africa: British Ideas and Action, 1780–1850* (Madison, Wis., 1964), and *idem, Death By Migration: Europe's Encounter With the Tropical World in the Nineteenth Century* (Cambridge, 1989), are two superb monographs by a leading Africanist. See also G. W. Hartwig and K. D. Patterson, eds., *Disease in African History: An Introductory Survey and Case Studies* (Durham, N.C., 1978).

On the formation of the new specialism, see Michael Worboys, "The Emergence of Tropical Medicine: A Study in the Establishment of a Scientific Specialism," in G. Lemaine et al., eds., *Perspectives on the Emergence of Scientific Disciplines* (The Hague, 1976), 75–98. The imperial aspirations behind the establishment of the London and Liverpool schools are described by Worboys, "Manson, Ross and Colonial Medical Policy: Tropical Medicine in London and Liverpool, 1899–1914," in Macleod and Lewis, *Disease, Medicine and Empire.*

G. Harrison, *Mosquitoes, Malaria and Man: A History of Hostilities Since 1880* (London, 1978), is a good account of malaria and of the Ross–Manson collaboration. Ronald Ross, *Memoirs* (London, 1923), provides better insight into the mind of this complex man than more recent biographies, although several articles by Eli Chernin explore important facets. See, for example, Chernin, "Sir Ronald Ross, Malaria and the Rewards of Research," *Medical History*, 32 (1988), 119–41. The older history of the field, H. H. Scott, *A History of Tropical Medicine*, 2 vols. (London, 1939), is still helpful.

For yellow fever, see William Coleman, *Yellow Fever in the North: The Methods of Early Epidemiology* (Madison, Wis., 1987), and J. M. Gibson, *Physician to the World: The Life of General William Gorgas* (Durham, N.C., 1950). For sleeping sickness, see Maryinez Lyons, *A Colonial Disease: A Social History of Sleeping Sickness in Northern Zaire, 1900–1940* (Cambridge, 1991). Koch's involvement with disease in Africa has been powerfully evoked by Paul Cranefield, *Science and Empire: East Coast Fever in Rhodesia and the Transvaal* (Cambridge, 1991). John Farley, *Bilharzia: A History of Imperial Tropical Medicine* (Cambridge, 1991), examines schistosomiasis eradication programs. Essays by R. C. Ileto and I. J. Catanach in Arnold, *Imperial Medicine*, deal with colonial concerns with cholera and plague, respectively. Peter Curson and Kevin McCracken, *Plague in Sydney: The Anatomy of an Epidemic* (Kensington, NSW, Australia, n.d.), is a good study of the early twentieth-century Australian experience of the plague pandemic. Guenter B. Risse, " 'A Long Pull, A Strong Pull, and All Together': San Francisco and Bubonic Plague, 1907–1908," *Bulletin of the History of Medicine*, 66 (1992),

260–86, looks at the San Francisco response. Rockefeller involvement in international health issues is critically analyzed by E. R. Brown, *Rockefeller Medicine Men: Medicine and Capitalism in America* (Berkeley, 1979). One locally felt dimension is described by N. Rogers, "Germs with Legs: Flies, Disease and the New Public Health," *Bulletin of the History of Medicine*, 63 (1990), 599–617.

Several of the essays in Coleman and Holmes, *The Investigative Enterprise*, describe specific German institutes and local arrangements. See, especially, Arleen M. Tuchman, "From the Lecture to the Laboratory: The Institutionalization of Scientific Medicine at the University of Heidelberg"; Timothy Lenoir, "Science for the Clinic: Science Policy and the Formation of Carl Ludwig's Institute in Leipzig"; and F. L. Holmes, "The Formation of the Munich School of Metabolism." Kathryn M. Olesko's concluding commentary in the volume, "On Institutes, Investigations, and Scientific Training," is bibliographically rich. For the physical sciences, there is David Cahan, *An Institute for an Empire: the Physikalisch-Technische Reichsanstalt, 1871–1918* (Cambridge, 1989).

The Institut Pasteur in Paris and a succession of others elsewhere in France, or in countries within the French sphere of influence, are beginning to receive serious historical attention. A Delaunay, *L'Institut Pasteur, des Origines à Aujourd'hui* (Paris, 1962), is a good narrative account. More recently, Anne Marie Moulin, *Le Dernier Langage de la Médecine: Histoire de L'Immunologie de Pasteur au SIDA* (Paris, 1991), is illuminating on the institutions as well as the science. See also *idem*, "Patriarchal Science, the Network of the Overseas Pasteur Institutes," in C. Jami, A. M. Moulin, and P. Petitjean, eds., *Science and Empires* (Boston, 1992).

Alter, *Reluctant Patron*, has a valuable analysis of private scientific philanthropy in late Victorian and Edwardian Britain. Several papers by Roy M. Macleod also examine relevant issues. See, especially, Macleod, "The Royal Society and the Government Grant: Notes on the Administration of Scientific Research, 1814–1914," *Historical Journal*, 14 (1971), 323–58; and *idem*, "Resources of Science in Victorian England: The Endowment of Science Movement, 1860–1900," in Peter Mathias, ed., *Science and Society, 1600–1900* (Cambridge, 1972), pp. 111–66. Harriette Chick, Margaret Hume, and Marjorie MacFarlane, *War on Disease: A History of the Lister Institute* (London, 1971), is dated. Just after World War I, the MRC created a State-funded medical research institute. See A. Landsborough Thomson, *Half a Century of Medical Research*, 2 vols. (London, 1973–5); and Joan Austoker and Linda Bryder, eds., *Historical Perspectives on the Role of the M.R.C.* (Oxford, 1989).

Victoria A. Harden, *Inventing the N.I.H.: Federal Biomedical Research Policy, 1887–1937* (Baltimore and London, 1986), examines the policies and laboratories that shaped the present research complex in Bethesda, Maryland. Also useful are Ralph C. Williams, *A History of the Public Health Service, 1798–1950* (Washington, D.C., 1951); Richard Shryock, *American Medical Research Past and Present* (New York, 1947); and George Rosen, *Preventive Medicine in the United States, 1900–1975* (New York, 1975).

Private philanthropy has also attracted much historical attention. Steven C. Wheatley, *The Politics of Philanthropy: Abraham Flexner and Medical Education* (Madison, Wis., 1988), looks at Flexner's career within the context of the Carnegie and Rockefeller Foundations. George W. Corner, *A History of the Rockefeller In-*

stitute, 1901–1953: Origins and Growth (New York, 1967), describes one of the key investments of the Rockefeller program. John Ettling, *The Germ of Laziness: Rockefeller Philanthropy and Public Health in the New South* (Cambridge, Mass., 1981), focuses on one of the early initiatives. Robert E. Kohler, *Partners in Science: Foundations and Natural Scientists, 1900–1945* (Chicago, 1991), is a fine study of the role of the foundations in the growth of the American science community.

Arthur M. Silverstein, *A History of Immunology* (New York, 1989), is a sound history of the main issues in the discipline since the late nineteenth century. Debra Jan Bibel, *Milestones in Immunology: A Historical Exploration* (Madison, Wis., 1988) presents a collection of primary sources with helpful editorial introductions. The literature on Pasteur and Koch, already noted, sets their ideas in context, and a new biography of Metchnikoff ably recounts the ideas of this complex man: Alfred I. Tansler and Leon Cherynak, *Metchnikoff and the Origins of Immunology: From Metaphor to Theory* (New York, 1991). Leonard Colebrook, *Almroth Wright: Provocative Doctor and Thinker* (London, 1954), is still useful and the essay by Ilana Löwy, " 'From Guinea Pigs To Man," The Development of Haffkine's Anti-cholera Vaccine," *Journal of the History of Medicine and Allied Sciences*, 47 (1992), 270–309, makes excellent use of the Haffkine papers in Jerusalem. Spink, *Infectious Diseases*, contains a concise discussion of diphtheria and its antitoxin; a fuller study is Paul Weindling, "From Medical Research to Clinical Practice: Serum Therapy for Diphtheria in the 1890s," in Pickstone, *Medical Innovations*, pp. 72–83. There are also descriptions in H. F. Dowling, *Fighting Infection: Disease Conquests of the Twentieth Century* (Cambridge, Mass., 1977); and J. H. Parish, *History of Immunization* (London, 1965). For Ehrlich, see Ernst Baümler, *Paul Ehrlich: Scientist for Life* (New York, 1984); and Jonathan Liebenau, "Paul Ehrlich as a Commercial Scientist and Research Administrator," *Medical History*, 34 (1990), 65–78.

For the older world of drug compounding, manufacturing, and merchandising, see E. Kremens and G. Urdang, *History of Pharmacy*, 4th ed., revised by G. Sonnedecker (Philadelphia, 1976); Roy Porter and Dorothy Porter, "The Rise of the English Drug Industry: The Role of Thomas Corbyn," *Medical History*, 33 (1989), 277–96; and L. Matthews, *History of Pharmacy in Britain* (Edinburgh and London, 1962). James Harvey Young, *The Toadstool Millionaires: A Social History of Patent Medicine in America before Federal Regulation* (Princeton, 1961), is both entertaining and instructive on the patent medicine scene in the United States. The AMA and *BMJ* campaigns against patent remedies are described in Young, *Toadstool Millionaires* and *idem, Medical Messiahs: A Social History of Health Quackery in Twentieth-Century America* (Princeton, N.J., 1967); and Bartrip, *Mirror of Medicine*.

For the pharmacological background to the research-based pharmaceutical industry, see C. D. Leake, *An Historical Account of Pharmacology to the Twentieth Century* (Springfield, Ill., 1975), and Miles Weatherall, *In Search of a Cure: A History of Pharmaceutical Discovery* (Oxford, 1990). For the development of the industry itself, see Jonathan Liebenau, *Medical Science and Medical Industry: The Formation of the American Pharmaceutical Industry* (London, 1987); *idem*, "Paul Ehrlich as a Commercial Scientist and Research Administrator," *Medical History*, 34 (1990), 65–78; J. Liebenau et al., eds., *Pill Peddlers: Essays on the History of the Pharmaceutical Industry* (Madison, Wis., 1990); and E. M. Tansey, "Science, Commerce and Authority: The Wellcome Physiological Research Laboratories and the Home Office 1900–1901," *Medical History, 23* (1989), 1–41. Key pharmacological discoveries are investigated by John Parascandola, "The Theoretical Basis of Paul Ehrlich's Chemotherapy," *Journal of the History of Medicine and Allied Sciences, 36* (1981), 19–43; and *idem,* "John J. Abel and the Early Development of Pharmacology at the Johns Hopkins University," *Bulletin of the History of Medicine, 56* (1982), 1–18 and *The Development of American Pharmacology: John J. Abel and the Shaping of a Discipline* (Baltimore, 1992). An evocative analysis of the translation of pharmacology and the other medical sciences into medical care in the United States is Charles Rosenberg's "The Theraputic Revolution: Medicine, Meaning and Social Change in Nineteenth-Century America," in Morris J. Vogel and Charles E. Rosenberg, eds., *The Therapeutic Revolution* (Philadelphia, 1979). John Harley Warner, *The Therapeutic Perspective* (Cambridge, Mass., 1986), brilliantly scrutinizes the complicated relationship between therapeutic choice and professional identity in mid-century America, at a time when orthodox doctors felt the challenge of the various medical sects most strongly.

Richard D. French, *Antivivisection and Medical Science in Victorian Society* (Princeton, N.J., 1975), is a splendid account of the antivivisection movement and the passage and implementation of the 1876 Cruelty to Animals Act in Britain, as well as the scientific community's strategies for dealing with it. The cultural background to Victorian attitudes to animals is expertly dealt with by Harriet Ritvo, *The Animal Estate: The English and Other Creatures in the Victorian Age* (Cambridge, Mass., 1987). Nicholaas Rupke, ed., *Vivisection in Historical Perspective* (London, 1987), is an excellent collection with essays on European countries and North America as well as Britain. The "Brown Dog Affair" has been luridly described in Coral Lansbury, *The Old Brown Dog: Women, Workers and Vivisection in Edwardian England* (Madison, Wis., 1985).

Geison, *Michael Foster and the Cambridge School of Physiology,* remains the standard account of British physiology during its formative period and neatly complements French's *Antivivisection.* Medvei, *History of Endocrinology,* describes the experimental and clinical work on the thyroid gland, and David Hamilton, *The Monkey Gland Affair* (London, 1986), assesses the excitement caused by the work on "rejuvenation." Brown-Séquard's life and career are fully described in Michael J. Aminoff, *Brown-Séquard: A Visionary of Science* (New York, 1993).

Otto Glasser, *Wilhelm Conrad Röntgen and the Early History of the Röntgen Rays* (London, 1933), is still valuable for the context and immediate reaction to Röntgen's work on x-rays. Ruth and Edward Brecher, *The Rays: A History of Radiology in the United States and Canada* (Baltimore, 1969), has material on popular as well as professional attitudes. Eve Curie, *Madame Curie,* trans. Vincent Sheean (New York, 1939), is one of a number of biographies elevating Pierre and Marie Curie to the pantheon of science.

CHAPTER 7. DOCTORS AND PATIENTS

Edward Shorter, *Bedside Manners: The Troubled History of Doctors and Patients* (New York, 1985), is a vivid account of its subject. George Rosen, *The Structure of American Medical Practice, 1875–1947,* ed. Charles E. Rosenberg (Philadelphia, 1983), has a useful description of a doctor's office around the turn of the century.

Peterson, *Medical Profession*, and Newman, *Evolution of Medical Education*, contain good discussions of the Victorian medical profession and its education. Jeffrey Berlant, *Profession and Monopoly* (Berkeley, 1975), is also valuable as a comparative study of the United States and Great Britain. Most analyses of the collective values of the modern medical profession draw on the insights of E. Freidson, *Profession of Medicine: A Study of the Sociology of Applied Knowledge* (New York, 1970). The comparative perspective of Abraham Flexner, *Medical Education: A Comparative Study* (New York, 1925); and *idem, Universities: American, English, German* (New York, 1930), makes his work still of relevance.

American educational and licensing issues are expertly analyzed in Paul Starr, *The Social Transformation of American Medicine*, as well as in Rothstein, *American Medical Schools*, and Ludmerer, *Learning to Heal*. For the "full-time" system, see W. Bruce Fye, "The Origin of the Full-Time Faculty System," *Journal of the American Medical Association*, 265 (1991), 1555–62. James G. Burrow, *AMA: Voice of American Medicine* (Baltimore, 1963), examines the Association's involvement in these debates.

Brian Abel-Smith, *The Hospitals, 1800–1948* (London, 1964), is a good survey of hospitals in Britain. John Woodward, *To Do the Sick No Harm: A Study of the British Voluntary Hospital System to 1875* (London, 1974), concentrates on the more prestigious voluntary hospitals. Geoffrey Rivett, *The Development of the London Hospital System, 1823–1982* (London, 1986), provides an excellent account of London hospitals. John V. Pickstone, *Medicine and Industrial Society: A History of Hospital Development in Manchester and its Region* (Manchester, 1985), offers another fine local analysis. A good history of a specialist hospital is Lindsay Granshaw, *St. Mark's Hospital, London: A Social History of a Specialist Hospital* (London, 1985). G. M. Ayres, *England's First State Hospitals and the Metropolitan Asylums Board* (London, 1971), is a pioneering study of State involvement in hospitals. See also Granshaw and Porter, *The Hospital in History*, and Hodgkinson, *The Origins of the National Health Service*.

Nursing history has become a vigorous subject in its own right. Celia Davies, ed., *Rewriting Nursing History* (London, 1980), provides a good sample of recent work in the field. Brian Abel-Smith, *A History of the Nursing Profession* (London, 1960), is still a useful survey. Susan Reverby, *Ordered to Care: The Dilemma of American Nursing, 1850–1945* (Cambridge and New York, 1987), examines the American scene. Florence Nightingale continues to provide a focus, even if much contemporary scholarship is at pains to demonstrate that nineteenth-century nursing cannot be seen simply as her brainchild. Monica Baly, *Florence Nightingale and the Nursing Legacy* (London, 1986), examines the uses to which the funds established in Nightingale's honor were put. F. B. Smith, *Florence Nightingale – Reputation and Power* (London, 1982), is a trenchant analysis of her devious personality.

Two magisterial works on American hospitals survey that institution: Charles E. Rosenberg, *The Care of Strangers: The Rise of America's Hospital System* (New York, 1987), and Rosemary Stevens, *In Sickness and in Wealth: American Hospitals in the Twentieth Century* (New York, 1989), between them provide a convincing account from 1800 to the present day. Morris Vogel, *The Invention of the Modern Hospital* (Chicago, 1980), and David Rosner, *A Once Charitable Enterprise: Hospitals and Health Care in Brooklyn and New York, 1865–1915* (Cambridge, Mass., 1982), are two exemplary local studies.

Hospital design is a feature of Thompson and Golden, *The Hospital*, and is covered in passing in Rosenberg, *Care of Strangers*. Jeremy Taylor, *Hospital and Asylum Architecture in England 1840–1914: Building For Health Care* (London, 1991), provides an architectural perspective on the subject. The King Edward's Hospital Fund for London has recently been expertly assessed by Frank Prochaska, *Philanthropy and the Hospitals of London* (Oxford, 1992). The classic study of medical specialization is George Rosen, *The Specialization of Medicine with Special Reference to Ophthalmology* (New York, 1933; reprinted 1972). See also Rosemary Stevens, *Medical Practice in Modern England: The Impact of Specialization and State Medicine* (New Haven, Conn., 1966), and, for Germany, Hans-Heinz Eulner, *Die Entwicklung der medizinischen Specialfächer an den Universitäten des Deutschen Sprachgebiet* (Stuttgart, 1970). Rosen, *Structure of American Medical Practice*, pp. 81–94, is good on the United States, and the essays in Russell C. Maulitz and Diana E. Long, eds., *Grand Rounds: One Hundred Years of Internal Medicine* (Philadelphia, 1988), offer case studies of the development of several of the medical specialties. J. T. Crissey and L. C. Parish, *The Dermatology and Syphilology of the Nineteenth Century* (New York, 1981), is a lively account of the ideas and personalities in these two disciplines. Ornella Moscucci, *The Science of Woman: Gynaecology and Gender in England, 1800–1929* (Cambridge, 1990), examines this specialism in England, and Judith Leavitt, *Brought to Bed: Childbearing in America, 1750–1950* (New York and Oxford, 1986), analyzes the cluster of issues surrounding the emergence of obstetrics as a medical specialty.

Probably no specialty has recently attracted as much historical scrutiny as psychiatry. For a sample of this literature, see Andrew T. Scull, ed., *Madhouses, Mad-doctors and Madmen* (Philadelphia, 1981); and W. F. Bynum, Roy Porter, and Michael Shepherd, eds., *The Anatomy of Madness*, 3 vols. (London, 1985–8). Each of these four volumes has a historiographical introduction. Roy Porter, "Madness and its Institutions," in A. Wear, *Medicine in Society*, is full of insight and has an extensive bibliography.

Much of the scholarship during the past couple of decades has been affected by Michel Foucault, *Madness and Civilization: A History of Insanity in the Age of Reason*, trans. R. Howard (New York, 1965), although there is now also a large literature analyzing Foucault's analyses. See, for example, P. Spierenberg, "The Sociogenesis of Confinement and its Development in Early Modern Europe," in P. Spierenberg, ed., *The Emergence of Carceral Institutions: Prisons, Galleys and Lunatic Asylums* (Rotterdam, 1984).

For eighteenth-century England, see Roy Porter, *Mind-Forg'd Manacles: Madness in England from the Restoration to the Regency* (London, 1987). Andrew Scull, *Museums of Madness: The Social Organization of Insanity in Nineteenth-Century England* (London, 1979), is a fine analysis of the later period. A completely revised edition has been published as *The Most Solitary of Afflictions: Madness and Society in Britain, 1700–1900* (New Haven, Conn., and London, 1993). Anne Digby, *Madness, Morality and Medicine* (Cambridge, 1985), is an excellent study of the York Retreat. The essays in S. Cohen and A. Scull, eds., *Social Control and the State* (Oxford, 1983), explore the value of the concept of social control in psychiatry and the social sciences generally.

Jan Goldstein, *Console and Classify* (Cambridge, 1987), provides expert analysis of the French psychiatric profession. It can be supplemented by Ian Dowbiggin, *Inheriting Madness: Professionalization and Psychiatric Knowledge in Nineteenth Cen-*

tury France (Berkeley, 1991), which scrutinizes the ways in which the concept of hereditary degeneration was used. Daniel Pick, *Faces of Degeneration: Aspects of a European Disorder c. 1848–1918* (Cambridge, 1989), offers a more general examination of the concept.

Gerald Grob, *Mental Institutions in America* (New York, 1973), and *idem, Mental Illness and American Society, 1875–1940* (Princeton, 1983), present a balanced account of the asylum in the United States. Nancy Tomes, *A Generous Confidence: Thomas Story Kirkbride and the Art of Asylum Keeping, 1840–1883* (Cambridge, 1984), is a fine study of one psychiatric institution and its medical superintendent.

Midwifery and its relationship to the medical profession can be approached through Jean Donnison, *Midwives and Medical Men* (London, 1977), and J. B. Litoff, *American Midwives: 1860 to the Present* (Westport, Conn., 1978). An instructive Dutch comparison is provided by M. S. van Lieburg and Hilary Marland, "Midwife Regulation, Education and Practice in the Netherlands during the Nineteenth Century," *Medical History, 33* (1989), 296–317. The historical problem of maternal mortality is definitively examined in Irvine Loudon, *Death in Childbirth: An International Study of Maternal Care and Maternal Mortality, 1800–1950* (Oxford, 1992). For Semmelweis, see K. Codell Carter's translation and excellent introduction to I. Semmelweis, *The Etiology, Concept and Prophylaxis of Childbed Fever* (Madison, Wis., 1983). See also Leavitt, *Brought to Bed.* For the death of Princess Charlotte, see Franco Crainz, *An Obstetric Tragedy* (London, 1977).

Moscucci, *The Science of Woman,* provides a modern gloss on the development of gynecology. It may be complemented by Ann Dally, *Women Under the Knife: A History of Surgery* (London, 1991). A powerful evocation of the difficulties nineteenth-century American men, including doctors, had in coming to terms with female sexuality may be found in G. J. Barker-Benfield, *The Horrors of the Half-Known Life* (New York, 1976).

Two recent fine monographs explore the entry of women into medicine: Regina Markell Morantz-Sanchez, *Sympathy and Science: Women Physicians in American Medicine* (New York and Oxford, 1985); and Thomas Neville Bonner, *To the Ends of the Earth: Women's Search for Education in Medicine* (Cambridge, Mass., 1992). Modern scholars would do well to exploit the pioneering work of Kate Campbell Hurd-Mead, *A History of Women in Medicine* (Haddam, Conn., 1938).

David G. Green, *Working-Class Patients and the Medical Establishment: Self-Help in Britain from the Mid-Nineteenth Century to 1948* (New York, 1985), examines the origins and operation of collective schemes for employing medical men. Jeanne L. Brand, *Doctors and the State* (Baltimore, 1965), Chapter VIII, assesses the same phenomenon, as well as many other areas where the late Victorian state in Britain touched medicine and medical care. Two good readable contemporary analyses of the issues are S. Squire Sprigge, *Medicine and the Public* (London, 1905); and Beatrice and Sydney Webb, *The State and the Doctor* (London, 1910). W. F. Bynum, "Medical Values in a Commercial Age," in Christopher Smout, ed., *Victorian Values* (London, 1993), provides a general context.

A number of works look at the Victorian origins of the modern British "Welfare State," of which a good example is Derek Fraser, *The Evolution of the British Welfare State: A History of Social Policy Since the Industrial Revolution* (London, 1973). Eric J. Evans, *Social Policy, 1830–1914, Individualism, Collectivism and the*

Origins of the Welfare State (London, 1978), is a useful collection of primary sources. W. J. Mommsen, ed., *The Emergence of the Welfare State in Britain and Germany* (London, 1981); G. A. Ritter, *Social Welfare in Germany and Britain*, trans. Kim Traynor (Leamington Spa, 1986); and E. P. Hennock, *British Social Reform and German Precedents: The Case of Social Insurance 1880–1914* (Oxford, 1987), look at the comparisons and contrasts between the British and German models. B. B. Gilbert, *The Evolution of National Insurance in Great Britain* (London, 1966), describes the background and implementation of the 1911 N.H.I. Act.

British and American experiences are compared and contrasted in Daniel Fox, *Health Policies, Health Politics: The British and American Experiences, 1911–1965* (Princeton, N.J., 1986). Ronald L. Numbers, *Almost Persuaded: American Physicians and Compulsory Health Insurance, 1912–1920* (Baltimore and London, 1978), examines a road not taken in the United States.

A good deal of recent scholarship on the social history of medicine tackles issues surrounding the patient. For the earlier period, the works of Roy and Dorothy Porter, referred to earlier, are outstanding. F. B. Smith, *The People's Health, 1830–1910* (London, 1979), contains many vignettes of patients' experiences. Elaine Showalter, *The Female Malady: Women, Madness and English Culture, 1830–1980* (New York, 1985); and Janet Oppenheim, *"Shattered Nerves": Doctors, Patients and Depression in Victorian England* (New York and Oxford, 1991), are two fine studies that emphasize female patients. From the extensive literature analyzing attitudes toward death and dying may be cited Philippe Ariès, *The Hour of Our Death*, trans. Helen Weaver (New York, 1981); John McManners, *Death and the Enlightenment* (Oxford, 1981); and Ralph Houlbrooke, ed., *Death, Ritual and Bereavement* (London, 1989).

For the life and illness of Alice James, see Leon Edel, ed., *The Diary of Alice James* (New York, 1964); Ruth Bernard Yenzell, *The Death and Letters of Alice James* (Berkeley, 1981); and Jean Strouse, *Alice James, A Biography* (London, 1981). All of these works misidentify the Sir Andrew Clark who diagnosed Alice James's breast lesion. There are several good biographies of William James that discuss his own health concerns. I have relied principally on Gay Wilson Allen, *William James* (New York, 1967).

CHAPTER 8. CONCLUSION: DID SCIENCE MATTER?

The most ardent advocate of the thesis that improvements in health in the nineteenth century must be looked for outside of formal medical care was the late Thomas McKeown, whose basic ideas changed but little over the thirty years he was devoted to the topic. His thesis was developed in several books, including McKeown, *The Role of Medicine: Dream, Mirage or Nemesis?* (Oxford, 1979); *idem, The Modern Rise of Population* (London, 1970); and *idem, The Origins of Human Disease* (Oxford, 1988).

Many historical demographers have been skeptical of McKeown's methods, and the overriding emphasis he placed on better nutrition as the prime force behind nineteenth-century population increases. The issues are cogently discussed in Richard Smith, "Medicine and Demography," in Bynum and Porter, eds., *Companion Encyclopedia*, pp. 1663–82. S. R. Szreter, "The Importance of

Social Intervention in Britain's Mortality Decline, c. 1850–1914: A Reinterpretation of the Role of Public Health," *Social History of Medicine*, 1 (1988), 1–38; and Anne Hardy, *The Epidemic Streets*, provide additional sharp criticism of the "McKeown thesis."

Sources of quotations

1. MEDICINE IN 1790

1. W. Cullen, *Institutions of Medicine*, in *Works*, ed. J. Thomson, 2 vols. (Edinburgh, 1827), I, p. 3.
2. Cullen, *Practice of Physic*, in *Works*, II, ed. J. Thomson (Edinburgh, 1827), p. 330.
3. Ibid., p. 239.
4. Ibid., p. 257.
5. Ibid., p. 266.

2. MEDICINE IN THE HOSPITAL

1. Tenon, quoted in E. H. Ackerknecht, *Medicine at the Paris Hospital, 1794–1848* (Baltimore, 1967), p. 16.
2. Fourcroy, quoted in Ackerknecht, *Medicine*, p. 32.
3. Ibid.
4. Cullen, *Lectures Introductory to the Course on the Practice of Physic*, in *Works*, I, p. 423.
5. J. B. Morgagni, *Seats and Causes of Diseases*, trans. B. Alexander (1769; reprinted 1980), vol. I, p. xxx.
6. M. Baillie, *Works*, ed. J. Wardrop (1825), vol. II, p. lxx.
7. Bichat, quoted in Ackerknecht, *Medicine*, p. 56.
8. All quotations from J. N. Corvisart, *An Essay on the Organic Diseases and Lesions of the Heart and Great Vessels* (Eng. ed. 1812; reprinted 1962).
9. Ibid., p. xiii.
10. R. T. H. Laennec, *A Treatise on the Diseases of the Chest*, trans. J. Forbes (1821; reprinted 1962), pp. 284–5.
11. Ibid., p. 282.
12. Ibid. (Forbes's Preface), pp. xiii–xiv.
13. P. C. A. Louis, *An Essay on Clinical Instruction*, trans. Peter Martin (London, 1834), p. 3.
14. J. Millar, quoted in U. Tröhler, "Quantification in British Medicine and Surgery 1750–1830, with Special Reference to its Introduction into Therapeutics" (Univ. of London Ph.D. Thesis, 1980), p. 111.
15. G. Andral, quoted in Ackerknecht, *Therapeutics: From the Primitives to the 20th Century* (New York, 1973), p. 106.

251

16. F. Broussais, quoted in Ackerknecht, *Medicine*, p. 69.
17. C. A. Wunderlich, *Wien und Paris* (1841; reprinted Bern, 1974), p. 23.
18. James Hope, *A Treatise on the Diseases of the Heart and Great Vessels*, third edition (London, 1839), p. xxxiv.

3. MEDICINE IN THE COMMUNITY

1. B. Disraeli, *Sybil*, as quoted in *Oxford Dictionary of Quotations*, 3rd ed. (Oxford and New York, 1979), p. 185, where the quotation on statistics is also given.
2. Sir Walter Scott, quoted in Harold Perkin, *The Origins of Modern English Society 1780–1880* (London, 1969), p. 179.
3. E. Chadwick, quoted in S. E. Finer, *The Life and Times of Sir Edwin Chadwick* (London, 1952), p. 298.
4. [W. Farr], *Second Annual Report of the Registrar-General of Births, Deaths, and Marriages in England* (London, 1840), p. 71.
5. W. Budd, quoted in C.-E. A. Winslow, *The Conquest of Epidemic Disease: A Chapter in the History of Ideas* (1943; reprinted Madison, Wis., 1980), p. 281.
6. [L. Shattuck], *Report of the Sanitary Commission of Massachusetts* (Boston, 1850), p. 10.

4. MEDICINE IN THE LABORATORY

1. James Bryce, quoted in J. T. Merz, *History of European Thought in the Nineteenth Century* (orig. pub. 1904–12; New York, 1965), I, p. 159.
2. C. Bernard, *An Introduction to the Study of Experimental Medicine* (Eng. trans., 1957), p. 43, citing "a contemporary poet."
3. L. Pasteur, cited in a slightly different formulation in *The Oxford Dictionary of Quotations*, 3rd ed. (Oxford and New York, 1979), p. 369.

5. SCIENCE, DISEASE, AND PRACTICE

1. R. Virchow, "Standpoints in Scientific Medicine" (1847), in L. J. Rather, ed., *Disease, Life, and Man: Selected Essays by Rudolph Virchow* (Stanford, Calif., 1958), p. 31.
2. L. Pasteur, quoted in L. Geison, "Louis Pasteur," in C. C. Gillispie, ed., *Dictionary of Scientific Biography* (New York, 1970–80), X, p. 364.
3. F. Löffler, quoted in T. D. Brock, *Robert Koch: A Life in Medicine and Bacteriology* (Madison, Wis., 1988), p. 180.
4. J. Erichsen, quoted by Holmes, entry "Hospitalism," in Richard Quain, ed., *A Dictionary of Medicine* (London, 1895), I, p. 874.
5. R. Graves, *Clinical Lectures on the Practice of Medicine*, ed. J. Neligan, 2 vols. (Sydenham Society, 1884), vol. I, p. 14. [First published 1848.]
6. J. S. Bristowe, *A Treatise on the Theory and Practice of Medicine*, 6th ed. (London, 1887), p. 124.

6. MEDICAL SCIENCE GOES PUBLIC

1. *The Lancet*, 1881, ii, p. 342.
2. P. H. Manson-Bahr and A. Alcock, *The Life and Work of Sir Patrick Manson* (London, 1927), p. 146.

7. DOCTORS AND PATIENTS

1. W. Lawrence, quoted in Rosemary Stevens, *Medical Practice in Modern England: The Impact of Specialization and State Medicine* (New Haven, Conn., 1966), p. 27.
2. Jean Strouse, *Alice James, A Biography* (London, 1981), p. 176.
3. Leon Edel, ed., *The Diary of Alice James* (New York, 1964), pp. 206–7.

8. CONCLUSION: DID SCIENCE MATTER?

1. John Simon, *English Sanitary Institutions*, 2nd ed. (London, 1897), pp. 465 and 464.
2. J. S. Bristowe, *Treatise on the Theory and Practice of Medicine*, 6th ed. (London, 1887), p. 449.

Index

254